Flint Family Cookbook

Flint Family Cookbook

Suzanne Flint

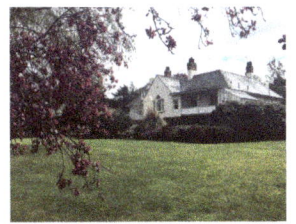

Copyright ©2025 by Roger Flint

All rights reserved. No part of this book may be reproduced or utilized in any form or by any means, electronic or mechanical, including photocopying, recording, online or through any information storage or retrieval system, except for brief excerpts for the purposes of reviewing the book, without the written permission of the author.

Enquiries should be directed to:

Roger Flint, MB ChB
36 Barnton Avenue
Edinburgh Scotland EH4 6JL
United Kingdom
roger-f@hotmail.co.uk

Book Design by Barry P. Chaiken

Published by Poplar Tree Media
Boston, MA USA

Printed in the United Kingdom.

Harback ISBN: 978-1-7367021-6-1

Dedication,

I have always loved being in the kitchen and creating meals for the family, which I hope they have enjoyed. Cooking helps me to relax and unwind from life's daily pressures.

Many years ago, I thought it would be a good idea to write down those meals that had given me particular pleasure. This food diary has grown into some 700 pages over two plastic binders. Obviously, this had come to the attention of Roger and Crispin, and unbeknown to me, Roger was looking for a way to have these recipes published.

Whilst in Boston, USA, Roger mentioned this to Barry. On Christmas 2024, I was presented with the draft proof of the Flint Family Cookbook, and I was quite overwhelmed. I, therefore, would like to dedicate this book to our dear son Roger, the prime instigator of the book, and to my loving husband Crispin, chief taster and critic, but also to Barry, without whom this book would not have been published.

I hope that you find some of the recipes enjoyable and not too testing to make and that you have as much pleasure as I have had in making them.

Meanwhile, I am working on Volume 2!

Love, Mum xx

Recipes

Soup — 1

Soup Basics — 3
Broccoli Soup — 5
Canary Soup — 7
Carrot Soup — 9
Cauliflower, Pear, and Blue Cheese Soup — 11
Classic Tomato Soup — 13
Creamy Smoked Haddock Soup — 15
French Onion Soup — 17
Ham Hock Pea and Mint Soup — 19
Mushroom Soup — 21
Red Pepper and Orange Soup — 23
Rustic Tomato and Basil Soup — 25
Spinach and Rosemary Soup — 27
Stilton, Onion, and Parsley Soup — 29

Salad — 31

Tuna Niçoise — 33

Fish — 35

Baked Salmon Terrine — 37
Crespellini — 39
Devilled Seafood — 43
Fish Pie — 45
Kedgeree — 49

Marinated Prawns with Chilli Dipping Sauce	51
Prawn Cocktail	53
Prawn and Ginger Noodle Stir-Fry	55
Roasted Fish with Sun-dried Tomato Tapenade	57
Salmon and Haddock Fishcakes	59
Smoked Trout, Avocado, and Tomato Timbales	61
Smoked Salmon Pâté	63
Speedy Seafood Curry	65
Spicy Prawns, Orange Sherry & Wild Rice Pilaf	67
Spicy Prawns with Tomato	69
South Indian Prawn Curry	71
Thai Yellow Fish Curry	73

Vegetable Mains   75

Vegetable Lasagne	77

Cheese   79

Cheese Fondue	81

Chicken   83

Balti Butter Chicken	85
Balti Chicken Pasanda	87
Chicken Basque	89
Chicken Korma	91
Chicken with Mozzarella, Prosciutto, and Sage	93
Chicken Tagine	95
Chicken with Tarragon	97
Chicken Tikka Masala	99
Coronation Chicken	103

Ham-wrapped Chicken with Chestnut Stuffing — 105
Italian Style Chicken — 107
Peppered Chicken with Tarragon and Parma Ham — 109
Roast Chicken Dinner — 111
Spatchcock Chicken — 119
Sweet and Sour Balti Chicken — 121

Ham — 123

Honey Glazed Ham - Boiled and Roasted — 125
Honey Glazed Ham - Slow Cooked — 127

Veal — 129

Wiener Schnitzel — 131

Beef — 133

Beef Burgers — 135
Beef Carbonnade — 137
Beef Stroganoff — 139
Beef Tagine — 141
Chilli Con Carne — 143
Cottage Pie — 145
Devilled Meatballs — 147
Goulash — 149
Lasagne — 151
Polish Nelson Steaks — 155
Ragu Modenese — 157
Roast Beef — 159
Spaghetti Bolognaise — 163
Stir-fry Beef — 165

Lamb 167

Lamb Tagine 169
Slow-Cooked Leg or Shoulder of Lamb 171

Vegetables 173

Boston Baked Beans 175
Bubble and Squeak Cakes 177
Confit D'Oignons 179
Gratin Dauphinoise 181
Herby Tabbouleh 183
Parsley Sauce 185
Parsnip Baked in Parmesan Cheese 187
Perfect Cauliflower Cheese 189
Persian Rice Salad 191
Pesto 193
Plum Chutney 195

Dessert 197

Apple Crumble 199
Apple Pie 201
Apricot Cheesecake 205
Bakewell Tart 207
Blackcurrant Mousse 209
Chocolate Fondant 211
Chocolate Hazelnut Cheesecake 213
Chocolate Rum Mousse 215
Chocolate Sauce 217
Chocolate Tears 219

Crepes Suzettes	223
Lemon Meringue Pie	227
Lemon Soufflé	231
Lemon Tart	235
Malt Chocolate Cheesecake	237
Maple Pecan Pie	239
Pastry – Almond	241
Pastry – Sweet	243
Pavlova with Berries	245
Pavlova with Lemon Topping	247
Port Wine Jelly	249
Squidgy Chocolate Log	251
Sticky Toffee Pudding	253
Tiramisu	257

Cake — 259

Carrot Cake	261
Chocolate Chip Brownies	263
No Flour Clementine Cake	265
Coffee and Walnut Cake	267
Coffee and Walnut Cake with Almonds	269
Fudge Icing	271
No Cook Chocolate Cake	273
Salted Caramel Brownies	275
Seville Orange Marmalade Cake	277
Sticky Gingerbread	279
Victoria Sponge Cake	281

Biscuits 285

- Eccles Cake — 287
- Empire Biscuits — 289
- Flapjacks — 291
- Mars Bar Slices — 293
- Millionaire's Shortbread — 295
- Nougat — 299
- Scones — 301
- Shortbread — 303
- Tiffin — 305

Jam 307

- Fresh Lemon Curd — 309
- Raspberry Jam — 311

Flint Family Cookbook

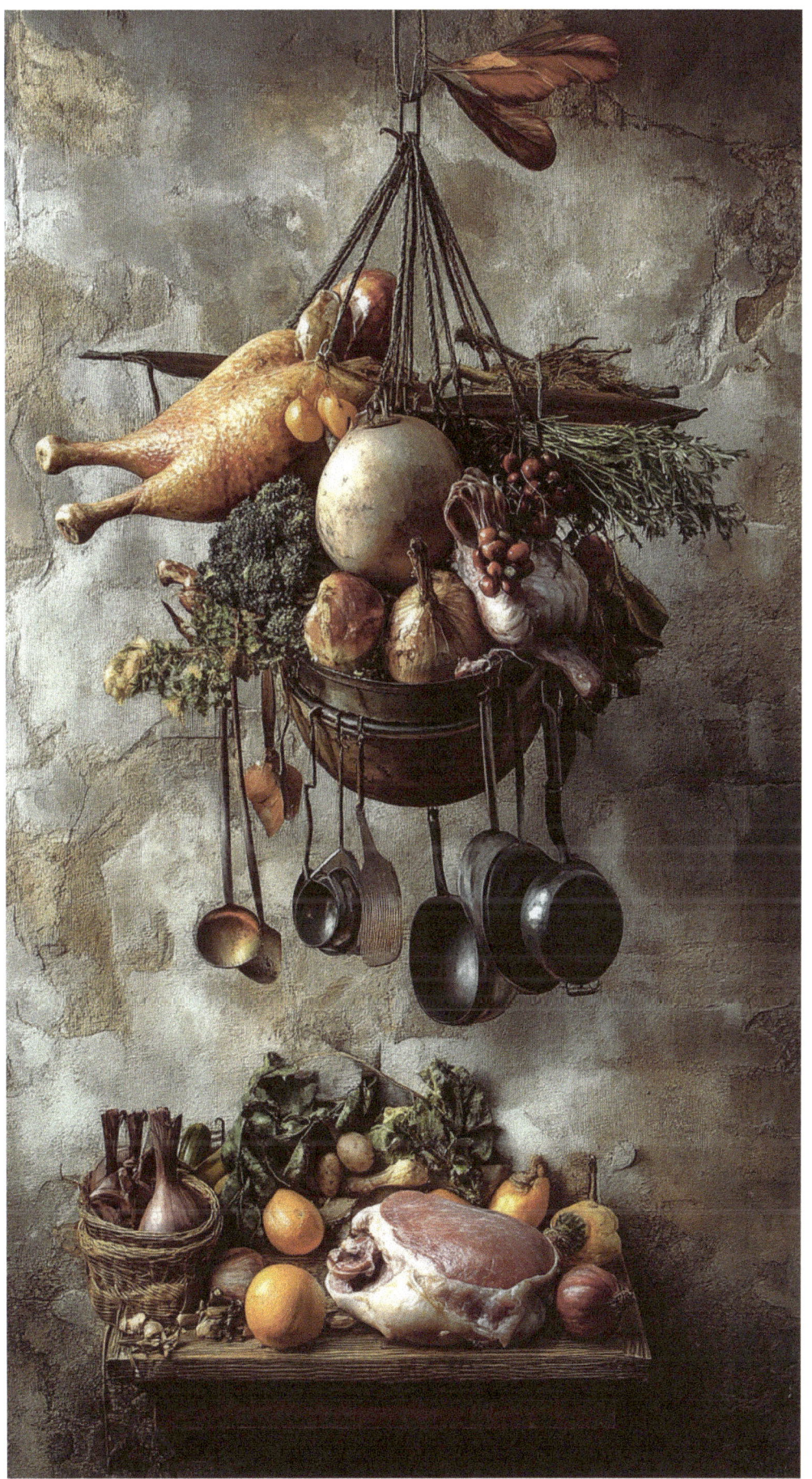

XIII

XIV

Flint Family Cookbook

Soup

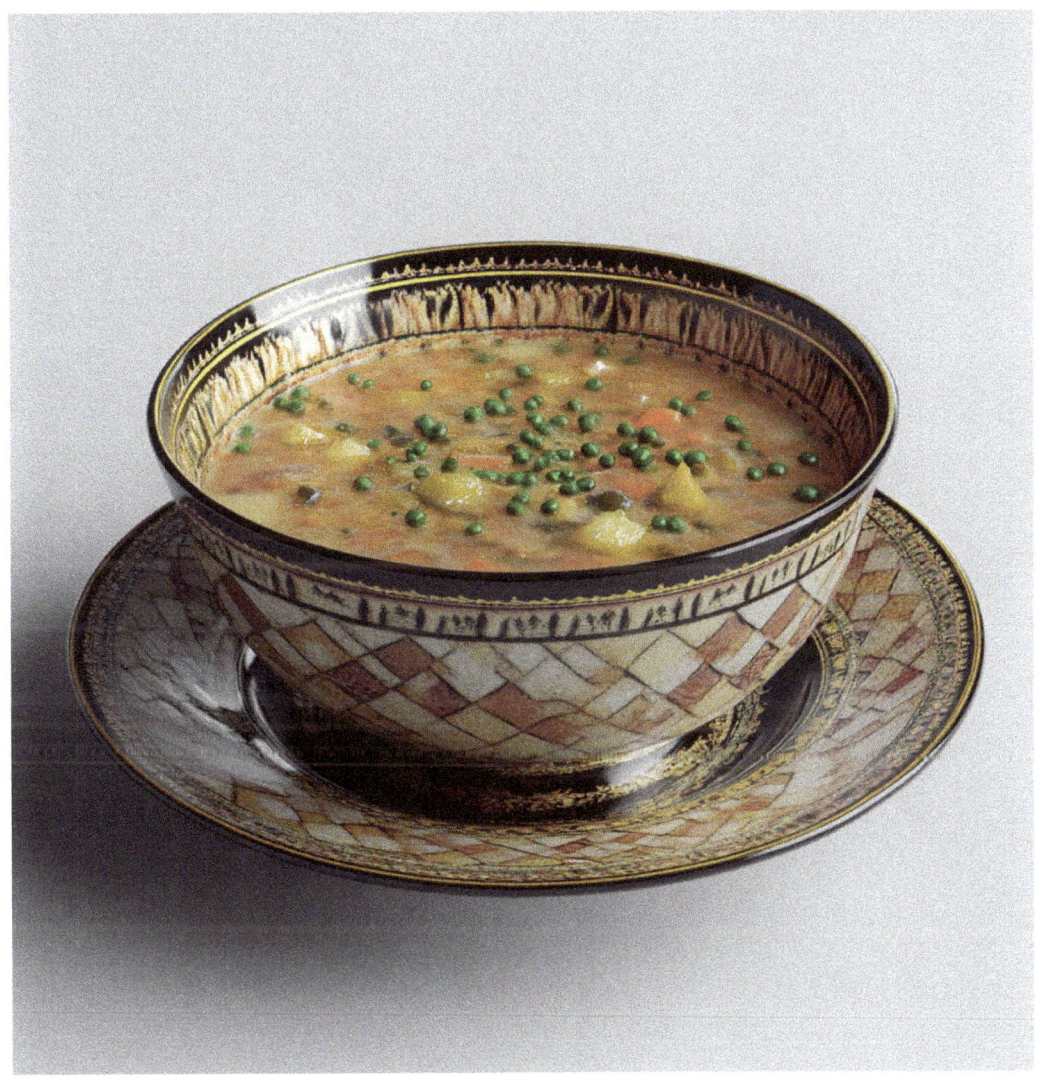

Soup

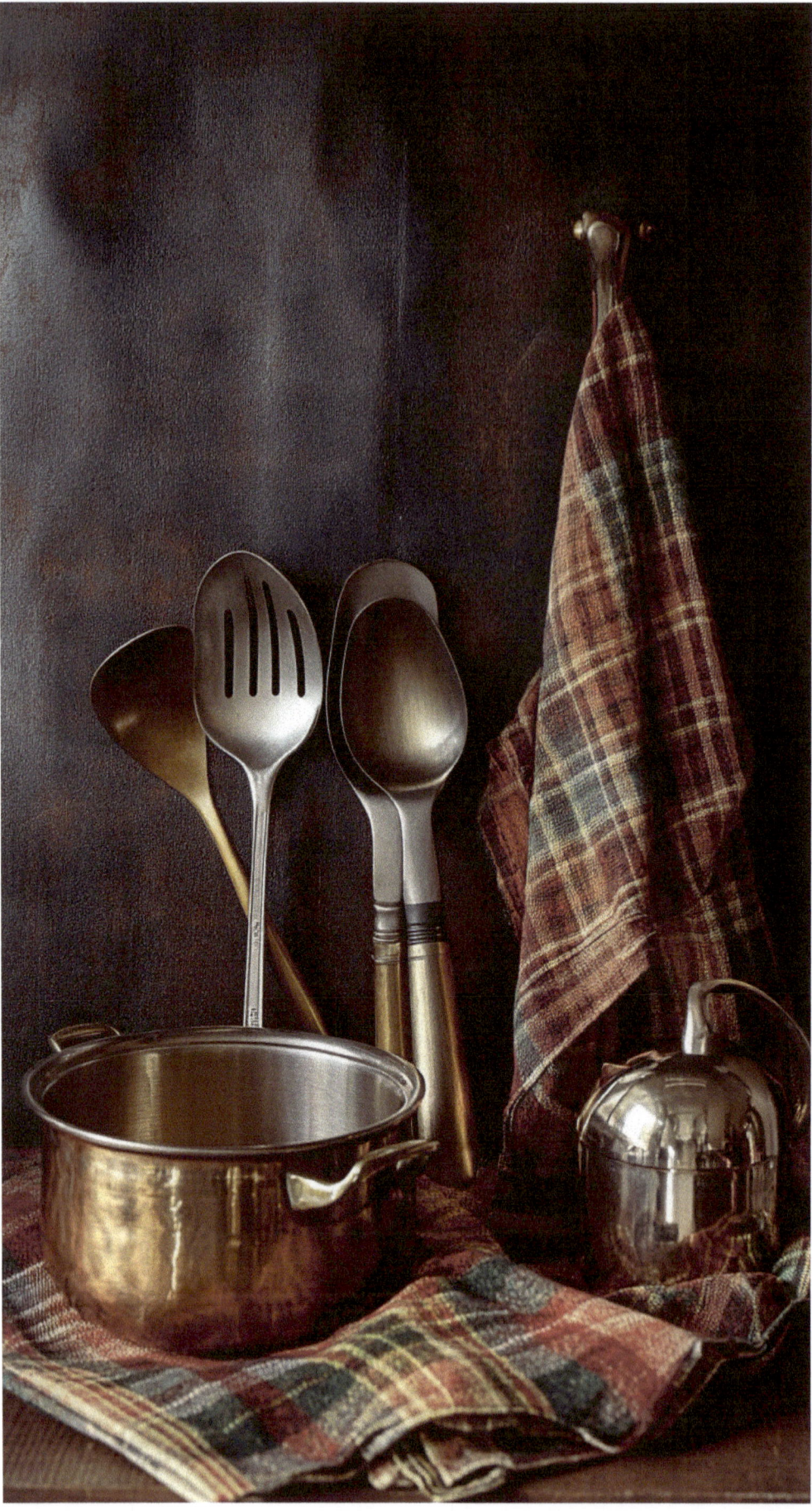

Soup Basics

Rules

1. Use a ratio of 25% onion to the main vegetable ingredient.
2. Cut the vegetables into the smallest pieces, 5mm (¼ in) dice. This reduces the cooking time.
3. Always add boiling water to the vegetables as this reduces the time the soup is off the boil, where it can stew and lose its freshness.
4. Once cooked, liquidise the soup and cool it as quickly as possible—this will keep its quality and flavour.
5. It is much easier to cook a big batch of soup. That way, you can freeze it in handy-size portions then once defrosted just reheat.

Approximate Cooking Time for Vegetables

Artichoke	35 minutes
Parsnips	50 minutes
Broccoli	10 minutes
Pea	3 minutes
Carrots	45 minutes
Spinach	5 minutes
Cauliflower	45 minutes
Tomato	20 minutes
Mushrooms	4 minutes
Watercress	2 minutes

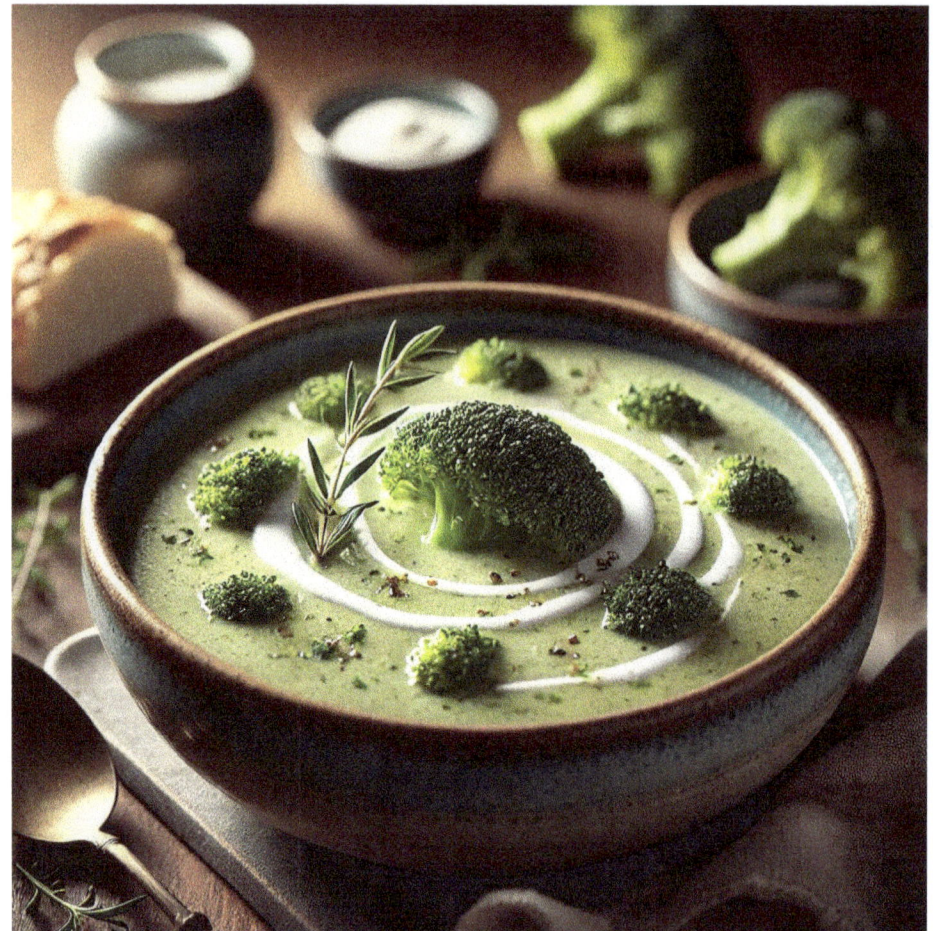

A Broth of Gentle Green

A simmered song, so soft, so sweet,
With butter's warmth and herbs discreet.
Leeks and celery, tenderly stewed,
A fragrant wisp, a mellow mood.

The stock enfolds the florets bright,
A verdant feast, a taste of light.
A swirl of cream, a final grace,
To warm the soul in cold embrace.

—*Inspired by Robert Louis Stevenson*

Broccoli Soup

Serves Six

Ingredients

50 g butter

60 g celery, finely chopped

125 g white part of the leek, finely chopped

3 onions, peeled and thinly sliced, can be used in place of the celery and leek)

3 rounded tablespoons plain flour

1.5 L hot chicken stock

800 g broccoli florets (125 g reserved for decoration)

Salt and pepper

Pinch of grated nutmeg

150 ml double cream (120ml for the soup & the rest for garnish)

2 rounded tablespoons finely chopped parsley/chives

6 sprigs of rosemary for decoration

Method

1. Melt the butter over low heat in a large saucepan. Add the celery and leeks (onions), and gently cook for 10 minutes, stirring occasionally until the vegetables are soft.

2. Stir in the flour and cook for another couple of minutes.

3. In another pan, place the chopped broccoli florets in the hot chicken stock, bring it back to the boil, and simmer for 12 minutes until tender. Drain the broccoli, reserving the stock. Run cold water over the broccoli to stop the cooking process.

4. Add the reserved stock a little at a time to the flour and vegetables, stir well, bring to a boil, then add the broccoli and liquidize with a stick blender.

5. When ready to serve, add the nutmeg and 100ml of cream and season to taste. Reheat gently to just below the boil, then serve with a swirl of cream and a sprinkle of finely chopped parsley on top and a sprig of rosemary for decoration.

6. Serve with warm brown rolls.

Soup

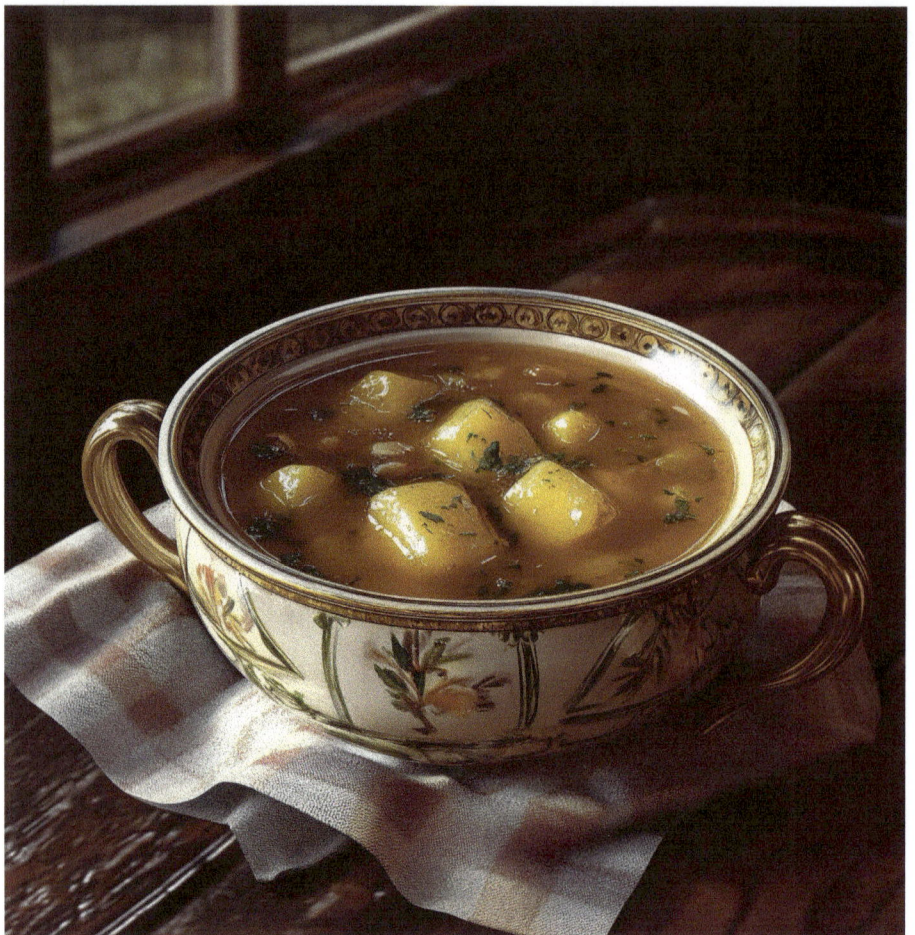

Ode to the Sea's Gift

Upon the coast where white waves break,
The silver catch is ours to take.
A haddock smoked in curling mist,
A taste the Highlander won't resist.

With onions soft and milk so sweet,
A broth to make the cold retreat.
A fisher's strength in every sip,
A taste of home upon the lip.

—Inspired by Sir Walter Scott

Canary Soup

Serves 6

Ingredients

250 g chickpeas (2 tins of chickpeas)

4 large potatoes

4 carrots

4 tomatoes

250 g green beans

2 courgettes

250 g diced pumpkin

2 Tbsp olive oil

1 onion

2 cloves garlic

1 tsp paprika

1 tsp crushed cumin seeds

1 pinch saffron

1 Tbsp wholemeal flour

2 L of boiling water or vegetable stock

Method

1. Soak the chickpeas overnight. Next day, cook them in a large saucepan with 2 litres of water and simmer for 2 hours. (Substitute tin chickpeas) Drain the chickpeas.

2. Meanwhile, peel and roughly chop potatoes, carrots, pumpkin, and tomatoes into bite-size pieces. Slice the courgettes and green beans. Add all the vegetables and the chickpeas to a large pan and pour over 1½ litres of boiling water/vegetable stock, mixing well.

3. Heat the oil in a frying pan, sauté thinly sliced onion, and finely chop the garlic, adding the spices and seasoning. When the onion is cooked, blend in the flour, cook for a few minutes, then add a little water, mix well, then add the onions to the stock and vegetables. Stir well, and bring all the ingredients to the boil.

4. Turn down the heat and simmer gently for an hour. It improves if allowed to stand a few hours before serving or is even better overnight and reheated.

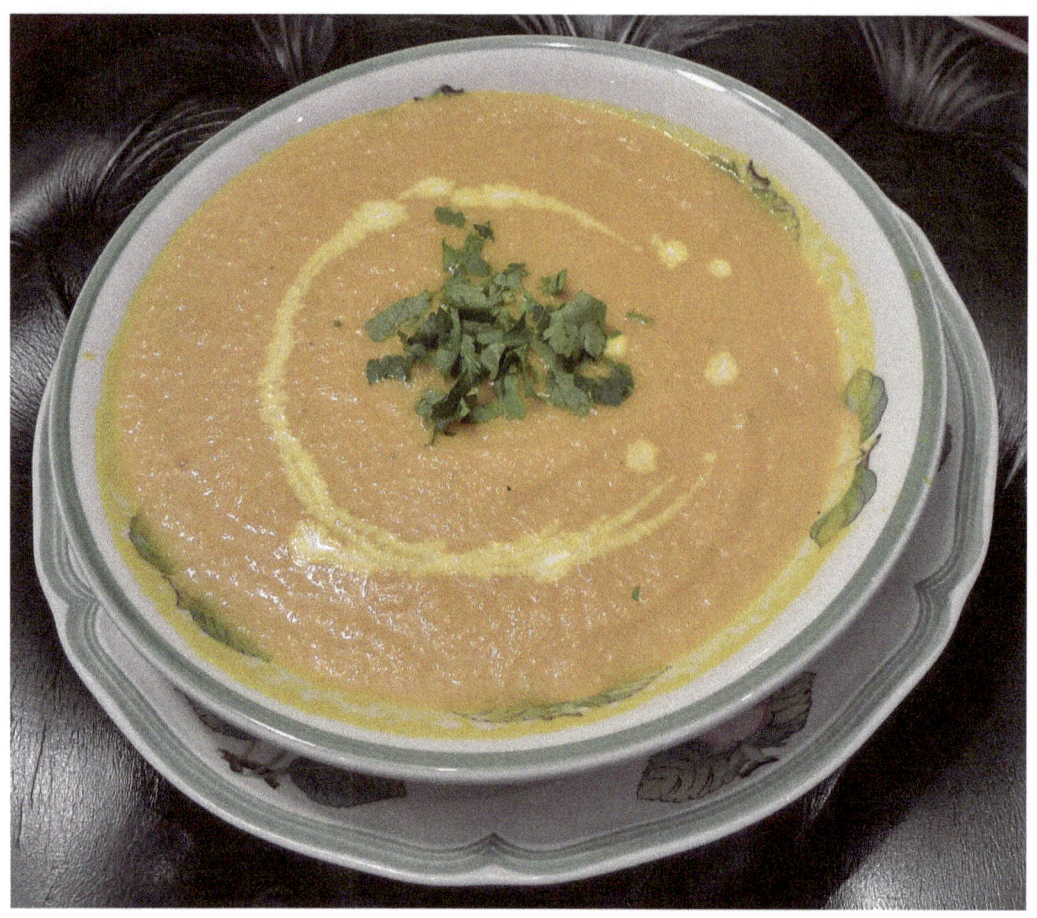

A Golden Glow

A pot of gold, so bright, so warm,
A simple charm, a rustic form.
With honey kissed and ginger's fire,
It wakes the heart, it lifts desire.

A humble bowl, yet rich and deep,
To soothe the soul, its comfort keep.
A swirl of cream, a gentle cheer,
A taste of sun through winter drear.

—Inspired by Contemporary Scottish Poets

Carrot Soup

Ingredients

80 g unsalted butter

150 g onion, thinly sliced

20 g root ginger

750 g carrots peeled and grated

1 Tbsp clear honey

1 tsp lemon juice

2 tsp Maldon salt

¼ tsp of white pepper

900 ml boiling water

Method

1. Melt the butter in a large saucepan. Add the onions and stir to coat. Don't let the onions go brown.

2. Using the flat edge of a heavy knife, crush the ginger (this releases the oil). Add this to the onions and let them sweat for ten minutes.

3. Add the grated carrot, honey, lemon juice and seasoning. Stir well. Pour in the boiling water and bring it back to the boil. Simmer for 45 minutes. (You may have to add a little more liquid during this time to allow for evaporation)

4. Remove the pan from the heat and liquidise the contents (with a hand-held blender or in the liquidiser) until smooth and creamy.

Decorate with a swirl of cream and some chopped parsley.

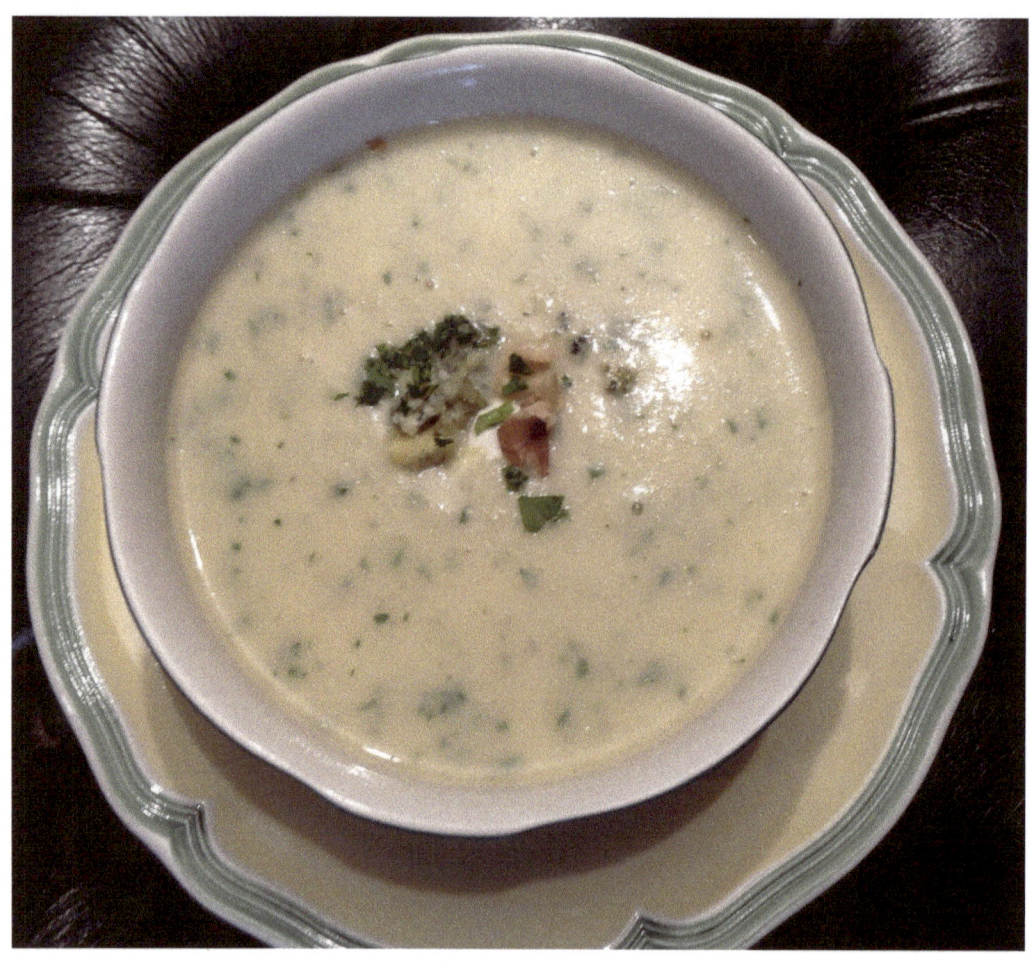

A Curious Blend

Upon the tongue, a dance so rare,
Of earth and fruit, a softened pear.
A cauliflower's snowy bloom,
Meets blue-veined bite, its fragrant plume.

A spoonful swirls in creamy white,
A walnut crunch, a sharp delight.
A dish both bold and light anew,
A poet's dream in golden hue.

—*Inspired by Robert Louis Stevenson*

Cauliflower, Pear, and Blue Cheese Soup

Serves 4

Ingredients

- 25 g butter
- 6 shallots diced
- 1 stick celery, finely chopped
- 1 large conference pear, peeled and cored and roughly chopped
- 1 cauliflower broken into florets (about 500 g)
- 1 L of vegetable stock (1 L of boiling water & 2 Knorr vegetable stock pots)
- 4 Tbsp of crème fraîche or double cream, reserve a small amount for the decoration
- 100 g British blue cheese, roughly chopped
- 3 Tbsp of flat-leaf parsley, plus extra for garnish

For the walnut decoration

- ½ tsp sea salt
- 1 tsp caster sugar
- 50 g walnuts roughly chopped

Method

1. Preheat the oven to 180°C.
2. Place the sea salt and sugar in a pestle and mortar for the walnut decoration and pound into a powder. Place the walnuts on a baking tray, sprinkle over the powdered salt and sugar, and toss well until evenly coated. Roast for 5-7 minutes until golden, then remove from the oven and set aside to cool.
3. For the soup, melt the butter in a large saucepan. Add the shallots and celery and cook for 5 minutes until they start to soften. Stir in the pears and cauliflower, toss together well, and then pour over the boiling stock. Simmer for 20 minutes until the cauliflower is tender.
4. Stir in the crème fraîche and most of the blue cheese (reserve a little for garnish). Simmer for 5 minutes more, then remove from the heat. Blend the mixture until smooth. Add the parsley.
5. Ladle the soup into serving bowls and sprinkle with the walnuts, reserved blue cheese, extra parsley, a swirl of crème fraîche and a little ground black pepper.
6. Serve with crusty bread.

To make ahead: Prepare the walnuts up to a week in advance and store them in an airtight container. Prepare the soup to the end of step 3, leaving out the crème fraîche and parsley. Pour into a rigid, freezer-proof container and leave to cool completely. Freeze for up to one month. To serve, defrost thoroughly before heating through until piping hot, then stir in the crème fraîche and parsley and garnish as step 4.

Soup

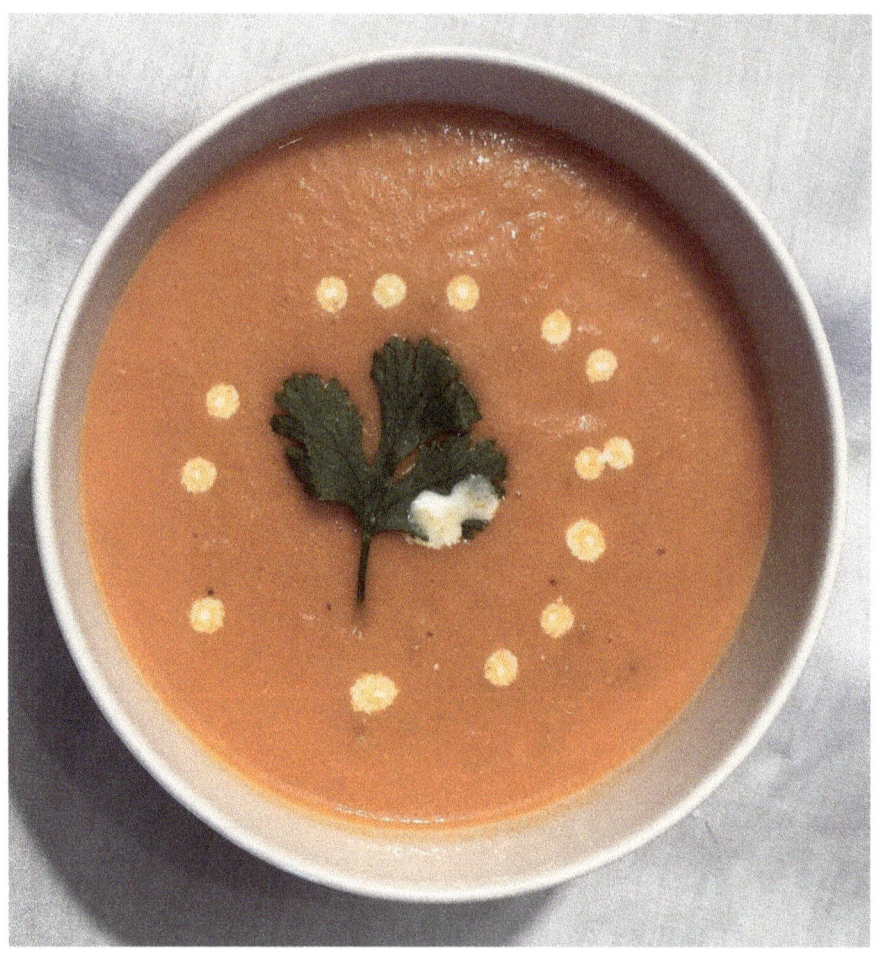

A Homely Tale

No feast so fine nor dish so grand,
Could match this bowl in loving hand.
The vine's red fruit, both ripe and sweet,
A summer's gift in warmth complete.

With every sip, the days return,
Of fireside tales and bread well-burned.
A taste of youth, a mother's grace,
A simple joy, a soft embrace.

—Inspired by John Buchan

Classic Cream of Tomato Soup

Serves 4-6

Ingredients

50 g butter

1 Tbsp olive oil

2 onions, finely chopped

2 celery sticks, finely chopped

2 carrots, finely diced

1 tsp sugar

2 garlic cloves, minced

20 ripe tomatoes, about 1.720 kg, skinned and roughly chopped, a mix of plum and classic.

1 jar of sun-dried tomatoes, finely chopped and well-drained

1 L hot vegetable stock

3 Tbsp double cream

Salt and pepper

Method

1. Heat the butter and olive oil in a heavy saucepan over medium heat. Add the onions, and sauté for 8-10 minutes, stirring frequently, until very soft but not coloured.
2. Next, add the celery and carrots and continue cooking gently without burning for another 10 minutes, stirring occasionally.
3. Add the garlic and sugar and saute for another 2 minutes, stirring all the time.
4. Add the tomatoes to the pan, stirring for 5 minutes to allow the flavours to combine.
5. Pour in the hot vegetable stock and simmer the soup for 25 minutes.
6. Blend the soup to a smooth puree using a hand-held blender. Add the double cream a teaspoon at a time until you are happy with the texture. Season with salt and pepper and serve.

Freeze up to 3 months before cream is added.

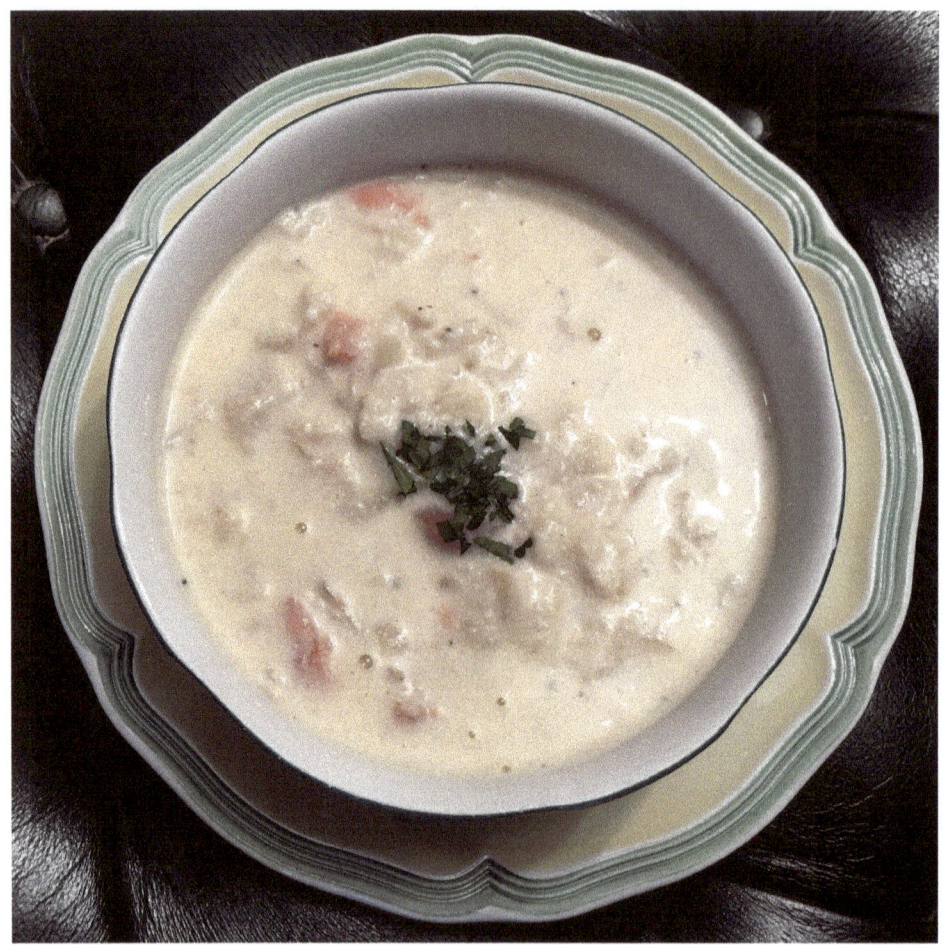

A Song of the Sea

A whisper rolls from ocean deep,
Where silver tides in silence sleep.
A fisher's prize, so firm, so white,
Now swirls in cream, a bold delight.

A hint of smoke, a drift of brine,
A broth so soft, so rich, so fine.
The cold recedes, the night stands still,
As warmth flows in, its hunger filled.

—*Inspired by Sir Walter Scott*

Creamy Smoked Haddock Soup

Serves 6

Ingredients

700 g smoked undyed haddock

1 L (mainly milk and a little water)

50 g butter

2 onions skinned and finely sliced

2 medium potatoes, chopped into 2 cm cubes

½ tsp freshly grated nutmeg

2 tomatoes, skinned, seeded, and chopped

Freshly ground black pepper

1 heaped Tbsp chopped parsley

Single cream to serve (optional)

Method

1. Skin the tomatoes by placing them in a bowl and pouring boiling water on top; leave for 2 minutes until the skins start to split. Remove each one from the water with a slotted spoon and carefully slip the skins off. Chop the tomatoes up and leave to one side.

2. Remove the bones from the centre of the fish. Put the fish into a saucepan with the milk and water. Bring the liquid slowly to just under the boil, then remove it from the heat and let the fish cool in the pan.

3. Melt the butter in another saucepan and add the onions. Cook over low heat for about 10 minutes, stirring occasionally to prevent sticking.

4. Place the chopped potatoes in another pan with some boiling water, turn down the heat, and cook until soft. Remove from the water. Place ¼ of the potatoes and ¼ of the onions with half the milk stock in which the fish was cooked. (Save the remainder of the milk.) Blend with a hand-held stick; this will produce a thick sauce.

5. Flake the fish, being careful to remove all the bones. Combine all the ingredients. Add the tomatoes. Heat the soup gently. Season with nutmeg and ground pepper. Just before serving, add some cream and parsley to decorate each bowl of soup.

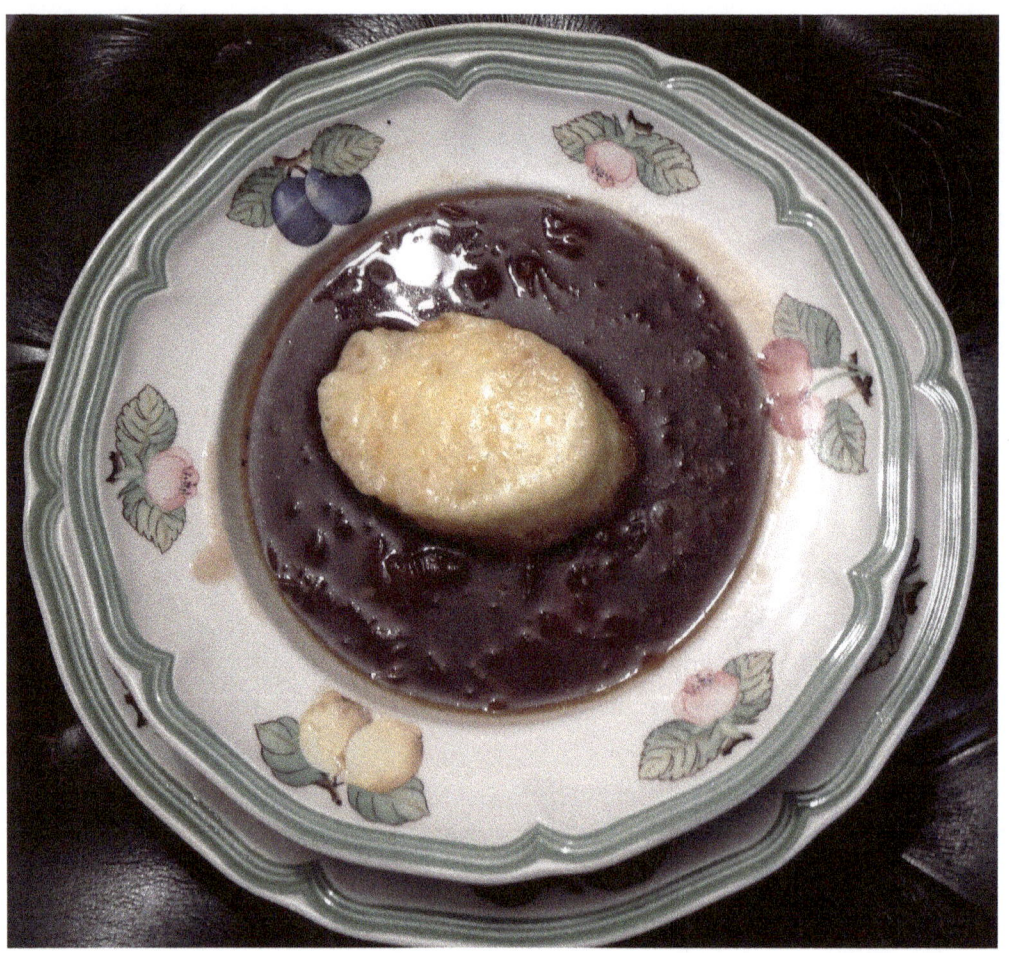

A Broth of Time and Patience

The onion hums, a tune so slow,
Through golden fire, its flavours grow.
A patient hand, a careful stir,
A scent to make the senses purr.

With wine's embrace and herbs so bright,
The broth is bold, the taste just right.
And on the top, a crusted dome,
A melted crown, a toast to home.

—*Inspired by Robert Burns*

French Onion Soup

Serves 6

Ingredients

700 g onions, thinly sliced

2 Tbsp olive oil

50 g butter

2 garlic cloves

½ Tbsp caster sugar

1.2 L of good beef stock (2 Knorr stock cubes)

275 ml dry white wine

3 bay leaves

1 sprig rosemary

Salt and milled ground pepper

French bread or baguette, cut into 2.5 cm diagonal slices

225 g gruyere cheese, grated

Dijon mustard (optional)

Method

1. Place the saucepan or casserole on high heat and mix the oil and butter. When this is very hot, add the onions and fry for 2-3 minutes. Lower the heat, cover with a lid, and cook for 10 minutes.

2. Remove the lid, sprinkle with the sugar, add the garlic, and season with salt and pepper. Then, fry over high heat for 2-3 minutes, stirring. Reduce the heat to low and cook for 15 minutes, occasionally stirring, until the onions are tender, golden, and caramelized.

3. Pour in the wine and boil for 2-3 minutes to allow the alcohol to evaporate. Add the stock and herbs, bring back up to the boil, and simmer over medium heat for 8-10 minutes.

4. Let the soup sit cold, preferably overnight. Skim off the fat. When you're ready to serve the soup, reheat it and taste it to check the seasoning. Preheat the grill to its highest setting, and warm the soup bowls in the oven.

5. Slice the baguette at an angle about 2 cm thick. Toast one side, turning it over when golden brown. Spread the untoasted side with mustard and top with Gruyere cheese. Place back under the grill until the cheese is golden brown and bubbling.

6. Remove the bay leaf and rosemary, fill the bowls with the soup, and top with the sliced baguette with melted cheese on top of the soup. Serve immediately.

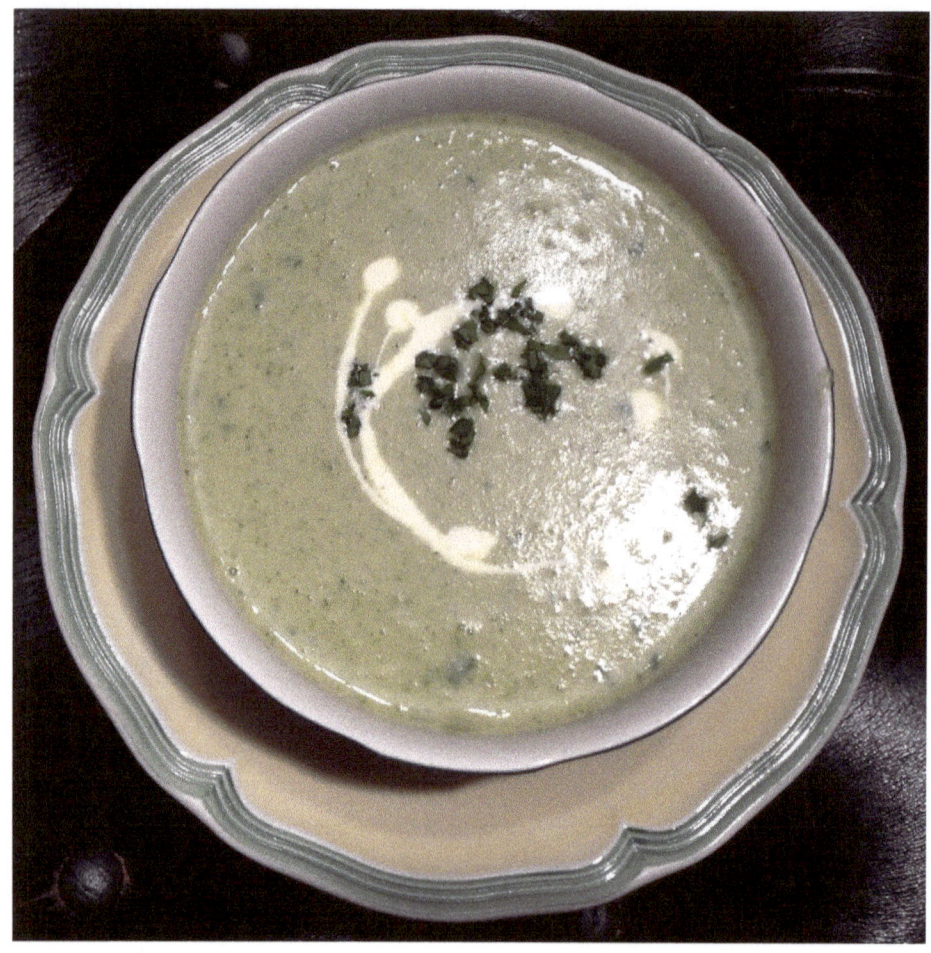

A Farmer's Feast

From rolling fields and gardens neat,
The ham is cured, the peas are sweet.
A broth of green, a minty breeze,
A taste of spring among the trees.

The spoon is dipped, the warmth unfolds,
A dish of toil, a tale retold.
A meal to mend, to cheer, to mend,
A sip of comfort to the end.

—*Inspired by Robert Burns*

Ham Hock, Pea, and Mint Soup

Serves 6

Ingredients

To cook the ham hock

1 ham hock (about 1 kg / 2 lb 4 oz)
1 large onion, thickly sliced
1 shallot, thickly sliced
1 head of garlic, cut in half horizontally
2 carrots cut into 2" chunks
1 stick of celery, cut into chunks
3 sprigs parsley
1 sprig thyme
6 whole peppercorns
1 bay leaf

For the soup

50 g butter
3 shallots, finely chopped
300 g potato, peeled and chopped
180 g cooked ham, diced
500 g frozen peas, defrosted
12 g fresh mint leaves, remove stalks, using 6 leaves for garnishing,
1 L ham stock, hot
150 ml double cream, reserve a little for garnish
Salt and black pepper
Garlic bread

Method

Ham Hock

1. For the ham hock, put the ham into a deep saucepan, add all the other ingredients, and cover with water. Bring slowly to the boil, then simmer for 1½–2 hours, then remove from the heat and allow to cool slightly.

2. Remove the ham hocks from the stock and shred the meat from the bone. (Keep warm.) Reserve the ham stock to make the soup.

Soup

1. Soften the shallots in the butter in a pan over low heat for 2–3 minutes. Add the potato and continue cooking, covered, for another 7–10 minutes or until the potato is tender. Pour over the hot stock and simmer for 10–15 minutes.

2. Add the peas and cook for 2–3 minutes. For the last 20 seconds of cooking, add the mint leaves. Whiz the soup using a stick blender until smooth. Stir in the diced ham.

3. Reheat the soup, add the cream, season with salt and pepper to taste. Garnish with cream and chopped mint.

4. Serve with garlic bread

One can also buy pulled ham hock in packets from Waitrose! Reheat in the microwave before adding to the soup.

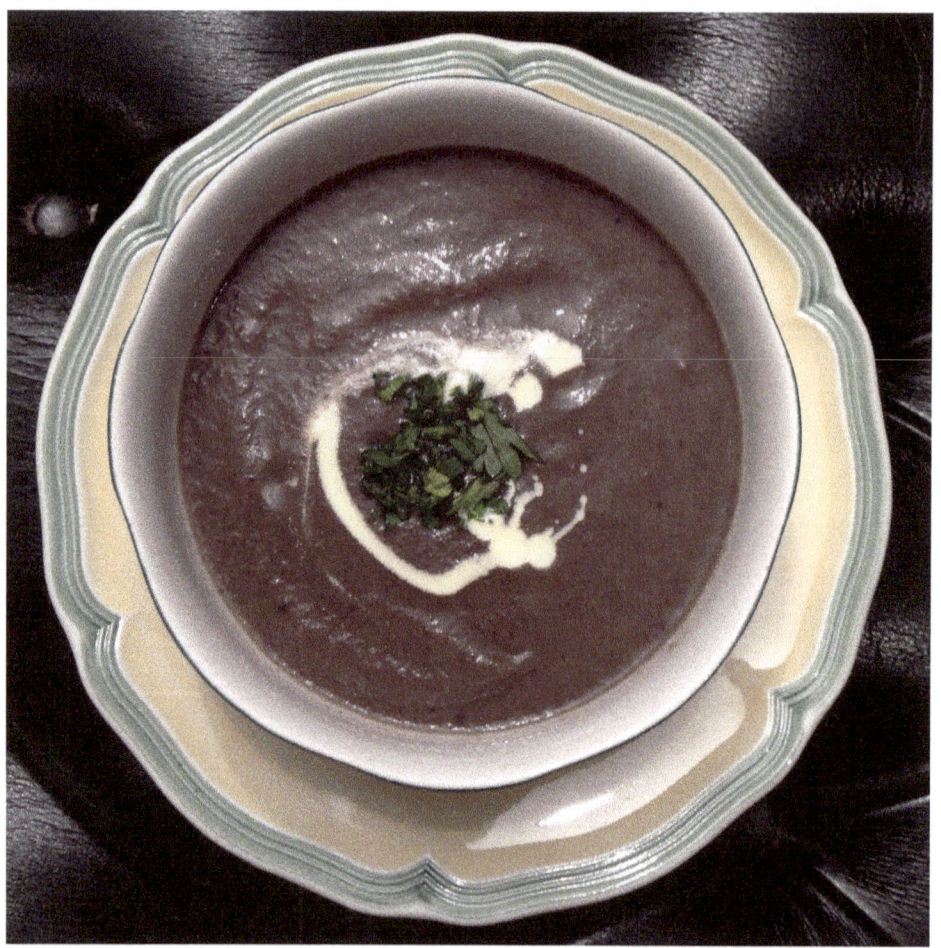

A Woodland Whisper

Through misty glen and shadowed shade,
The quiet mushrooms softly laid.
A scent of earth, of moss, of pine,
A bowl that hums of ancient time.

A velvet sip, a lingering glow,
A taste of secrets forests know.
With parsley fresh and cream so light,
It warms the heart through winter's night.

—*Inspired by Contemporary Scottish Poets*

Mushroom Soup

Serves 4

Ingredients

30 g butter

1 onion, finely chopped

2 celery sticks, finely chopped

2 garlic cloves, crushed

450 g mixed mushrooms, roughly chopped

200 g potatoes, peeled and cubed

1 L of hot vegetable stock

2 Tbsp finely chopped fresh parsley

Salt and freshly ground black pepper

Horseradish cream or cream to serve

Method

1. Melt the butter in a heavy-bottomed pan. Add the onion, celery, garlic, and potato stir to coat well when it starts to foam. Then, cover the pan with a lid and sweat the vegetables on a gentle heat for 10 minutes.

2. Add the stock, bring to a boil, and then simmer for 10 minutes or until the potato and onions are completely cooked. Add the mushrooms and boil the soup with the lid off for 2-3 minutes until tender. Do not overcook.

3. Using a stick blender, whiz the soup until smooth. Add the chopped parsley and season to taste with salt and pepper. Serve immediately, stirring a little horseradish cream (for extra kick) or cream into each bowl

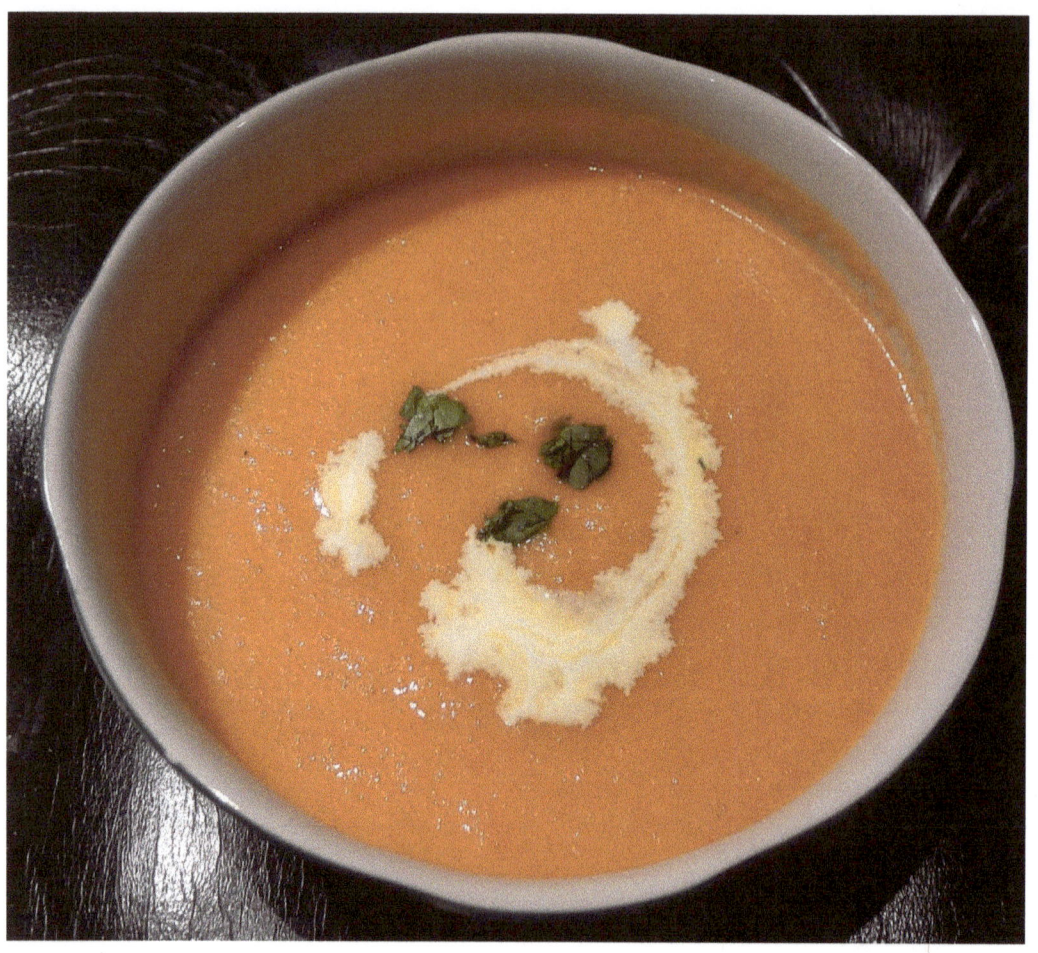

A Fire and Sun Delight

A pepper's flame, an orange's shine,
A bowl of warmth, a sip divine.
A hint of spice, a whisper sweet,
A dance of heat and citrus neat.

It sings of lands both bright and bold,
Where fruit and sun their flavours hold.
A spark of zest, a daring tune,
A taste of dusk, a sip of noon.

—*Inspired by Robert Louis Stevenson*

Red Pepper and Orange Soup

Serve 4-6

Ingredients

50 g unsalted butter
450 g onions, peeled and finely sliced
600 g red peppers, cored and seeded weight
85 ml dry sherry
1 orange rind finely grated
1 Tbsp of caster sugar
1 level tsp of ground coriander
½ L of freshly squeezed orange juice with bits
Seasoning
Garnish
Lightly whipped cream plus fresh coriander

Method

1. Melt the butter in a saucepan, add the onions, and cook until softened, stirring now and again with a wooden spoon.

2. Having removed the stalks and the seeds from the peppers, slice them finely in a food processor, this produces a more moist result than chopping by hand. Also, less liquid is added during the cooking process.

3. Add the peppers and all the remaining ingredients to the onions, stir, cover, and simmer gently for 40-60 minutes.

4. Liquidise until smooth, then pour through a mouli or sieve into the rinsed-out pan.

5. Reheat and correct the consistency by adding more water or orange juice and season to taste.

6. Serve in warm bowls. Garnish with a teaspoon of whipped cream and a leaf of fresh coriander.

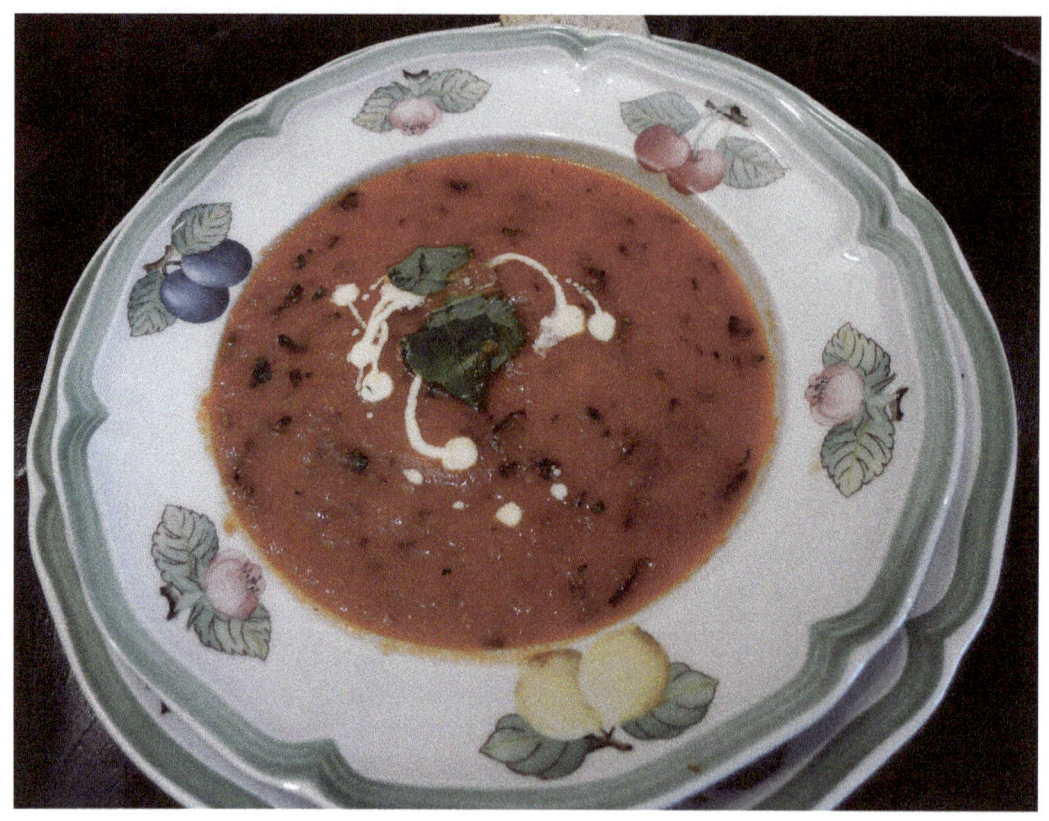

A Taste of Summer's Light*

Through garden green and summer bright,
The vines bear fruit in golden light.
A crimson burst, a fragrant bliss,
A spoonful warm, a sunlit kiss.

With basil's charm and bread so near,
A rustic joy, a taste sincere.
A bowl of ease, both rich and mild,
A memory sweet, a moment wild.

—*Inspired by John Buchan*

Rustic Tomato and Basil Soup

Serve 4-6

Ingredients

3 Tbsp of olive oil

2 red onions, peeled and diced

2 shallots, chopped

6 garlic cloves, peeled and diced

300 ml (½ pint) white wine

150 ml (¼ pint) water

12 plum tomatoes, quartered (they must be very ripe, or 2 400 g cans chopped plum tomatoes instead)

One Knorr chicken stock cube

½ loaf of ciabatta bread

15 g (½ oz) fresh basil

Sea salt and freshly ground black pepper

Single cream for decoration

Method

1. Skin the tomatoes by putting them in boiling water for 3 minutes, peel the skin away, then chop.

2. Heat the olive oil in a large pan, and cook the onions, shallots, and garlic for a few minutes to soften them slightly.

3. Add the wine, water, stock cube, and all the tomatoes. Bring to a boil and season with lots of salt and pepper.

4. Cook for 1 hour until reduced. Let it cool and liquidise very briefly. The more it is liquidised, the smoother the soup. Add finely chopped basil, taste, and season.

5. Serve with warm ciabatta bread, a swirl of cream, and a few torn basil leaves.

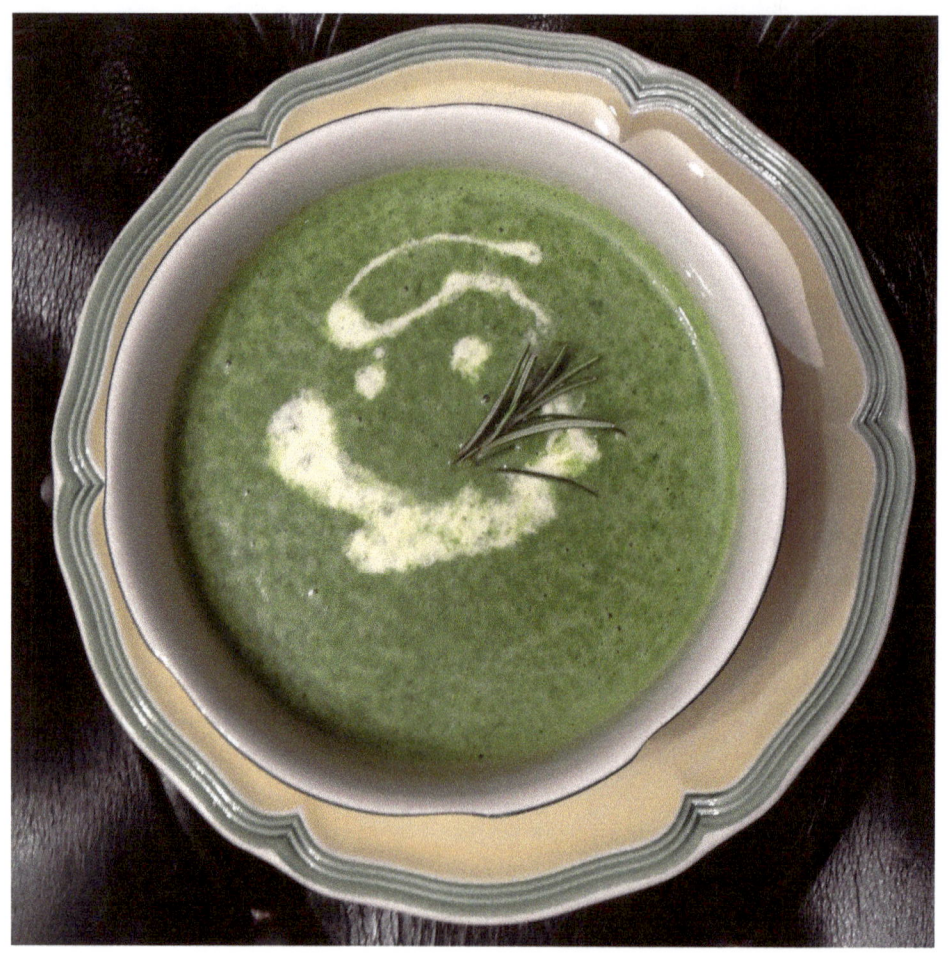

A Herb's Embrace

The wind may howl, the frost may creep,
Yet in this bowl, the warmth runs deep.
With leaves so dark and broth so bright,
It shields the soul in winter's night.

A sprig of green, a whisper low,
A taste the wandering heart will know.
A sip, a breath, a moment free,
A spoonful steeped in memory.

Inspired by Contemporary Scottish Poets

Spinach and Rosemary Soup

Serves 6

Ingredients

50 g butter

110 g onion, finely chopped

150 g potato, diced

Salt and freshly ground black pepper

450 ml hot vegetable or chicken stock

450 ml creamy milk (¼ cream and ¾ milk)

350 g spinach, destalked and chopped

1 Tbsp chopped fresh rosemary

2 Tbsp single cream to garnish

Sprig of rosemary to garnish

Method

1. Melt the butter in a heavy-bottomed pan. Add the diced onion and potato and stir to coat well when it starts to foam. Season well with salt and pepper, then cover the pan with a lid and sweat the vegetables gently for 10 minutes.

2. Add the stock and milk, bring to a boil, and then simmer for 5 minutes or until the potato and onions are completely cooked. Add the spinach and boil the soup with the lid off for 2-3 minutes or until tender. Do not overcook. Add the chopped rosemary, then whiz the soup with a stick blender and reheat gently.

3. Serve in warm bowls garnished with a swirl of cream and a sprig of rosemary with a flower on it in season, as it looks very pretty. This is good with crusty bread or cheese scones.

If freezing this soup, use only a small amount of rosemary as the flavour intensifies when frozen.

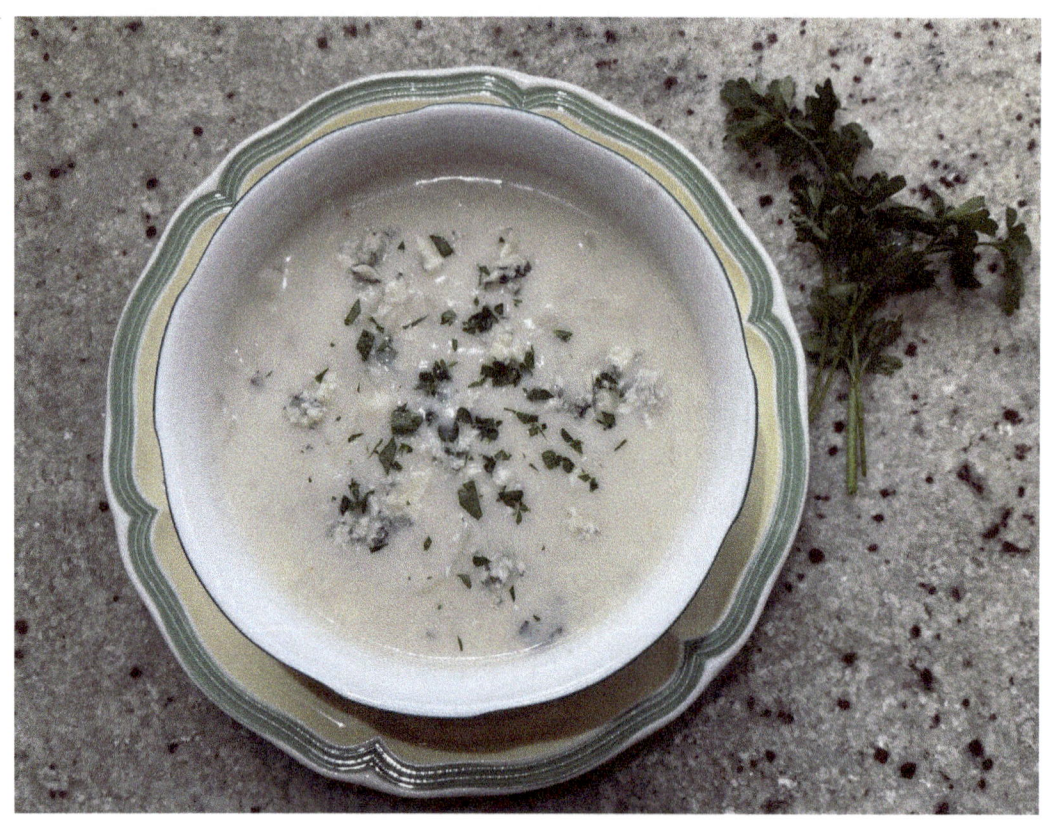

A Bold and Noble Brew

A broth of strength, a soup of might,
Where Stilton's tang meets onion's bite.
A hearty pour, a pot well-stirred,
A meal that needs no fancy word.

A warming touch, a curl of steam,
A dish both rich and bold in dream.
With parsley bright and nutmeg deep,
It wakes the soul from autumn's sleep.

—*Inspired by Sir Walter Scott*

Stilton, Onion, and Parsley Soup

Serves 6

Ingredients

600 ml milk
1 bay leaf
1/4 tsp grated nutmeg
90 g butter
3 medium onions, peeled and thinly sliced
75 g plain flour
170 g Stilton cheese, crumbled
1.2 L chicken stock
Salt and pepper
Single cream 150 ml (1/4 pint), optional
3 Tbsp parsley, finely chopped
Warm brown rolls

Method

1. Warm the milk with the bay leaf and grated nutmeg, bring almost to the boil. Remove from the heat. Cover and allow to cool for at least 20 mins.

2. Melt butter in a saucepan, add the onions, and cook gently over a low heat, stirring from time to time, for about 10 minutes, until the onions are soft and transparent.

3. Stir in the flour and cook for another couple of minutes.

4. Remove the bay leaf from the milk. Then very gradually add the milk and chicken stock over a low heat stirring all the time until combined, turn the heat up and bring to the boil.

5. Once it has boiled turn down the heat and simmer for 10 minutes.

6. Pull the saucepan off the heat and stir in the crumbled Stilton ,stirring until it has melted.

7. Season to taste with salt, and lots of black pepper.

8. You can make the soup up to this stage in advance but do not reboil or it will be become thin.

9. When ready to serve the soup gently stir in the cream (optional) add finely chopped parsley. If you add the parsley too soon, it will lose its bright, fresh colour in the heat of the soup.

10. Serve with warm brown rolls.

Soup

Flint Family Cookbook

Salad

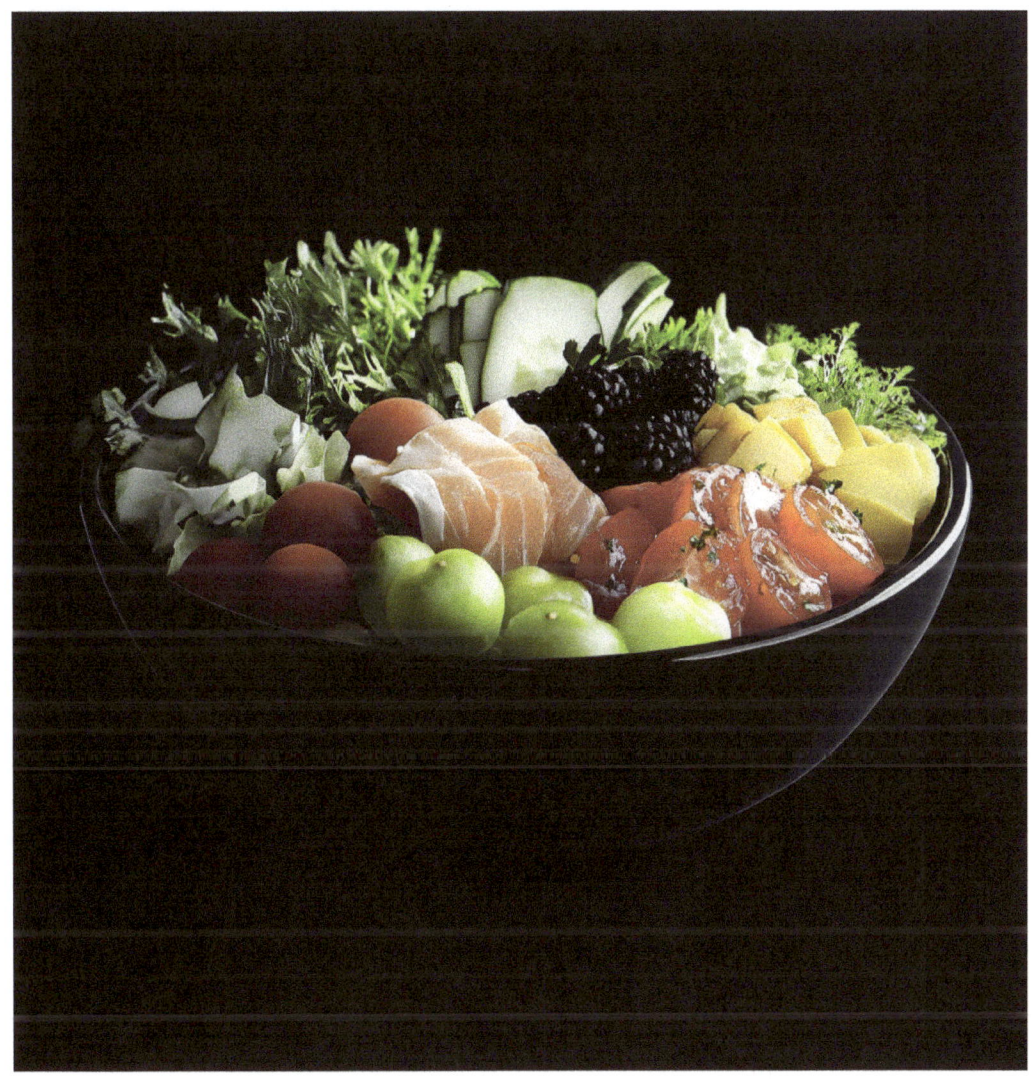

Salad

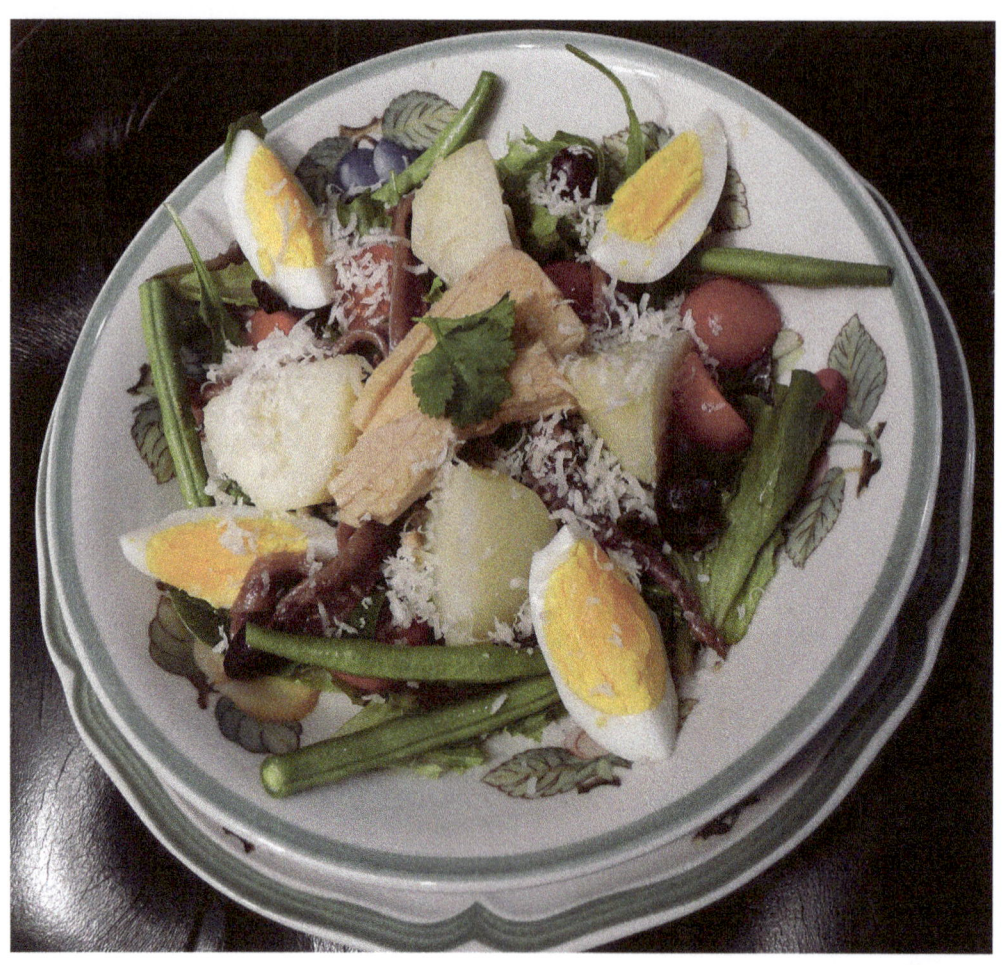

A Feast of the Mediterranean

Beneath the sun, so warm, so bright,
A dish is made in golden light.
The briny kiss of olives black,
The ocean's gift, the tuna's track.

With eggs so soft and greens so fair,
A burst of taste is waiting there.
A tang of mustard, tarragon's cheer,
A feast that sings of summer's year.

So lift your fork, embrace the day,
A meal to whisk the heart away.

—*Inspired by Robert Louis Stevenson*

Tuna Niçoise

Serves 4

Ingredients

225 g new potatoes with skins left on

225 g green beans, trimmed

4 eggs, hard-boiled

500 g tuna fish drained weight (2-3 tins)

225 g cherry tomatoes halved

1 bag of mixed lettuce

50 g Greek black pitted Kalamata olives

1 jar anchovy fillets

Dressing

7 Tbsp olive oil

2 Tbsp tarragon vinegar

1 Tbsp Dijon mustard

1 clove of garlic, peeled and halved, salt and pepper.

4 Tbsp grated parmesan cheese

Method

1. Scrub the potatoes until they are clean. Then, place it in a pan of cold, salted water. Bring to the boil and then simmer for 15 minutes until tender. Drain and put to one side. Cook the beans in boiling water for 4 minutes until tender, drain and place to one side. Cut the potatoes into large chunks.

2. Bring the eggs to a boil in cold salted water, turn down the heat, and simmer for 6 minutes. Run the eggs under cold water for 3 minutes before removing the shell. Quarter the softly boiled eggs, halve the tomatoes and drain the tuna fish.

3. Place the dressing ingredients in a screw-top jar and shake vigorously to blend. Put the lettuce in a bowl, pour 2 Tbsp of dressing over the leaves, and stir gently.

4. Divide the dressed lettuce and salad ingredients into 4 bowls. Any remaining dressing can be served with garlic bread.

5. Decorate with finely grated Parmesan cheese.

Salad

Flint Family Cookbook

Fish

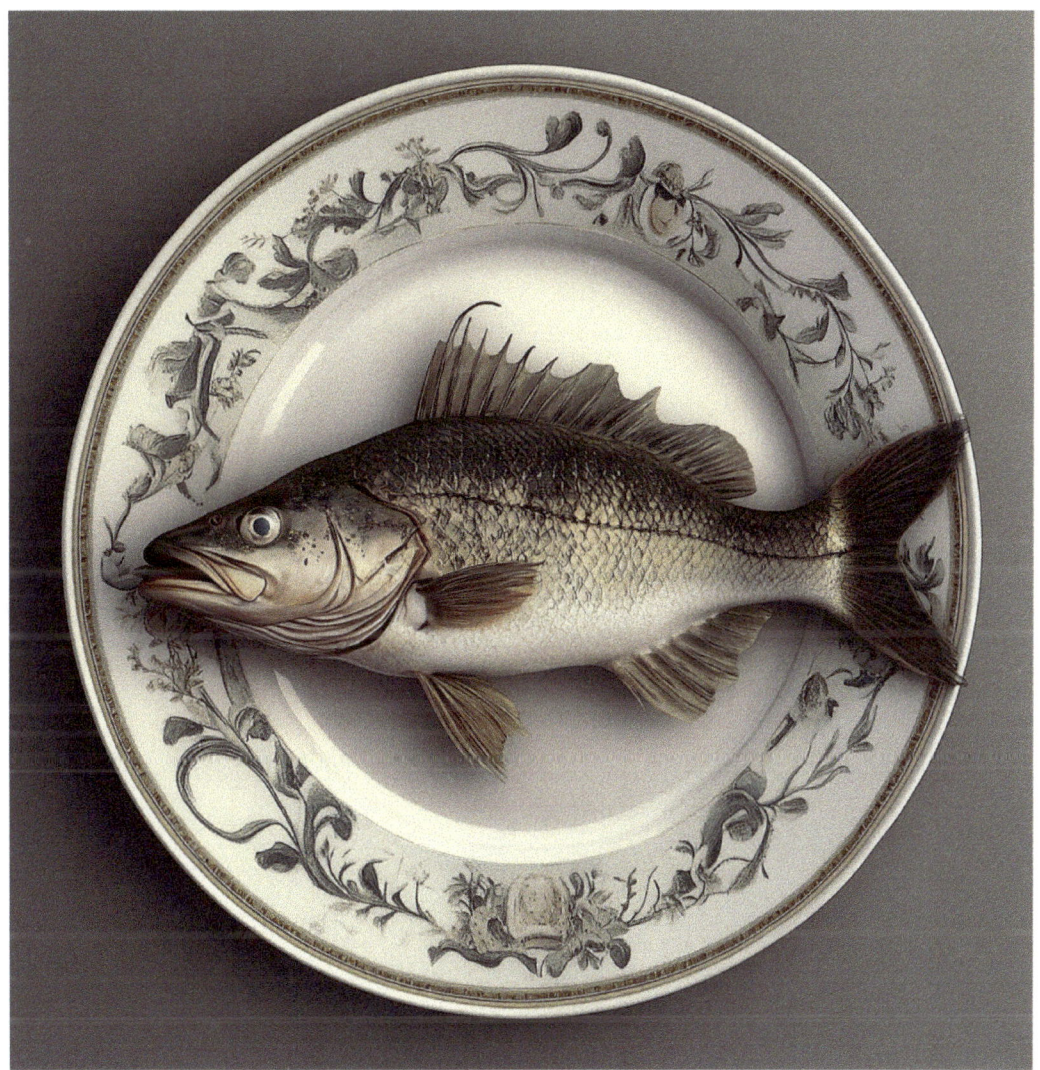

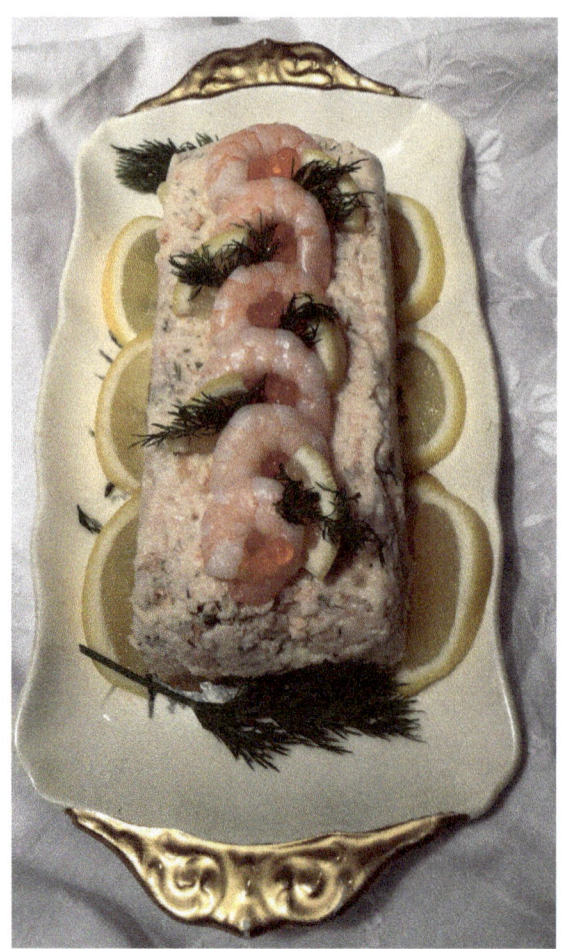

A Delicate Feast

Upon the plate, a coral hue,
A dish both rich and light anew.
The sea's embrace in layers fine,
With dill's fresh kiss and lemon's shine.

A spoonful soft, a savoury dream,
With roe that glows in golden gleam.
A terrine chilled, so light, so pure,
A taste the heart shall long endure.

—*Inspired by Robert Louis Stevenson*

Baked Salmon Terrine

Serves 6

Ingredients

1 small shallot, peeled
280 g pack salmon fillets, skin removed
200 g large prawns, plus extra to decorate
150 ml double cream
1 egg
1 Tbsp cornflour
¼ lemon, zest and juice
20 g pack dill, fronds chopped, some sprigs reserved to decorate
Rye bread to serve

Salmon roe dressing
50 jar salmon caviar
150 ml crème fraîche

Method

1. Prep the oven to 160°C. In a food processor, pulse the shallot a few times to chop. Add the raw salmon and pulse again until evenly chopped but still in quite large pieces. Add the prawns, cream, egg, cornflour, lemon juice, and zest, season, and whizz until evenly combined (you still want some coarse bits in there). Fold through the chopped dill and set aside.

2. Line a small, deep terrine or baking dish (about 600 ml in volume) with parchment paper. Add the salmon mixture. Cover the top with another sheet of baking parchment and pat down.

3. Put the dish inside a larger, deep roasting tin and place on the oven shelf. Carefully pour boiling water from the kettle into the tin so that it comes halfway up the sides of the dish. Bake for 45-55 minutes, until just set (it should have a slight wobble). The cooking time will vary depending on your dish, so check it after 20 minutes.

4. Meanwhile, combine the salmon roe and creme fraîche for the dressing, season and set aside.

5. Remove the mould from the hot water and cool completely before chilling for at least 2 hours (preferably overnight). Turn the terrine out onto a board and remove the parchment. Decorate with more prawns and the reserved dill sprigs.

6. Serve with rye bread, the salmon roe dressing, and lemon wedges, if liked.

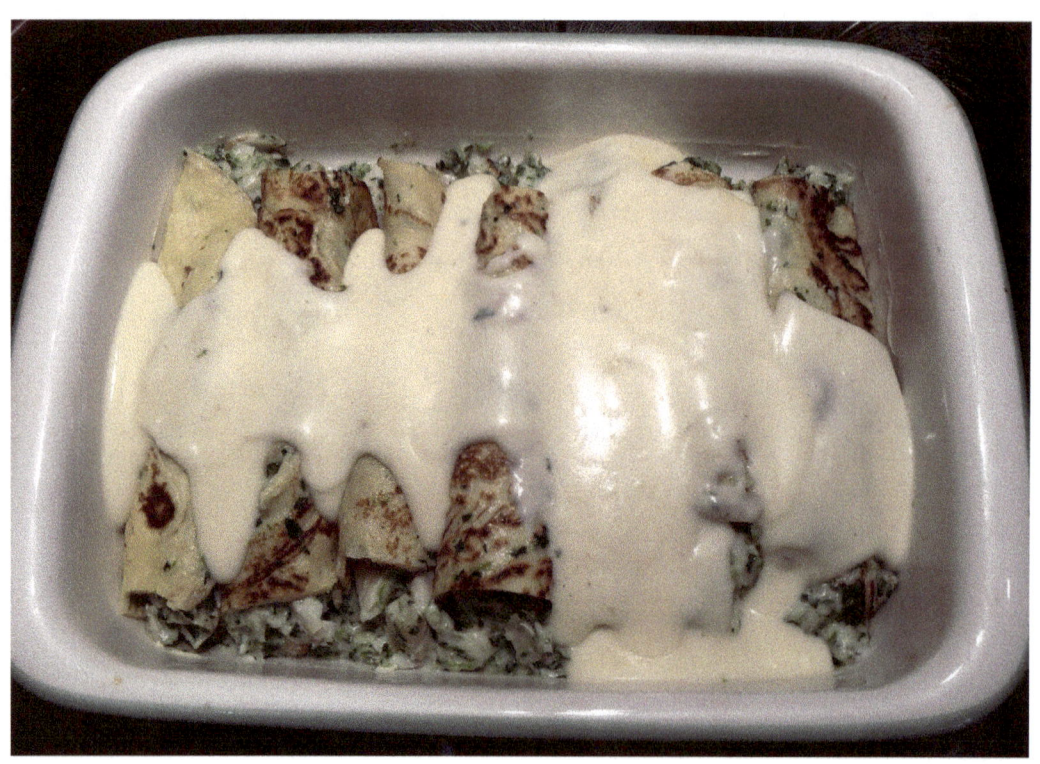

A Whisper of the Sea

A tender fold, so warm, so light,
A golden crepe, a soft delight.
With haddock's smoke and cheese so bold,
A tale of hearth and hands of old.

A sip of wine, a swirl of cream,
A meal to suit a poet's dream.
With every bite, the waves roll near,
A taste of comfort, rich and clear.

—*Inspired by John Buchan*

Crespellini

On a special occasion, the pancakes' sauce can be made with dry white wine instead of milk, and prawns, mussels, or scallops can replace the smoked fish. The dish can be made up to the baking stage 24 hours before. Keep covered in the fridge.

Serves 4

Ingredients

4 pieces of smoked haddock (900 g)
1 bay leaf
1 medium onion, peeled and sliced
A few black peppercorns
1 pt of milk
350 g fresh spinach cooked, drained and chopped or 225 g (8 oz) of frozen spinach thawed and drained

Pancake batter- makes about 12
110 g plain flour
Pinch of salt
2 eggs beaten
200 ml milk
75 ml water
1 Tbsp of melted butter
Vegetable oil or butter for frying

Sauce
½ pt of milk
75 g (3 oz) butter
75 g (3 oz) plain flour
150 g (5 oz) Gruyère cheese, grated
½-1 level tsp grated nutmeg
Salt and freshly ground pepper

Method

1. Put the fish in a saucepan with the bay leaf, onion slices, and peppercorns. Add the milk to cover the fish, adding a little water if there is not enough milk.

2. Slowly bring it to just below the boil. Remove from the heat, cover and **leave** until cold.

3. To make the pancakes, sieve the flour and salt in a mixing bowl and make a well in the centre. Pour in the beaten eggs and mix on a low setting until smooth.

4. Gradually beat in the milk to form a smooth batter. Continue beating until the batter is smooth and bubbly, with the consistency of single cream. Finally, beat in 1 Tbsp of melted butter.

5. Make the pancakes using a lightly oiled 6 / 7" (150mm) pan.

6. Pour a little oil or butter into the pan to grease it. Heat until it smokes slightly, tipping and tilting the pan so the base and sides are covered with a thin film. Pour off any excess.

7. Aiming for the centre of the pan, pour enough batter from a small jug to cover the base of the pan thinly.

8. As you pour the batter, quickly tip the pan so that it runs over the base before it cooks.
9. Cook until the pancakes dry and change colour and the underside is golden brown. To check the underside's colour, lift up a corner of the pancake with a spatula. If the pancake seems sticky, let it cook a little longer.
10. Slide the spatula under the centre of the pancake and flip it over. Cook until the side of the pancake that is now underneath is also coloured golden brown.
11. Slide the pancake out of the pan onto a plate lined with greaseproof paper and lay another sheet over it. Make the pancakes this way until all the batter is used up.
12. Note on making pancakes
13. When making pancakes, be prepared for the first couple to fail until the pan reaches the correct degree of heat and oiliness. At first, you have to cook the pancakes over high heat, but turn down the heat as the pan gets hotter.
14. When rolling or folding pancakes, remember that the side that was cooked first looks better, and this should be shown on the outside when folded. Unfilled pancakes can be stored stacked between layers of greaseproof paper.
15. Wrapped in polythene, they will keep for a week in the fridge and for two months in the freezer.
16. Preheat the oven to 190°C

Method – The Cheese Sauce

1. Drain the milk from the fish into a measuring jug, and add up to 850 ml (1½ pt) of fresh milk to make the cheese sauce. Melt the butter in a saucepan over low heat; add the flour and cook, stirring, for 1-2 minutes.
2. Remove from the heat and gradually blend in the milk. Return to the heat and bring it to a boil, stirring constantly. Simmer until thickened and smooth, then add the cheese with the nutmeg and season with salt and pepper. Stir until the cheese has melted, then remove from the heat.
3. To finish the filling, put the cooked/drained spinach in a bowl. Flake the fish, discarding all skin and any bones, and add it to the spinach. Then, add one-third of the cheese sauce to the spinach and adjust the seasoning.
4. Divide the filling equally between the 12 pancakes (about a heaped Tbsp of filling in each) and roll them up into cigar shapes around the filling.
5. Place three pancakes, with the joins underneath, in each of the four buttered gratin dishes or lay all the pancakes in one layer in a large shallow ovenproof dish.
6. Pour over the remaining cheese sauce.
7. Bake in the oven for 30-40 minutes or until bubbling.
8. Serve with crusty bread and a green salad.

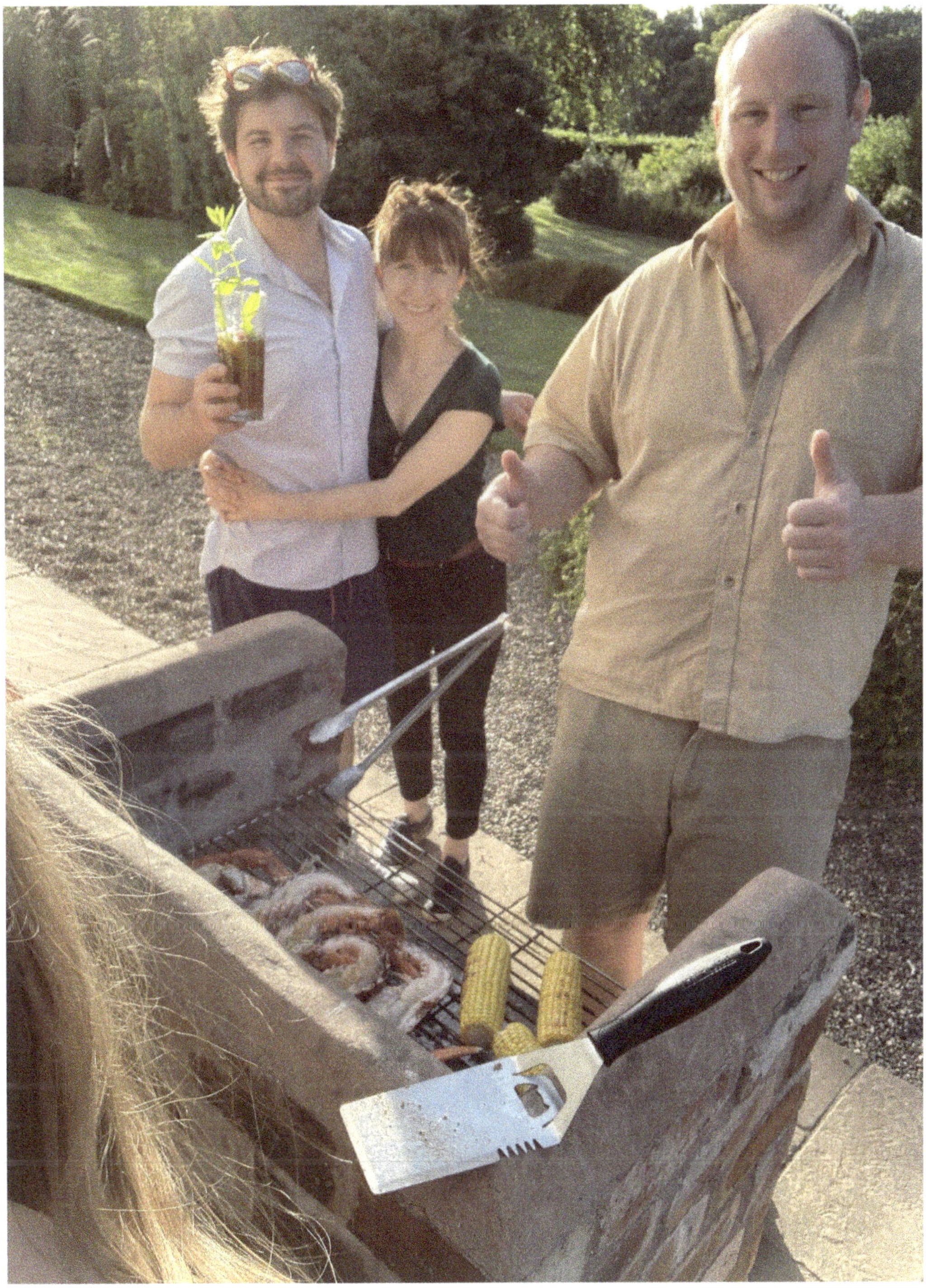

Fish

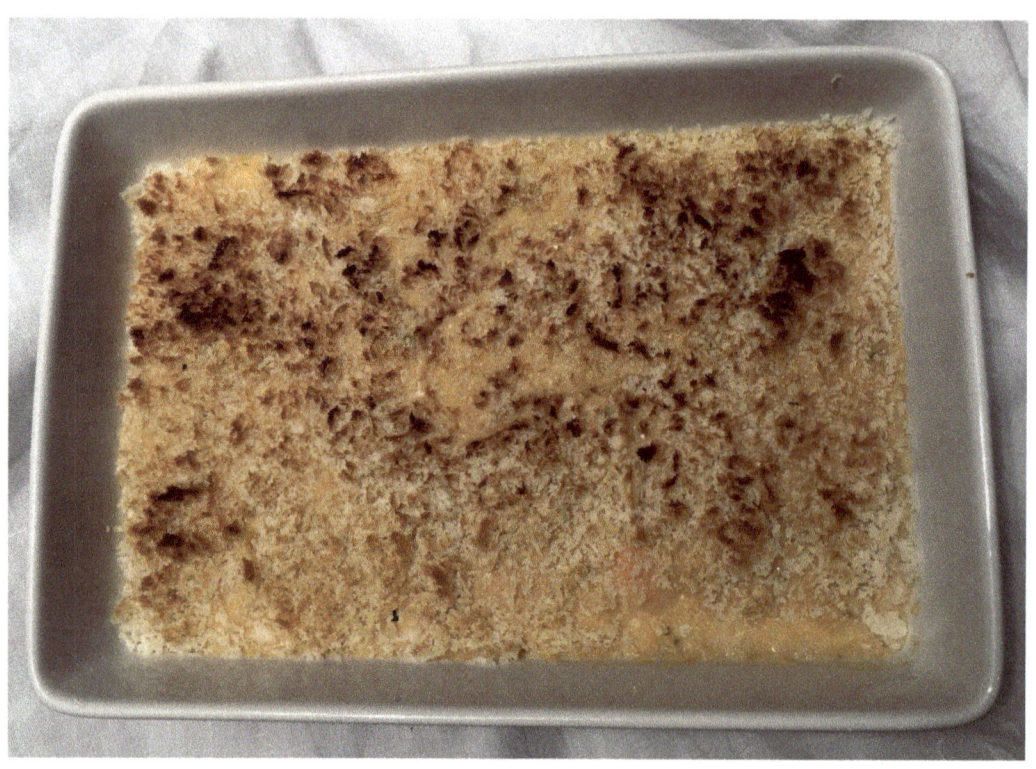

42

A Bold and Briny Bite

A fire within the ocean's prize,
With spice that wakes and butter wise.
The prawns and crab, the haddock bright,
A devil's touch, a deep delight.

With sherry's glow and mustard's might,
The broth is fierce yet rich in light.
A dish to stir the daring soul,
To lift the heart, to make it whole.

—*Inspired by Sir Walter Scott*

Devilled Seafood

Serves 8

Ingredients

- 900 g haddock
- Milk and water as required
- 450 g shellfish (prawns, scallops, crab)
- 225 g butter
- 9 rounded Tbsp flour
- 325 ml milk
- 225 ml evaporated milk
- 225 ml beef consommé
- 1 Tbsp lemon juice
- 1 Tbsp Worcestershire sauce
- 4 Tbsp tomato ketchup
- 1 Tbsp horseradish sauce
- 1 garlic clove, skinned and finely chopped
- 1 rounded tsp English mustard
- 1 tsp of salt
- 1 tsp soya sauce
- Dash of red pepper sauce (Tabasco)
- 4 rounded Tbsp finely chopped parsley
- 225 ml sherry
- Bread crumbs and extra butter to finish

Method

1. Put the haddock in a saucepan with milk and water to cover. Bring slowly to the boil, then remove from the heat and cool. Flake from the bones and skin when the fish is cool enough to handle.

2. Melt the butter in a saucepan. Stir in the flour and cook for a couple of minutes. Gradually add all the other ingredients, stirring until the sauce boils. (If it is too stiff for your liking, add more milk.)

3. When it has boiled, remove the saucepan from the heat and stir in the flaked fish and the shellfish. Simmer gently until everything is hot.

4. Butter an ovenproof dish and pour the devilled seafood into it. Sprinkle the bread crumbs over the surface and dot with butter. Put the dish under a hot grill to brown the breadcrumbs. Serve with rice and a green salad.

Fish

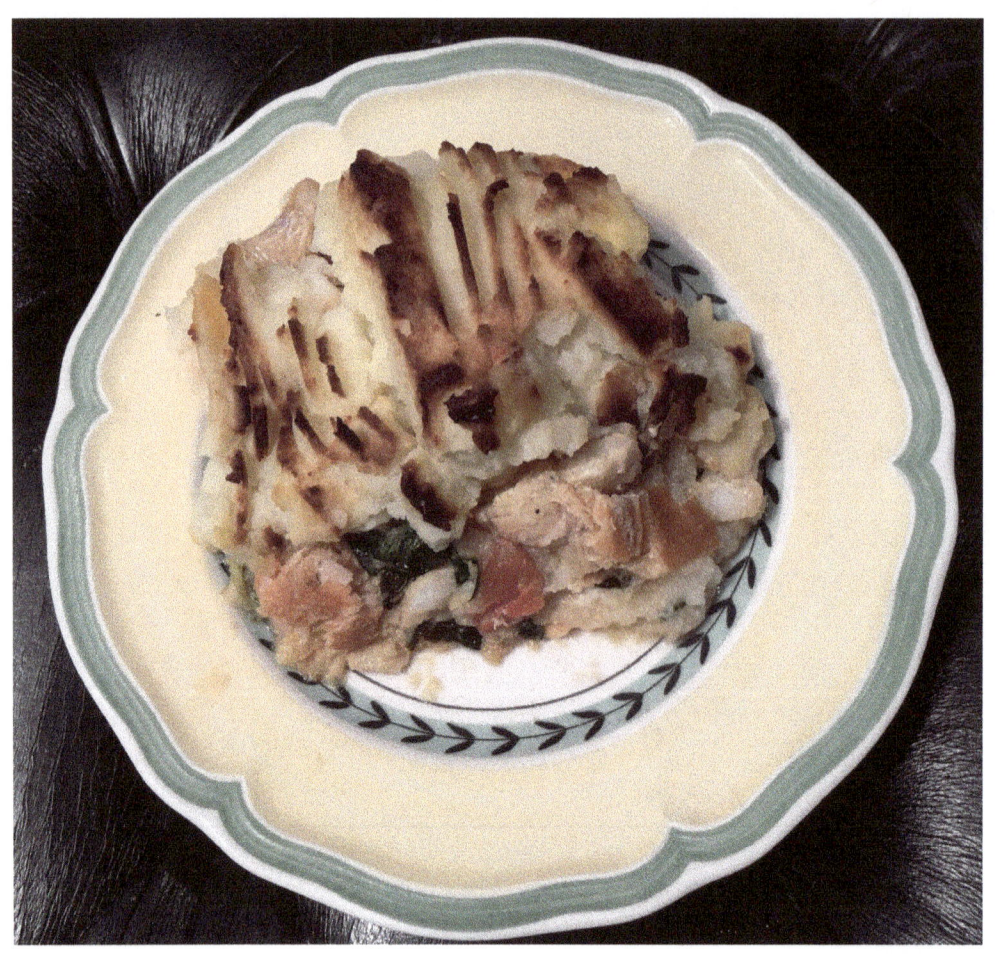

A Hearthside Tale

The winds may wail, the cold may bite,
Yet here within, the hearth burns bright.
With golden crust and ocean's fare,
A meal of love, a home's repair.

The haddock mild, the salmon sweet,
The prawn's embrace, the mash complete.
A dish to soothe, a heart's delight,
To warm the soul through winter's night.

—*Inspired by Robert Burns*

Fish Pie

Serves 6

Ingredients

- 1 kg potatoes (add cream or butter to make the mash)
- 1 carrot, peeled
- 2 sticks of celery
- 150 g good cheddar cheese
- 250 ml double cream
- 1 lemon
- ½ a fresh red chilli, remove pips or 1 tsp of mustard
- 6 g of flat-leaf parsley
- 750 g of any mixed fish (e.g., 300 g salmon fillets, skin off bones removed, 300 g undyed haddock fillets, skin off and bones removed, 150 g king prawns, raw, peeled)
- Sea salt and freshly ground black pepper
- Olive oil

Optional

- 2 Tbsp crème fraîche.
- 2 ripe tomatoes chopped
- 2 hard boiled eggs quartered
- 1 large handful of fresh cooked spinach or 4 oz frozen spinach thawed & chopped.

Method

1. Preheat the oven to 200°C and boil a large pan of salted water.
2. Peel the potatoes, cut into 2cm chunks.
3. Once the water is boiling, add your potatoes and cook for around 12 minutes, until soft.
4. Put the eggs into boiling water and cook for 8 minutes. Run under cold water, and cut each egg into small pieces. Meanwhile, put a box grater in a large, deep baking tray.
5. Grate the carrot and finely chop the celery & onion, fry gently in some olive oil until soft.
6. Add the cream and bring up to a boil (it will start to thicken)
7. Grate the Cheddar cheese on the coarse side of the grater. Add to onion mixture.
8. Finely grate the zest from the lemon; add to the onion mixture.
9. Finely grate or chop your chilli or mustard. Add to onion mixture
10. Finely chop the parsley leaves and stalks and add these to the mixture
11. Cut the salmon and smoked haddock into bite-size chunks and add the prawns to the other ingredients.

12. Squeeze over the lemon juice, drizzle with olive oil and add a good pinch of salt and pepper.
13. Do it now if you want to add tomatoes, crème fraîche or spinach. Mix everything together really well. Place in an ovenproof dish with approximately 3" sides, and pop the hard-boiled eggs on top. Your potatoes should be ready by now, so drain them in a colander and return them to the pan.
14. Add some cream or butter and a pinch of salt pepper
15. Mash until smooth, or use a potato ricer, then spread evenly over the top of the fish.
16. Place in the preheated oven for around 40 minutes or until cooked through, crispy and golden on the top
17. Serve piping hot with green beans.

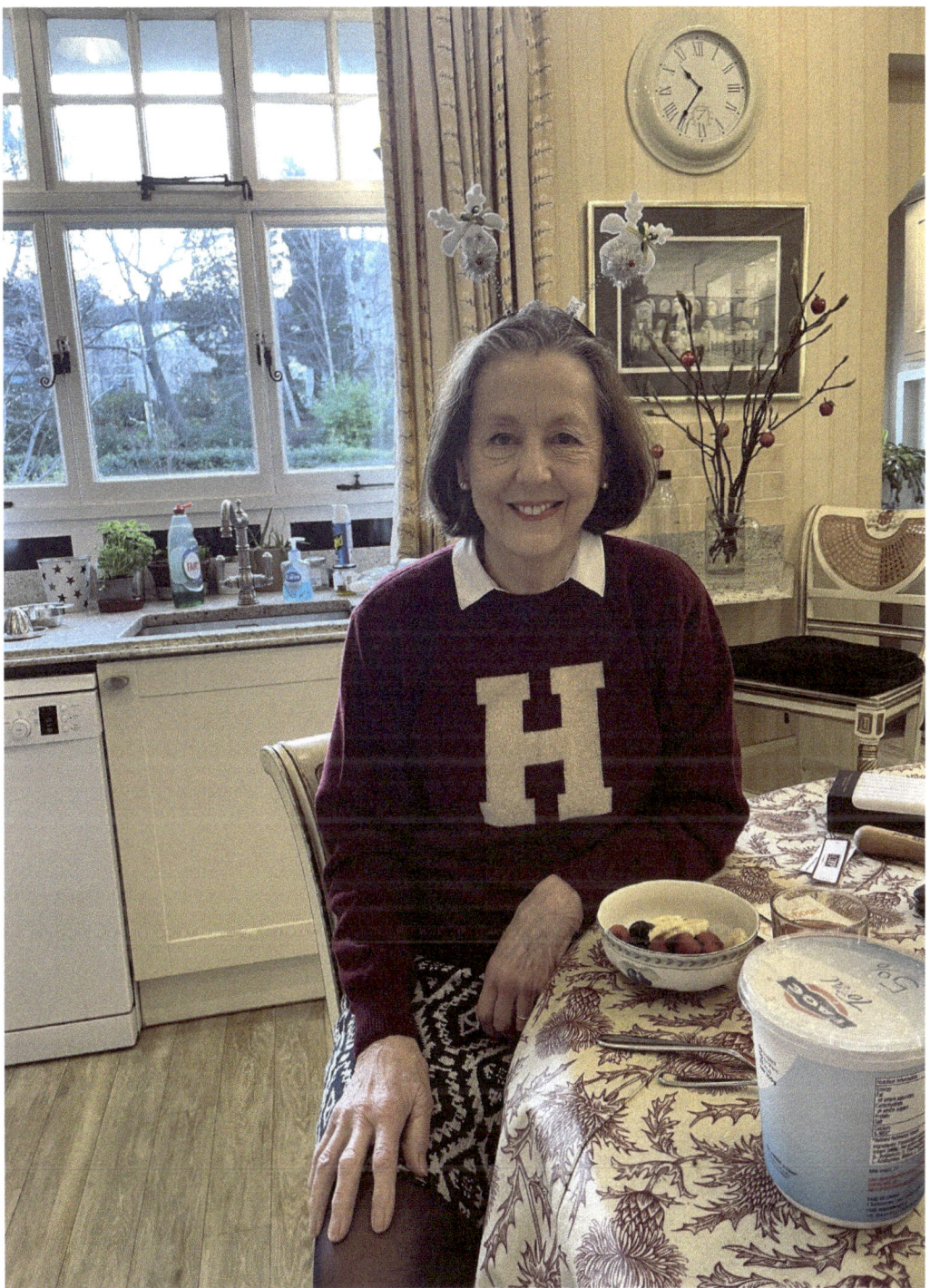

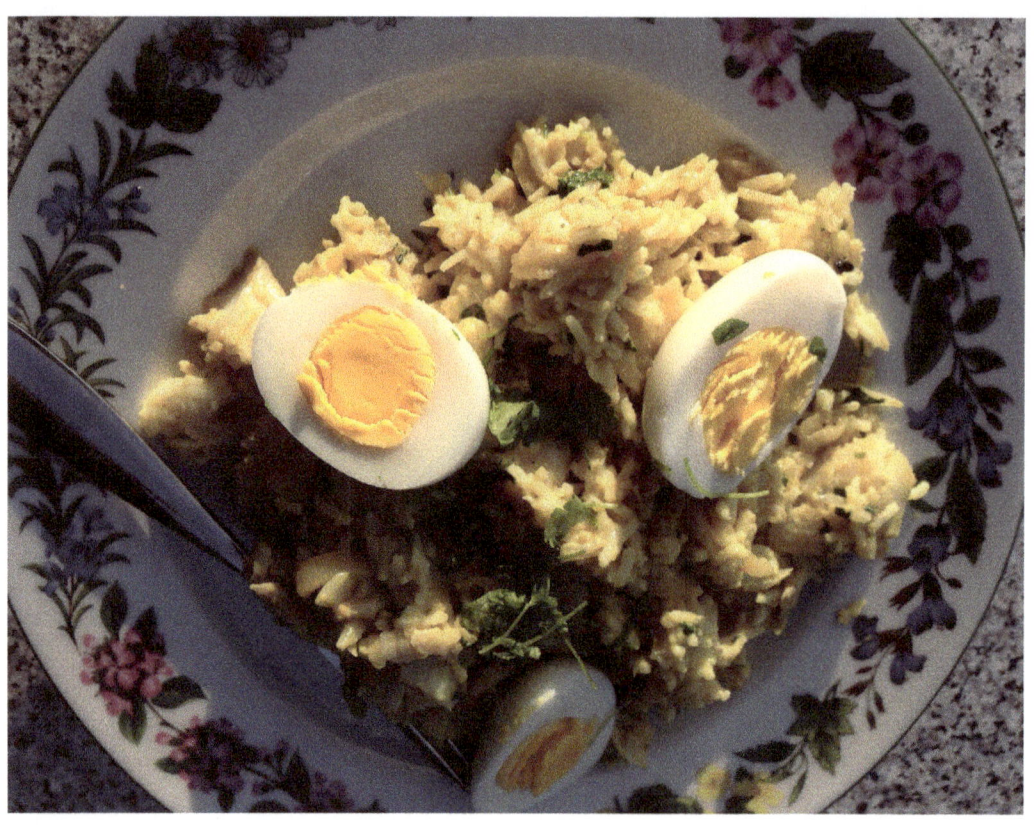

A Spice of Lands Afar

*A traveller's tale, a dish so bright,
With golden rice and spice just right.
The haddock's kiss, the curry's glow,
A feast that hums with fires below.*

*A touch of cream, a twist of lime,
A plate that speaks of sea and time.
A dish once made for kings and crew,
Now shared with hearts both old and new.*

—*Inspired by Robert Louis Stevenson*

Kedgeree

Serves 4

Ingredients

- 2 onions thinly sliced
- Salt & pepper
- Cayenne pepper
- 4 pieces of smoked undyed haddock fillets (remove bones before cooking)
- 300 g basmati rice
- 3 cardamom pods, split
- ½ cinnamon stick, about 3 cm (1¼") long
- 2 bay leaves
- 1 Tbsp of curry powder
- 4 large free-range eggs
- 40 g butter
- 4 Tbsp of double cream
- 3 heaped Tbsp of chopped parsley
- ½ lemon, juice only

Method

1. Put the haddock with the bay leaf in a large frying pan and pour over enough water to cover the fish. Simmer, cover, and cook on low heat for 5 minutes until opaque and cooked through. Remove the pan from the heat, drain in a colander set over a bowl, reserve the cooking liquor, discard the bay leaf, and place to one side.

2. Put the rice in a sieve and hold it under cold running water until the water runs clear. This removes starch and prevents clumping, making the rice lighter and fluffier. Pour the cooking liquor into a medium saucepan and stir in the rice. Cover with a lid and bring to the boil. Reduce the heat and gently simmer the rice for 10 minutes, then drain.

3. Meanwhile, break the eggs into simmering salted water in a small pan and cook for 3 minutes. Remove them from the water with a slotted spoon and place them on one side.

4. Meanwhile, heat 20 grams of butter in a large nonstick frying pan over medium heat and fry the 2 sliced onions slowly for 5 minutes, stirring occasionally. Then, add the chopped cardamom pods, cinnamon stick, and curry powder. Stir in the drained cooked rice into the onions and cook until hot.

5. Remove the cinnamon stick from the rice and carefully stir in the remaining butter, cream, parsley and fish. Season with salt and cayenne pepper, and add the lemon juice. Heat through over low heat, stirring gently once or twice so you don't break up the fish.

6. Pop the eggs on top and serve.

7. If not serving immediately, tip the kedgeree into a warm dish and dot with a few butter cubes. Cover with foil and keep warm in a low oven for up to 20 minutes before serving.

The poached eggs could be changed to soft-boiled eggs and cut into quarters.

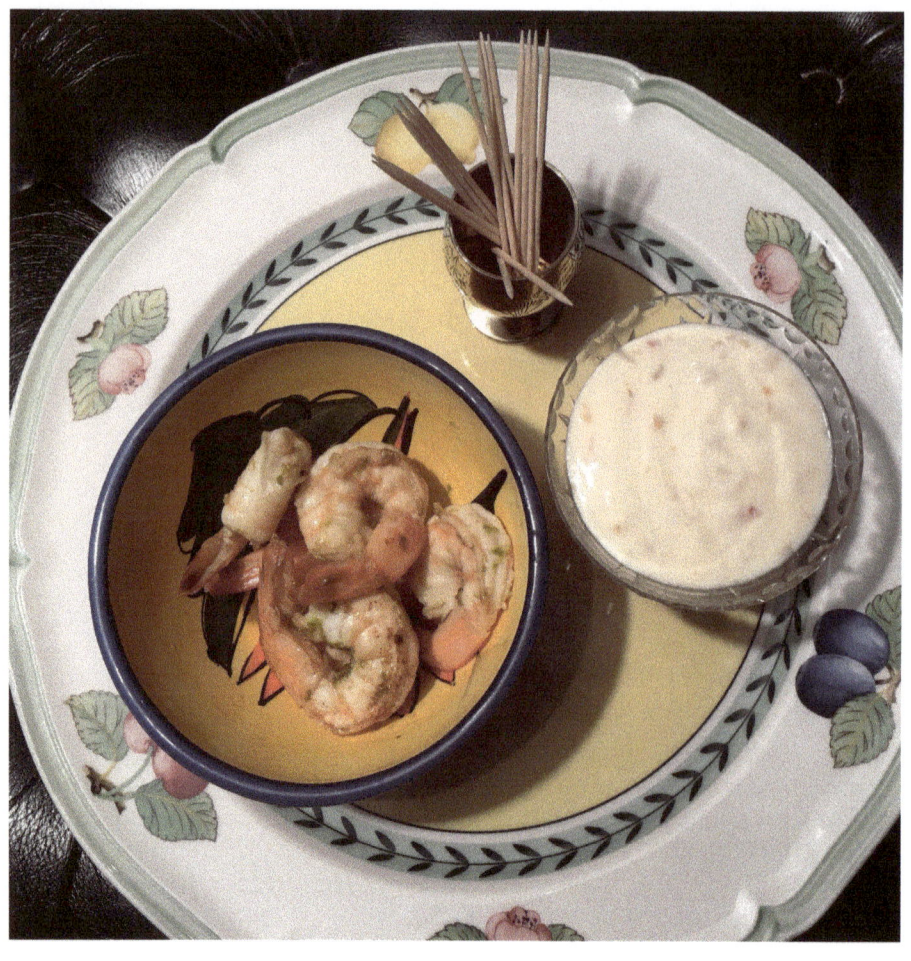

A Zestful Dance

A whisper bright, a fiery kiss,
A prawn's embrace, a tangy bliss.
With lime and heat in bold embrace,
A lively step, a playful grace.

A dip of cream, a cooling shade,
A balance struck, a flavour made.
A dish that sings in citrus cheer,
A bite of joy, both bright and clear.

—Inspired by Contemporary Scottish Poets

Marinated Prawns with Chilli Dipping Sauce

Serves 12

Ingredients

2 garlic cloves, crushed
½ red chilli, very finely chopped
Grated rind and zest of 2 limes
2 Tbsp olive oil
24 king prawns
15 g butter
For the dip
150 ml sour cream
2-3 Tbsp sweet chilli sauce
Cocktail sticks

Method

1. Place the garlic in a bowl with the chilli, lime zest, juice, and one tablespoon of the oil. Marinate the prawns in the marinade for 1 hour.

2. Meanwhile, make the dip. Mix the sour cream and chilli sauce together and serve in a little bowl alongside the prawns.

3. Heat the remaining oil and butter in a frying pan until hot and foaming. Fry half the prawns for 2-3 minutes over a high heat, turning once or twice until pink. Remove with a slotted spoon and set aside. Add the remaining prawns to the pan and cook in the same way. Return the other prawns to the pan and add any remaining marinade to the bowl. Heat for 30 seconds, then serve the prawns with the sauce and cocktail sticks.

Fish

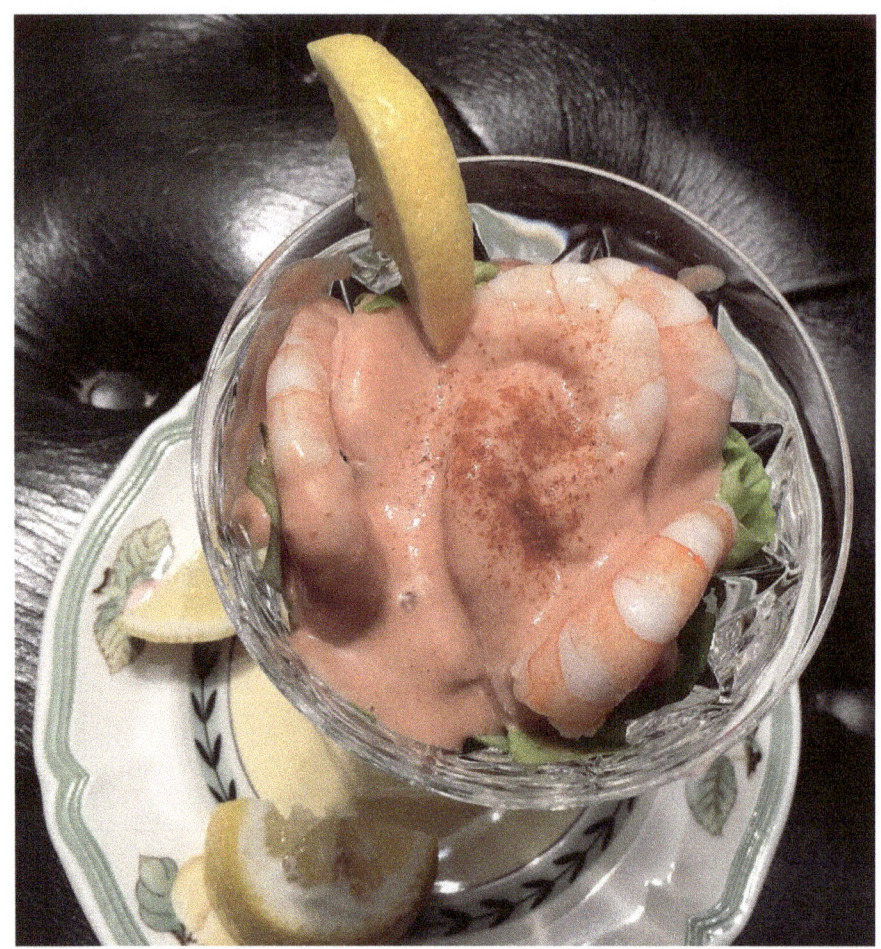

A Classic Charm

A dish of old, yet fresh anew,
With tender prawns in crimson hue.
A velvet sauce, both rich and light,
A touch of spice, a bold delight.

With lettuce crisp and lemon bright,
It wakes the tongue in pure delight.
A dish refined, yet simple still,
A taste that lingers, soft and chill.

—Inspired by John Buchan

Prawn Cocktail

Serves 6

Ingredients

450 g shelled cooked prawns

284 ml double cream or mayonnaise

2 Tbsp of double concentrate tomato puree

2-3 tsp lemon juice to taste

1 Tbsp Worcestershire sauce

½ garlic clove, skinned, crushed with salt

Freshly ground black pepper

1 crisp lettuce, washed and drained (or a packet of prepared salad)

1 lemon cut into six pieces

Cayenne pepper

Method

1. Whip the cream until soft peaks, or if using mayonnaise, add the tomato puree, lemon juice, Worcestershire sauce, garlic and plenty of black pepper. Taste for seasoning. This can be done in advance and kept in a covered bowl until you can assemble the cocktails in the evening.

2. Just before serving, shred the lettuce finely and put enough in each glass dish to fill it to about one-third. Keep six large prawns to one side. Stir the rest of the prawns into the cream and divide evenly between the serving dishes. Pop a prawn on the top.

3. Sprinkle with a pinch of cayenne pepper; put a wedge of lemon alongside each one. Serve with brown bread and butter.

When using double cream, it will be slightly thicker.

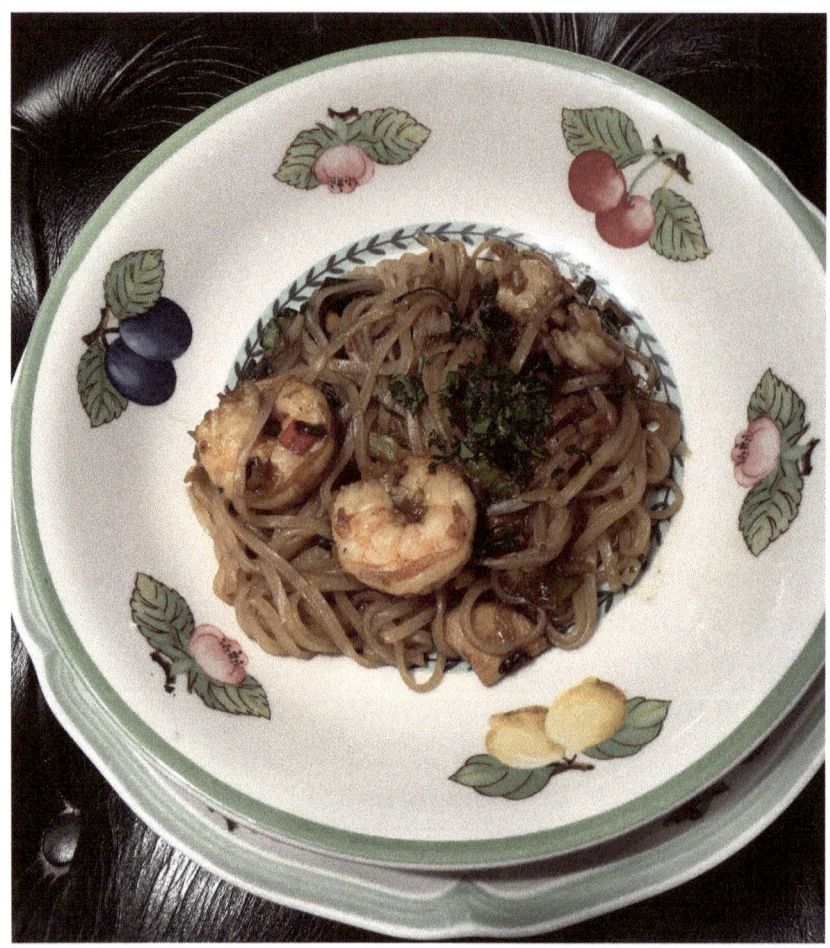

A Dance of Heat and Sea

A flame of spice, a prawn's soft grace,
A whisper bold, a lively pace.
With ginger's spark and noodles light,
A dish that sings of pure delight.

The greens still crisp, the broth aglow,
A feast that sets the heart to flow.
A touch of fire, a hint of sweet,
A dance of flavours, fierce yet neat.

—*Inspired by Contemporary Scottish Poets*

Prawn and Ginger Noodle Stir-Fry

Serves 4

Ingredients

- 150 g white noodles
- 100 g beansprouts
- 3 Tbsp olive oil
- 250 g sugar snap peas / or broccoli
- 1 small red chilli, deseeded and finely chopped
- 8 spring onions, thinly sliced
- 100 g chestnut mushrooms, thickly sliced
- 3 cm fresh root ginger, peeled and thinly sliced
- 2 fat garlic cloves finely chopped
- 225 g pak choi, thinly sliced, keeping the white and green parts separate
- 400 g raw king prawns
- Salt and freshly ground black pepper

For the sauce

- ½–¾ Tbsp Chinese five-spice powder
- 2 Tbsp soy sauce
- 3 Tbsp runny honey
- 2 tsp white wine vinegar
- 1 Tbsp sherry

To serve

- Juice of ½ lemon
- 2 Tbsp chopped coriander

Method

1. Cook the noodles according to the pack instructions, drain them, and refresh them in cold water.

2. Heat the oil in a large, nonstick frying pan or wok. Add the chilli, spring onions, garlic, mushrooms, sugar snap peas, ginger, and white parts of the pak choi and fry over high heat, stirring for about 4 minutes until the vegetables are nearly cooked but still crisp.

3. Add the beansprouts and cook for a further 30 seconds.

4. Add the prawns and fry for a further minute or until starting to turn pink. Tip the noodles into the pan and add the green leaves of the pak choi, then fry for another minute, stirring to combine.

5. Mix the sauce ingredients together in a small bowl until smooth. Pour the sauce over the noodle mixture in the pan and add any seasoning if necessary.

6. Once the prawns are completely pink, transfer them to individual bowls, squeeze over the lemon juice, scatter with chopped coriander, and serve immediately.

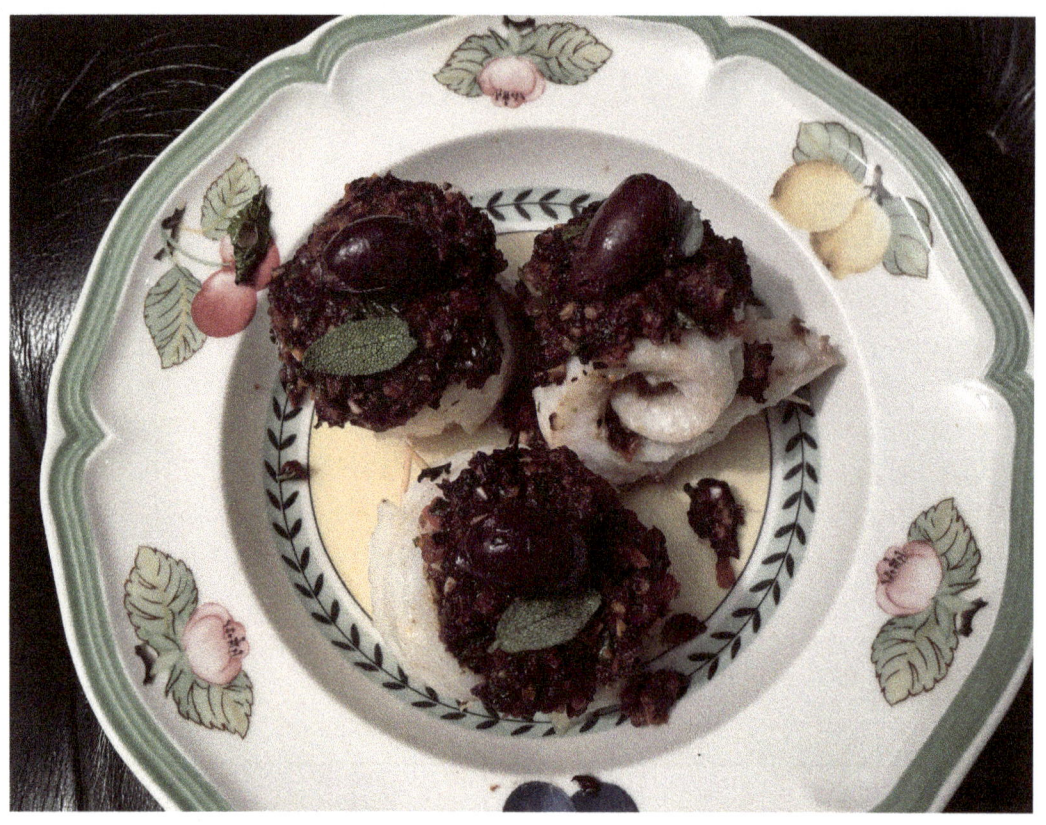

A Highland Feast

Upon the flame, the fish is laid,
With olives dark and basil swayed.
A crust of gold, a briny deep,
A meal the hills and shores would keep.

The sun-dried kiss, the pepper's cheer,
A dish both bold and bright, sincere.
A bite of warmth, a taste of home,
A song of sea, a meal well known.

—*Inspired by Sir Walter Scott*

Roast Fish with Sun-dried Tomato Tapenade

Serves 6

Ingredients

6 tail-end pieces of haddock, weighing 175-200 g each, skin removed

For the tapenade

300 g jar sun-dried tomatoes drained, pressed between double layers of absorbent kitchen paper to remove some excess oil

185 g tin pitted black olives in brine, drained and rinsed

2 15 g packets of basil leaves only

1 tsp green peppercorns in brine, rinsed and drained (36 peppercorns)

2 fat garlic cloves, peeled

50 g tin anchovies, drained

2 Tbsp of capers drained and pressed between double layers of absorbent kitchen paper

Freshly milled black pepper

Method

1. Preheat oven to 180°C

2. Reserve 6 whole olives and 6 medium basil leaves from the ingredients list. To make the tapenade (which can be made 2-3 days ahead), all you do is place the remaining ingredients in a food processor, then blend them together to a coarse paste.

3. It's important not to over-process so that the ingredients retain some of their identity.

4. When you are ready to cook the fish, wipe the fillets with kitchen paper, then fold them by tucking the thin end into the centre and then the thick end on top of that so you have a neat, slightly rounded shape. A cocktail stick helps hold the shape and is removed before serving.

5. Place the fish on an oiled baking sheet or dish, then divide the tapenade mixture equally between them, using it as a topping. Press it on with your hands quite firmly. Now, lightly rough the surface with a fork. Dip the reserved basil leaves in olive oil and place one on top of each piece of fish, following that with a little oil.

6. Place the baking tray on a high shelf in the oven. Bake the fish for 20-25 minutes, then serve immediately.

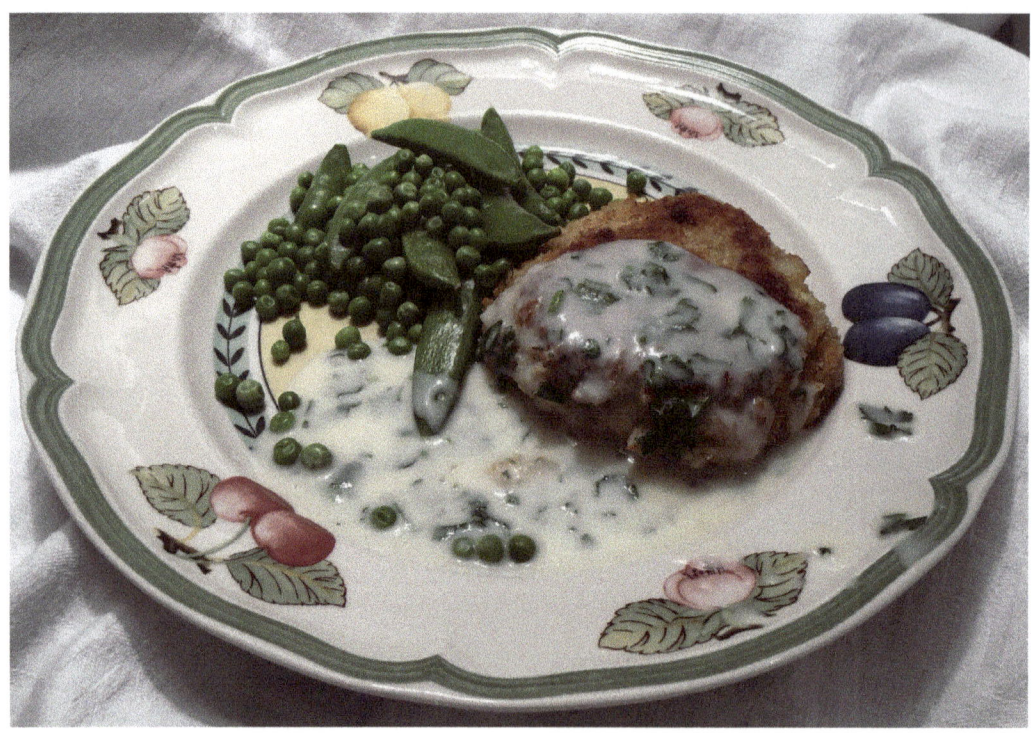

A Fisher's Reward

The tide rolls in, the boats return,
With silver catch in baskets stern.
A flake of fish, a golden crust,
A bite of sea, both firm and just.

With herbs so bright and butter's care,
A meal that sings of ocean air.
A humble dish, yet rich and free,
A taste of toil, a gift from sea.

—*Inspired by Robert Burns*

Salmon and Haddock Fishcakes

Makes 8

Ingredients

170 g tin of boneless and skinned salmon or a portion of fresh salmon

600 g smoked undyed haddock fillets when bones removed

To poach the fish

400 ml milk

1 onion, roughly chopped

1 sliced carrot,

1 bay leaf,

4 peppercorns

2 cloves

Fish cake

350 g dry mashed potatoes

75 g melted butter

1 onion, finely diced

25 g butter to sauté the chopped onion

1 Tbsp Worcestershire sauce

1 tsp of Dion mustard

2 hard-boiled eggs, chopped

3 Tbsp chopped parsley

2 Tbsp chopped dill

Salt and freshly ground black pepper

Plain flour for coating

2 eggs, beaten, for dipping

400 g breadcrumbs from white or brown bread

85 g butter or sunflower oil for frying

Method

1. Remove the bones from the haddock. Chop the haddock into bite-size pieces. Place the haddock and fresh salmon in a large frying pan with milk, onion, carrot, bay leaf, peppercorns, and 2 cloves. Simmer very gently until cooked.
2. When the fish is cooking, gently cook the onion over low heat until transparent.
3. With a slotted spoon, remove the fish from the milk, sieve the milk, and keep it for the parsley sauce. When the fish is cold, mix gently with the potatoes, melted butter, onion, Worcestershire sauce, eggs, parsley, and dill in a bowl until well combined. At this stage, add the tin of salmon.
4. Season to taste. If the mixture is too dry, add some of the poaching milk.
5. Divide the mixture into 8 portions, each approximately 140 grams. Shape into patties. Dip into the flour, then the egg, and finally the breadcrumbs, reshaping. Refrigerate for 2 hours to firm up.
6. Pan fry for 2 minutes on each side, and then cook in a medium oven at 170°C for 15 minutes.
7. Serve with parsley sauce, peas and lemon slices

The fish cakes can be made using only undyed smoked haddock; increase the amount of haddock accordingly. See the parsley sauce recipe.

Fish

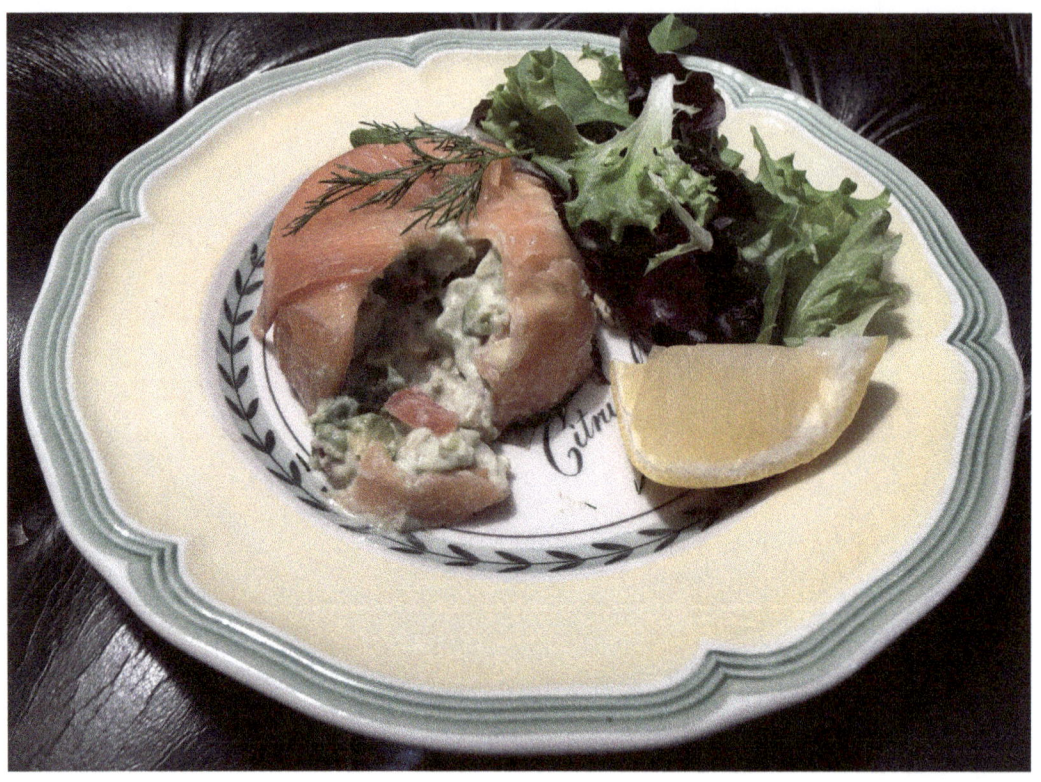

60

A Delicate Layer

A tower bright, a creamy fold,
With trout so fine and herbs of old.
A burst of red, a summer's cheer,
A dish both light and bold, sincere.

With citrus sharp and texture true,
A taste of earth, a skyward view.
A plate of grace, of balance fair,
A dish to serve with tender care.

—Inspired by Robert Louis Stevenson

Smoked Trout, Avocado, and Tomato Timbales

Serves 8

Prepare ahead the day before and keep in the fridge.

Ingredients

400 g cold smoked trout slices

2 good handfuls of mixed leaves to garnish

For the filling

3 medium ripe avocados, peeled, stoned and cut into tiny diced pieces

Juice of 1 lemon

2 spring onions, finely chopped

2-3 tomatoes, deseeded and cut into tiny diced pieces

4 Tbsp full-fat mayonnaise

4 Tbsp full-fat cream cheese

1 tsp Dijon mustard

Salt and freshly ground pepper

Method

1. To make the filling, add the diced avocados to a bowl and mix with the lemon juice, spring onions, and half the diced tomatoes. In a separate bowl, mix together the mayonnaise, cream cheese, and mustard, season with salt and pepper, and stir into the avocado mixture.

2. Wet the inside of eight oval or round ramekins and line with enough cling film so that some overhangs the sides. Line the base and side of each ramekin with a single layer of smoked trout, leaving a little overhanging on the sides.

3. Divide half the avocado mixture between the ramekins and press down with the back of a spoon. Scatter with the remaining diced tomatoes to give a red layer, and press down. Top with the remaining avocado mixture, pressing down with the back of a spoon and smoothing the tops.

4. Fold over the overhanging bits of smoked trout, cling film, and press down lightly. Chill in the fridge for at least 6 hours or, ideally, overnight. There is no need to weigh down the tops of the timbales while they are chilling. They will hold their shape well enough when they are turned out.

5. To serve, unwrap the cling film from the top of each dish and upend the timbales onto an individual plate, removing the ramekin and the cling film. Garnish each plate with a few dressed leaves and serve chilled with brown bread or rolls.

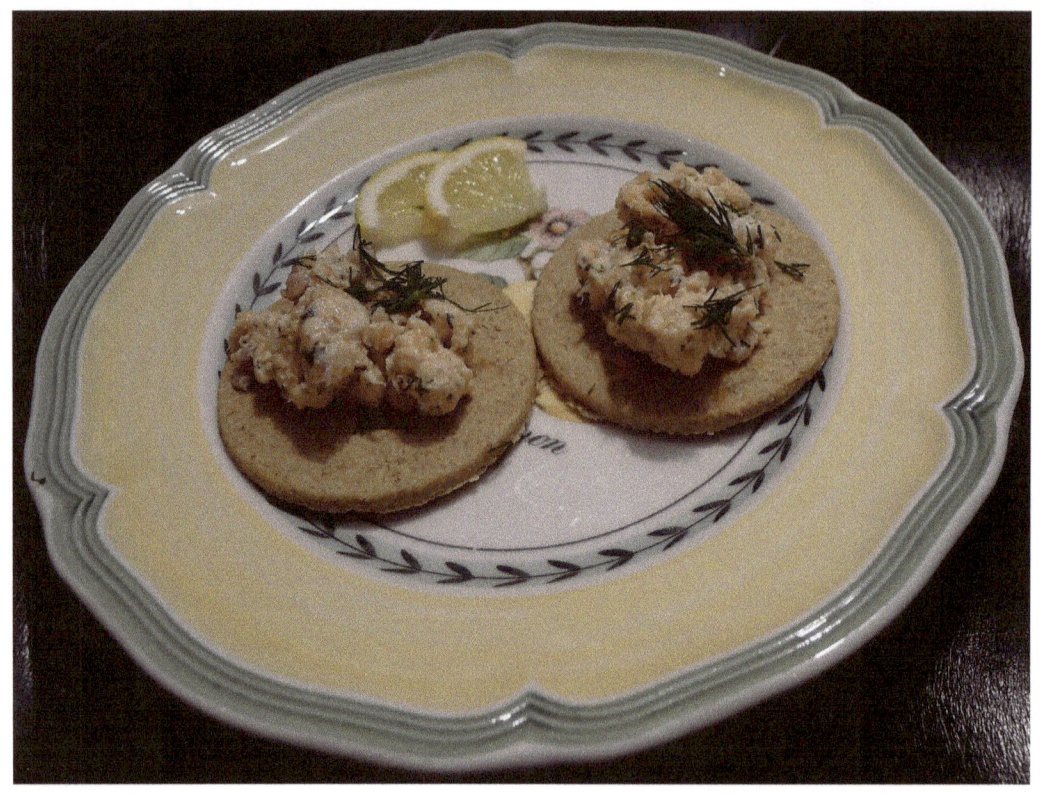

A Spread of Velvet Gold

A salmon's song, so soft, so bright,
With cream and herbs, a pure delight.
A dish to spread on oatcake fine,
A taste that hums with salt and brine.

A simple joy, yet rich and deep,
A flavour bold, a memory steeped.
With lemon's kiss and dill's embrace,
A dish of ease, of quiet grace.

—*Inspired by Contemporary Scottish Poets*

Smoked Salmon Pâté

Serves 4-6

Ingredients

255 g smoked salmon

110 g cream cheese (Philadelphia)

2 Tbsp double cream

½ lemon, juice only

Pinch of sugar

Salt and freshly ground pepper

2 Tbsp chopped dill/chives (plus some extra to sprinkle over the top)

1 lemon thinly sliced for decoration

Method

1. All ingredients (except the salt and pepper) are to be combined in a food processor and blitzed for a few seconds until blended.

2. Taste, then season with pepper and salt (but go easy on the salt, as the smoked salmon will be salty already). Blitz for a few seconds.

3. Substitute lime and coriander instead of lemon and chives for a change

4. Serve with oatcakes and sliced lemon and topped with a sprinkle of chopped herbs.

5. One could line a small ramekin with smoked salmon, fill it with the pate, fold over the flaps of the smoked salmon, put it in the fridge overnight, turn it upside down, decorate, and serve on special occasions.

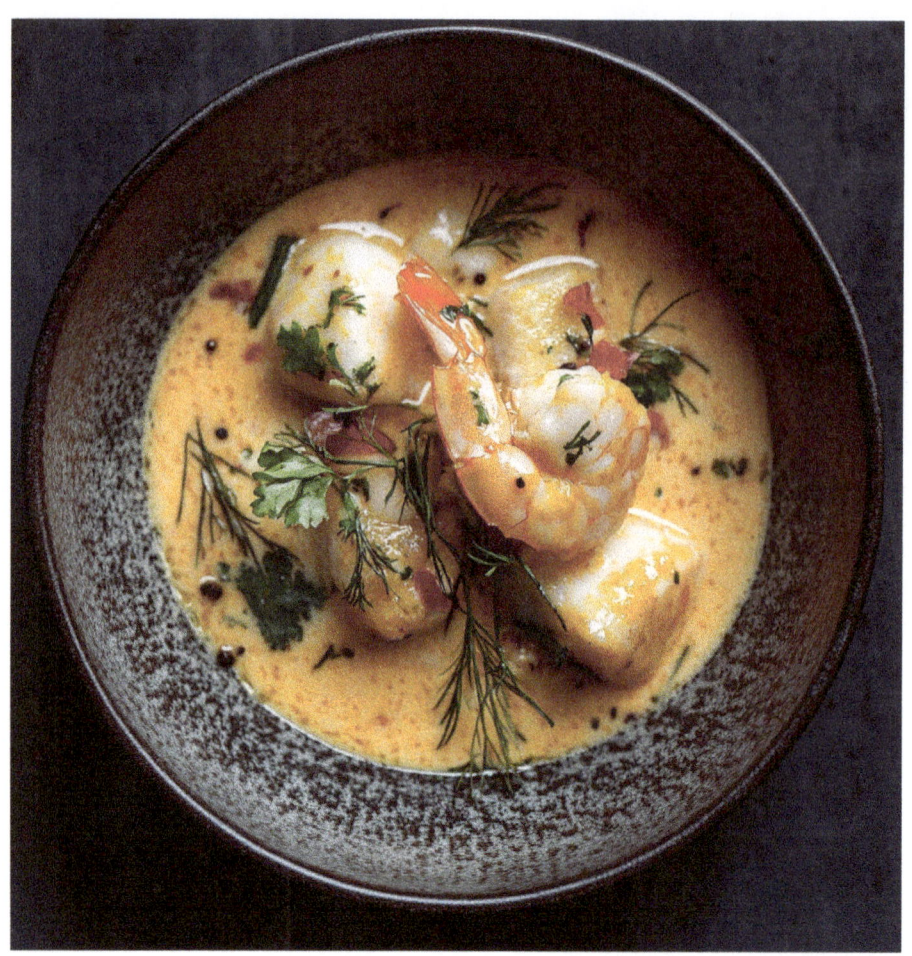

A Rush of Waves and Fire

A curry bright, a sea's embrace,
A broth of spice, a hurried pace.
With coconut and prawns so bold,
A dish that tells a tale retold.

A flash of lime, a hint of sweet,
A meal that lifts the weary feet.
A taste of heat, a touch of breeze,
A gift from both the land and seas.

—Inspired by Contemporary Scottish Poets

Speedy Seafood Curry

Serves 4

Ingredients

2 Tbsp vegetable or sunflower oil

1 finely sliced onion

2 cloves of garlic, finely chopped

2 Tbsp Thai red curry paste (M & S)

800 g monkfish, prawns or whatever you want

400 ml of full-fat coconut milk

200 ml fish stock

Juice of one lime

1-2 Tbsp Thai fish sauce

125 g mange touts, sliced lengthways

3 Tbsp freshly torn coriander

Method

1. Heat the oil and fry the sliced onion in a large nonstick pan until transparent. Add the finely chopped garlic and fry for another two minutes.

2. Add the curry paste and cook for 1-2 minutes.

3. Add the monkfish /prawns and stir well to coat in the curry paste. Add the coconut milk, stock, lime juice and fish sauce. Stir all the ingredients together and bring just to the boil.

4. Add the mange touts and simmer for 5 minutes until the mange touts and fish are tender. Stir in the coriander and check the seasoning, adding salt and freshly ground black pepper to taste. Serve with plain boiled rice.

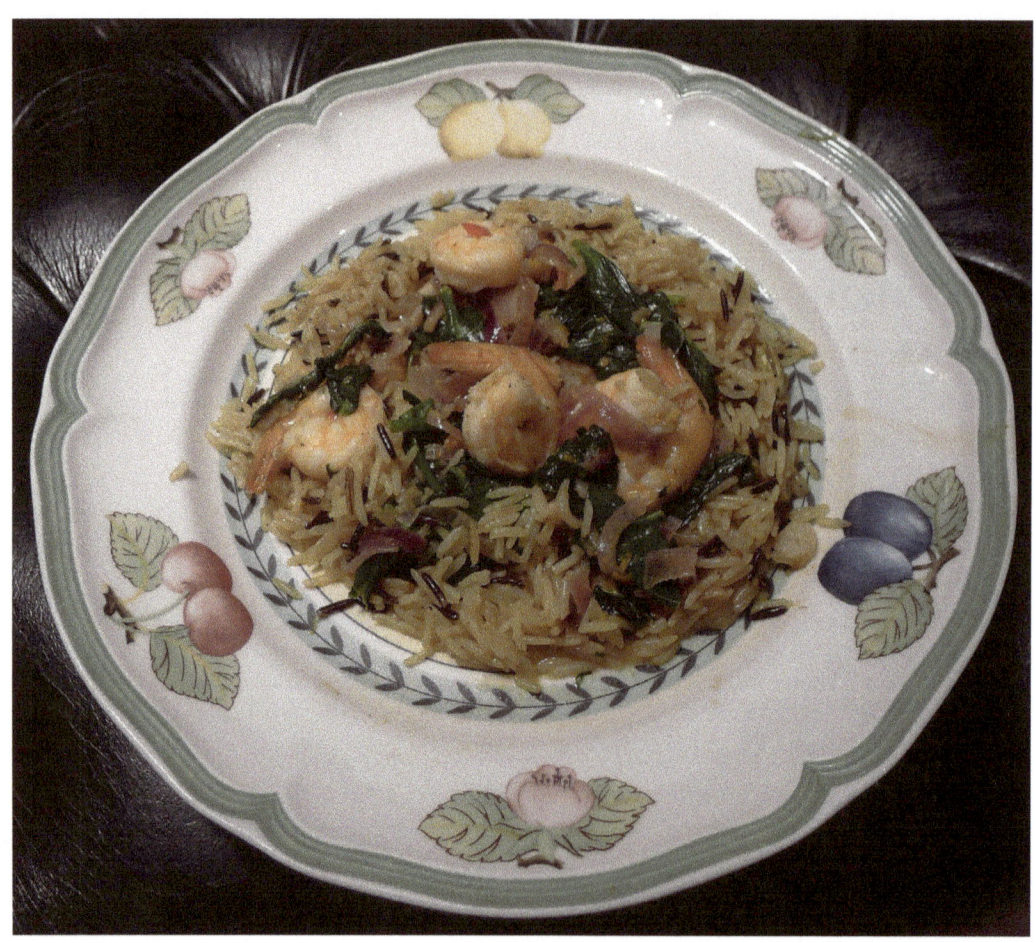

A Feast of Fire and Gold

A prawn so bold, a sauce so bright,
With citrus glow and spice's bite.
A dance of flame, a liquid cheer,
A meal to toast, to bring good cheer.

The sherry's warmth, the orange light,
A dish that glows through winter's night.
With rice so soft and herbs so free,
A meal of zest and revelry.

—*Inspired by Robert Louis Stevenson*

Spicy Prawns, Orange Sherry & Wild Rice Pilaf

Serves 4

This makes a great lunch or light supper dish, complimented perfectly by the basmati and wild pilau rice.

Ingredients

- 2 Tbsp olive oil
- 25 g butter
- 400 g raw tiger prawns
- 2 garlic cloves, peeled and finely chopped
- ¼ chilli, deseeded and thinly sliced (optional)
- 1 small red onion, thinly sliced
- Juice and pared zest of 2 oranges
- Sea salt and black pepper
- Generous splash of dry sherry
- 250 g spinach leaves

Wild rice

- 1 Tbsp oil
- 2 shallots, chopped
- 200 g basmati and wild rice
- 1 tsp garam masala
- 6 cardamom pods
- 500 ml hot chicken stock
- 1 tsp salt
- Small bunch of coriander roughly chopped

Method

1. Preheat the oven to 180°C.
2. To make the Pilau rice.
3. Heat the oil in an ovenproof pan and gently fry the shallots until soft and lightly golden. Tip in the rice, garam masala, and cardamom pods and stir for a minute to toast the spices. Pour in the stock, bring the liquid to a boil, and then cover the pan with a lid. Carefully transfer the pan into the oven for 15-20 minutes until the rice absorbs most of the liquid. Remove the pan from the oven, leaving the lid on, and let the rice sit for 5 minutes while you cook the prawns.
4. Heat a large frying pan with the oil and butter. Add the garlic, onion, chilli, orange zest, and some seasoning. Fry for 2 minutes.
5. Add a good splash of sherry, pour in the orange juice, boil, and reduce until you have a syrupy sauce. Add the prawns and cook until they have turned pink. Throw the spinach into the pan for 30 seconds, just until the spinach has wilted.
6. Fluff up the rice with a fork and stir the coriander through. Serve on a warm plate.

Fish

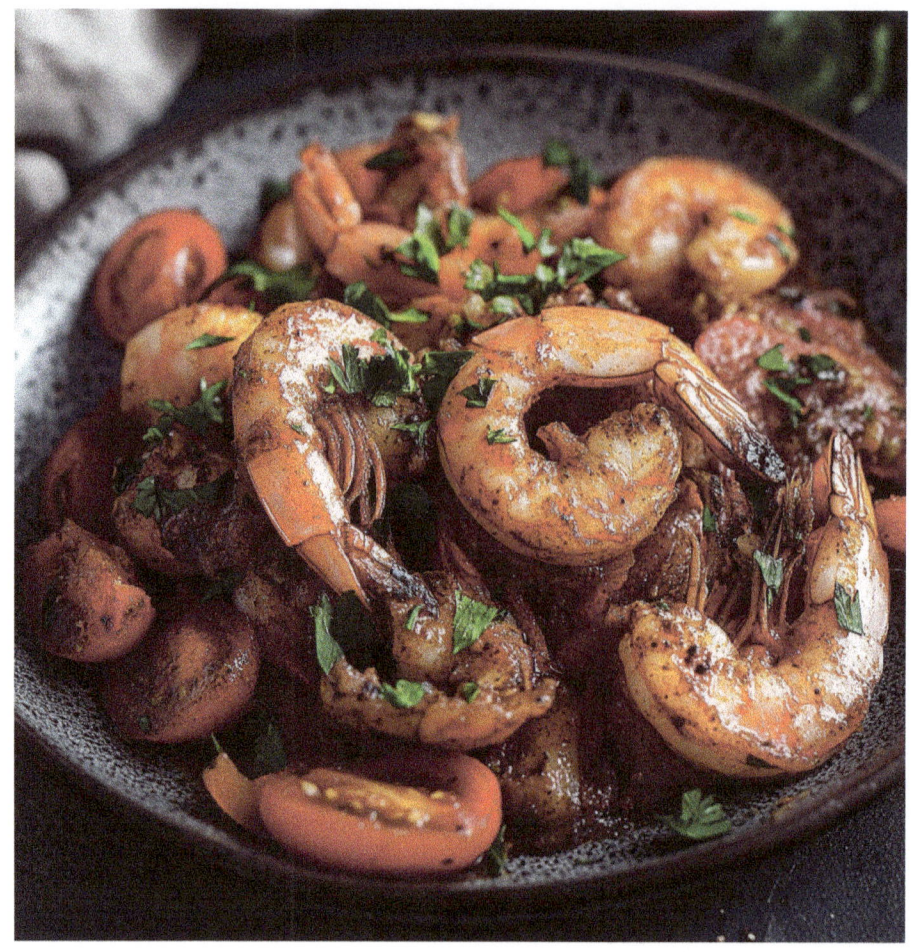

Dance of Fire and Sea

A fragrant stir, a golden hue,
The cumin hums, the cardamom true.
A sizzle bright, the garlic sings,
A dish of warmth, of spice, of kings.

The tomatoes melt, the sauce runs deep,
A simmered tale, a taste to keep.
With prawns so plump and rice so light,
A feast of colour, bold and bright.

—*Inspired by Robert Louis Stevenson*

Spiced Prawns with Tomato

Serve 3

Ingredients

400 g defrosted and well-drained prawns, save liquid to add to sauce

450 g tomatoes peeled and chopped

1½ Tbsp groundnut oil

1 large onion, halved and sliced

2 cloves garlic, crushed

½ tsp cumin seeds

1 tsp coriander seeds

3 cardamom pods

1 tsp grated fresh root ginger (10 g)

1 rounded tsp ground turmeric

½ tsp chilli powder

1 heaped Tbsp of tomato puree

50 g sun-dried cherry tomatoes chopped

¼ pt juice from the frozen prawns/chicken stock

Salt and pepper

Method

1. Heat the oil in a large frying pan. Add the onion slices and fry gently for approximately 10 minutes or until softened and golden.

2. In the meantime, place the whole spices in a dry frying pan and roast them over gentle heat for 5 minutes to draw out their aroma. Allow them to cool, then crush them with a pestle and mortar (or this can be done in a small basin using the end of a rolling pin). Then add all the spices and garlic to the onion and stir until everything is well heated.

3. Add the prepared tomatoes, tomato puree, sun-dried tomato liquid from the prawns / or chicken stock, salt, and pepper. Bring to the boil and simmer gently for 30 minutes, uncovered. By this time, much of the excess liquid will have evaporated, and the tomatoes will have reduced to the consistency of a thick sauce.

4. Add the prawns warm through fully and serve with spiced pilau rice (see recipe)

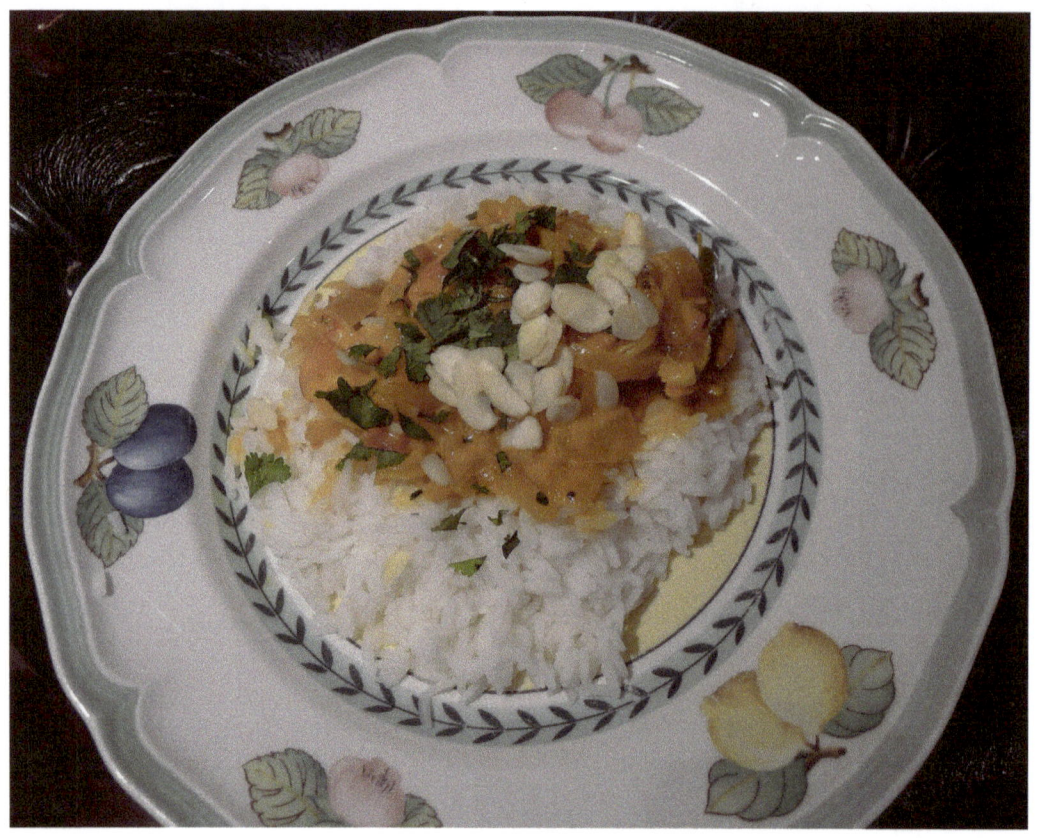

A Journey in Spice

A simmered dream, a saffron tide,
Where coconut and chilli bide.
A prawn so pink, a sauce so deep,
A curry rich, a joy to keep.

A hint of lime, a whisper low,
A dish that lets the warm winds blow.
A meal that lingers, bold yet mild,
A taste both fierce and reconciled.

—*Inspired by Contemporary Scottish Poets*

South Indian Prawn Curry

Serves 4

The sauce can be made the day before adding the prawns—cool, cover and chill.

Ingredients

- Vegetable oil
- Pinch of cumin seeds
- ½ tsp brown mustard seeds
- Pinch of fenugreek seeds or ¼ tsp of ground fenugreek
- 4 cloves garlic, peeled and chopped
- 5 cm piece fresh ginger, peeled and chopped
- 10 curry leaves (optional)
- 2 onions, peeled and chopped
- Zest and juice of 1 lime
- 1 Tbsp ground coriander
- 1 tsp turmeric
- 2 fresh red chillies, chopped
- 180 g tin chopped tomatoes
- 400 ml tin coconut milk
- 2 200 g packs of raw, peeled king prawns
- 1 large handful of flaked almonds, toasted
- Small bunch of fresh coriander leaves
- Sea salt

Method

1. Heat a wide pan over medium heat and add a splash of sunflower oil. Throw in the cumin, mustard, and fenugreek seeds (leave the ground fenugreek until later, if using). When they start to pop (about 1-2 minutes), add the garlic, ginger, curry leaves, and onions.

2. Cook gently for 10-15 minutes or until the onions turn soft and golden. Add the lime zest, ground coriander, turmeric, ground fenugreek, half the chilli, the tomatoes and 2 Tbsp of water.

3. Cook gently for 10 minutes until you have a paste, then add the coconut milk. Bring to a boil, add the prawns, bring back the heat and simmer for 5 minutes until pink.

4. Season with sea salt, add the lime juice, transfer to bowls, and sprinkle over the almonds, remaining chilli, and coriander.

Fish

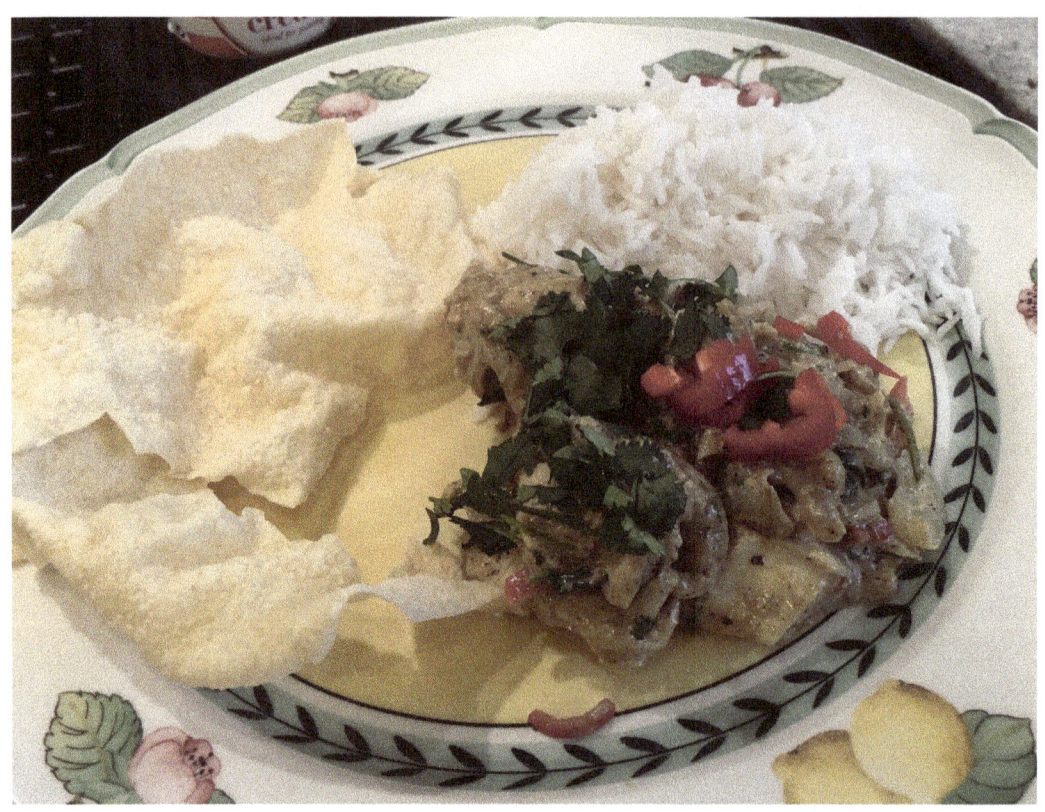

A Bowl of Distant Shores

A curry bright, both bold and mild,
With spices rich and flavours wild.
The sea's own gift, the fish so fair,
A dish of warmth, a scented air.

A touch of crab, a taste of lime,
A bowl that spans both space and time.
With jasmine rice and herbs anew,
A feast for both the old and new.

—*Inspired by Robert Louis Stevenson*

Thai Yellow Fish Curry

Serves 4

Ingredients

3 Tbsp sunflower oil

2 onions finely sliced

100 g brown crab meat

400 ml can of coconut milk

1 Tbsp creamed coconut

Juice of 1 lime

2 Tbsp palm sugar

2 Tbsp white crab meat

300 g tiger prawns (shell and heads removed)

350 g hake or other firm white fish skinless and boneless cut into bit size pieces

Large bunch of fresh coriander chopped

Steamed jasmine rice to serve

For the curry paste.

1 red chilli, pips removed

4 garlic cloves

1 lemon grass sticks, outer leaves removed, roughly chopped

2 shallots, roughly chopped

20 g fresh ginger, chopped

1 Tbsp Thai shrimp paste

1 Tbsp medium curry powder

2 tsp ground turmeric

2 tsp ground coriander

2 tsp ground cumin

1 Tbsp fish sauce

Method

1. Whizz the curry paste ingredients with 150 ml water in a mini food processor. Set aside.

2. Heat the oil in a large, deep frying pan over medium heat. Add the onions and fry for 12 minutes or until they start to soften. Add the curry paste and brown crab meat and cook for a further 10 minutes.

3. Add the coconut milk, creamed coconut, lime juice, and sugar. Simmer for 5 minutes, then add the white crab meat, prawns, and hake.

4. Simmer for 5–8 minutes until the seafood is cooked through. Very gently and occasionally stir to avoid breaking up the fish. Add the coriander and serve with steamed rice.

Fish

Flint Family Cookbook

Vegetable Mains

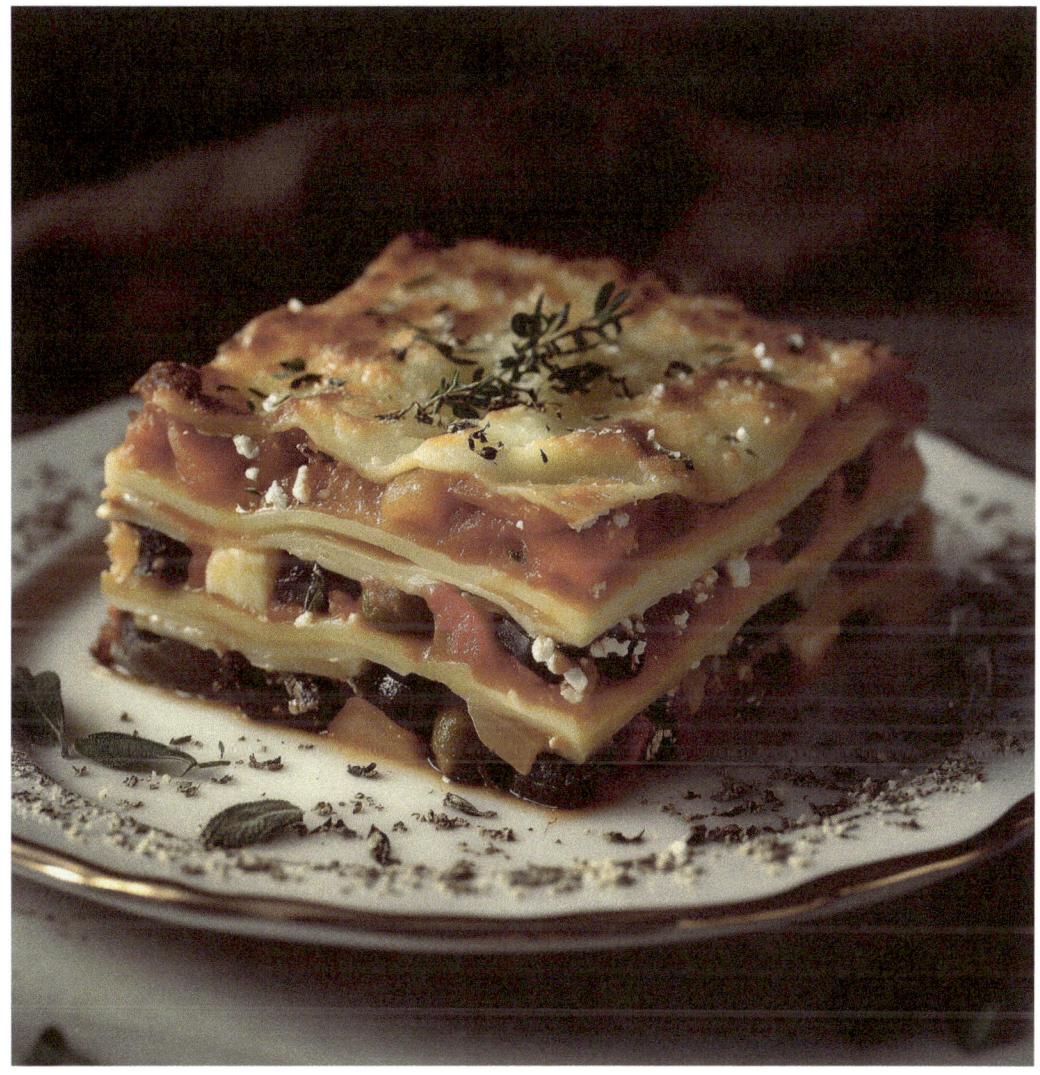

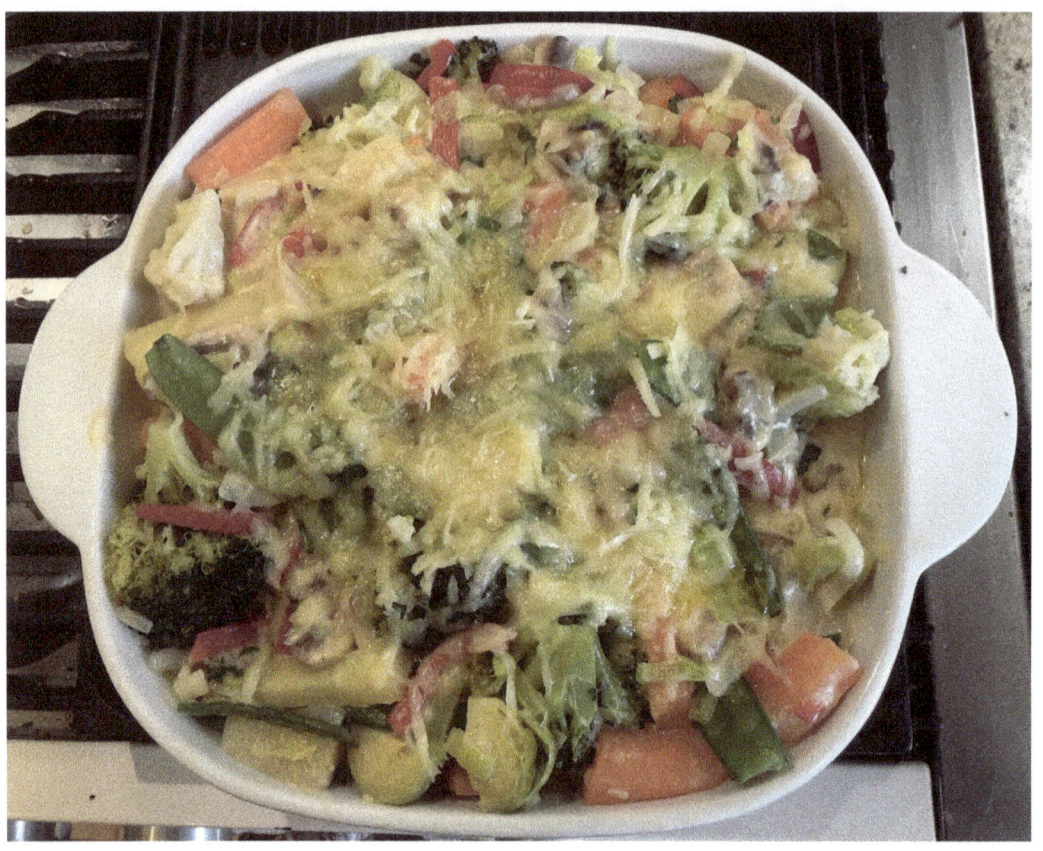

Layers of Comfort

In golden dish, so warm, so deep,
A harvest's gift in layers steep.
The earth's own roots, both firm and sweet,
With tender greens, a feast complete.

A sauce so rich, with spice just right,
A cloak of warmth, a soft delight.
The cheddar melts, the edges glow,
A dish of love, both crisp and slow.

So take your fork, embrace the cheer,
A meal to hold the seasons near.

—Inspired by John Buchan

Vegetable Lasagne

Serves 8-10

Ingredients

- 350 g green lasagne (the ready-to-bake variety, which needs no pre-cooking)
- 1 small cauliflower, washed and broken into florets
- 500 g carrots, scraped and cut into 1"/2.5cm strips
- 500 g parsnips, scraped and cut into 1"/2.5cm strips
- 1 red pepper, halved, deseeded and cut into thin strips
- 250 g green haricot beans, ends cut off and cut into 2.5 cm (1") length
- 250 g Brussels sprouts washed and trimmed,
- 75 g butter
- 2 Tbsp sunflower oil
- 2 medium onions, skinned and thinly sliced
- 2 garlic cloves, skinned and finely chopped
- 4 leeks, washed, trimmed and fairly thinly sliced
- 250 g mushrooms, wiped and sliced
- 75 g flour
- 2 rounded tsp mustard powder
- 1.2 L milk or milk and chicken stock mixed
- Salt, freshly ground black pepper and freshly grated nutmeg
- 250 g cheddar, grated (keep 50 g aside for sprinkling on top of the lasagne)
- 2 Tbsp finely chopped parsley

Method

1. Steam the cauliflower, sprouts, beans, carrots, parsnips and strips of red pepper. Then, quarter the cooked sprouts.

2. Heat the butter and oil together in a large saucepan. Add the onions and sauté for about 5 minutes until soft and transparent. Stir in the garlic and leeks. Sauté for another 5 minutes, stirring occasionally, so the leeks cook evenly. Then, stir in the mushrooms and cook for a couple of minutes before stirring in the flour and mustard. Gradually stir in the milk (or milk and stock), stirring continuously until the sauce boils—season with salt, freshly ground black pepper and nutmeg. Stir in 175 g of the grated cheese.

3. Add the steamed vegetables to this sauce and stir in the chopped parsley. Butter a large, shallow, ovenproof dish and put in a layer of vegetable sauce. Cover with a layer of pasta, 2 to 3 sheets thick. Layer up like this, finishing with a vegetable sauce layer. Sprinkle with grated cheese.

4. At this stage, you can cover it and keep it in the fridge for up to 2 days before baking. Or bake in the oven at 180°C for 40-45 minutes, until the sauce is bubbling, the cheese on the top is melted, and golden brown and the lasagne feels soft when you stick a knife into it.

Serve with a green salad tossed in vinaigrette and warmed garlic bread-buttered rolls.

Vegetable Mains

Flint Family Cookbook

Cheese

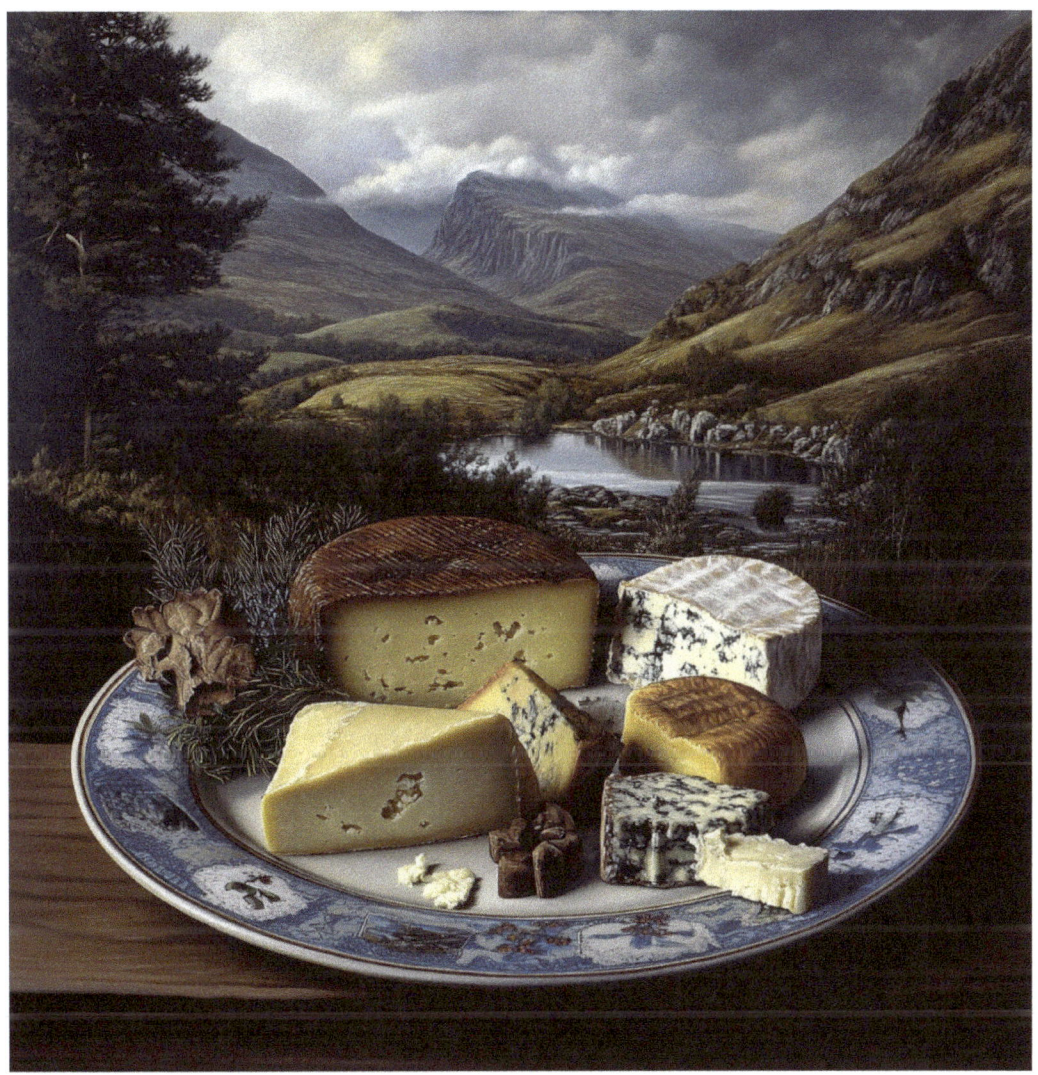

Cheese

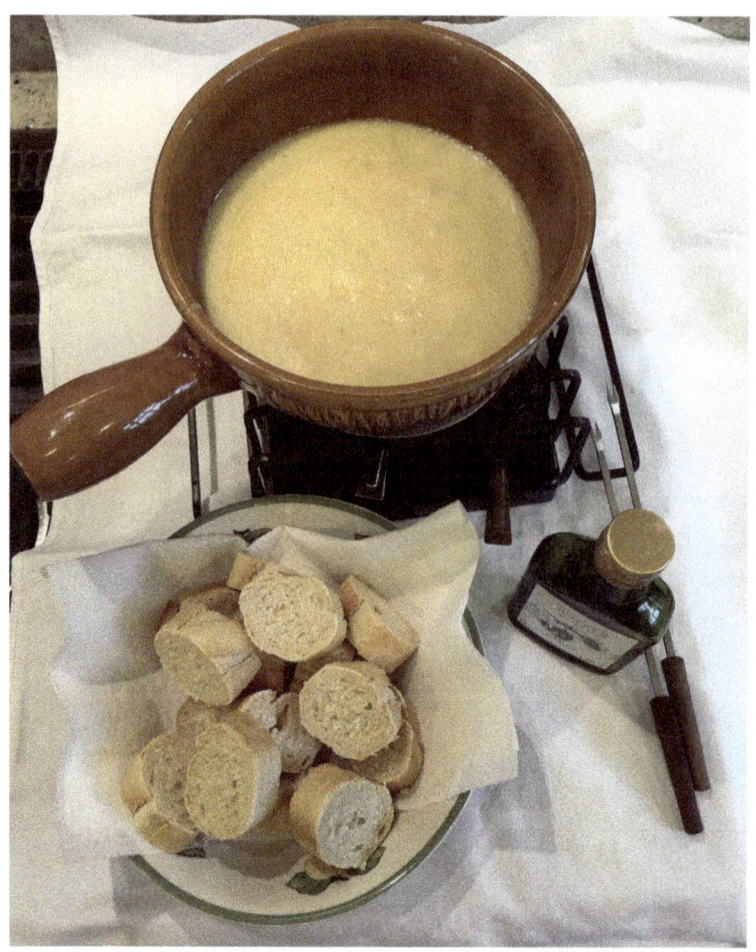

A Pot of Golden Cheer

A bubbling pot, so rich, so bright,
With wine's embrace and garlic's bite.
The melting tide of Gruyère deep,
A swirl of warmth, a joy to keep.

With bread to dip and Kirsch's cheer,
A feast to bring both far and near.
A pot of gold, so smooth, so fine,
A toast to love, to food, to wine.

—Inspired by Robert Burns

Cheese Fondue

Serves 2

Ingredients

2 garlic cloves, crushed

300 ml (½ pint) Riesling wine

400 g cheese (½ gruyere and ½ emmental) grated

2 level tsp of cornflour

Pepper

Pinch of nutmeg

Tiny squeeze of lemon juice

3 Tbsp of Kirsch

Method

1. Pour a little wine into the pot and cook the garlic over a low flame for a few minutes. Then, pour the rest of the wine and warm the liquid.

2. Add the cheese gradually and continue to heat, stirring, until the cheese has melted.

3. Blend the cornflour and seasoning with the kirsch to a smooth paste. Add it to the fondue and continue cooking for 2-3 minutes. When the fondue reaches a smooth consistency, it is ready to serve.

4. Serve with small cubes of crusty bread, white silver skin onions and small baked potatoes.

I don't think I would cook more than twice this amount at once, you might be best to start again.

Cheese

82

Flint Family Cookbook

Chicken

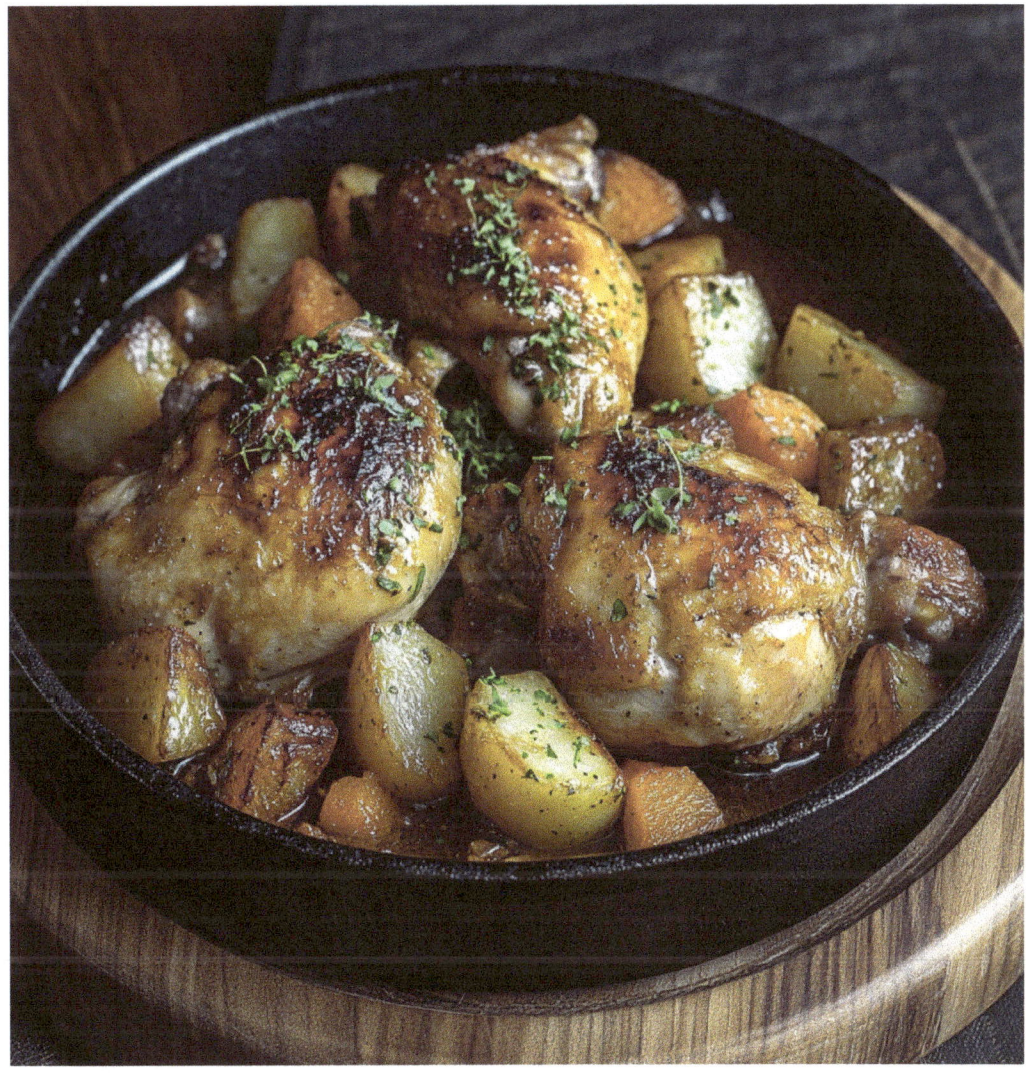

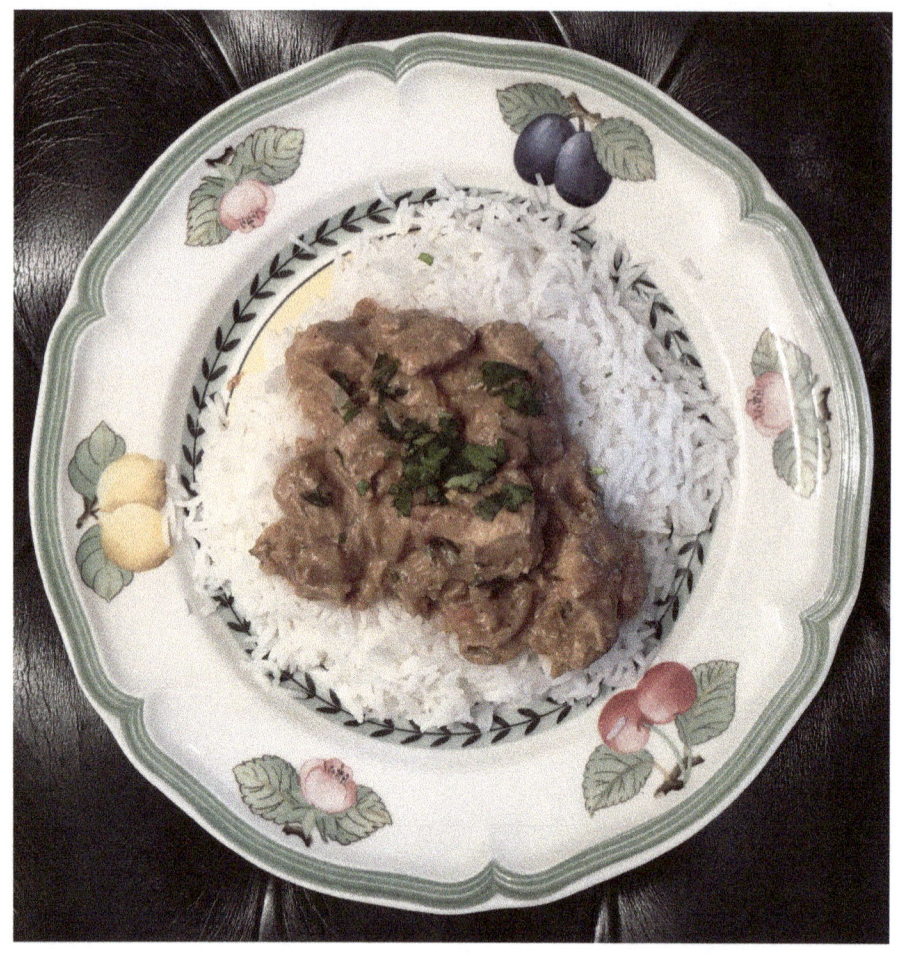

A Silk of Spice

A golden broth, so smooth, so deep,
Where butter sways and spices steep.
The cardamom hums, the bay leaves sing,
A warming touch in winter's cling.

A swirl of cream, a saffron glow,
A feast of fire, both rich and slow.
A dish to stir the heart anew,
A sip of warmth, a tale in brew.

—*Inspired by Robert Louis Stevenson*

Balti Butter Chicken

Serves 4

Ingredients

- 200 ml Greek full-fat yoghurt
- 50 g ground almonds
- ½ tsp chilli powder
- 3 bay leaves
- ¼ tsp ground cloves
- ¼ tsp ground cinnamon
- 2 tsp garam masala
- 6 cardamom pods crushed, remove the husks
- 1 tsp garlic pulp
- 1 tsp ginger pulp
- 200 g tin chopped tomatoes
- 1¼ tsp salt
- 1 kg chicken breast, skinned boned and cubed
- 75 g butter
- 1 Tbsp olive oil
- 2 medium onions
- 2 Tbsp chopped coriander
- 4 Tbsp single cream

Method

1. Put the yoghurt, ground almonds, all the dry spices, ginger, garlic, tomatoes and salt into a mixing bowl and blend thoroughly.
2. Melt half the butter and oil in a large, deep frying pan. Add the onions and fry for about 3 minutes. Add the garlic and ginger and fry gently for another 2 minutes. Tip the onions into the yoghurt mixture. Blend with a hand-held stick blender.
3. Melt the rest of the butter in the frying pan, and fry the chicken in batches. When lightly browned, tip into the yoghurt mixture until all the chicken has been sealed. Pour the mixture back into the frying pan and cook gently for 20 minutes until thoroughly cooked.
4. Stir in about half of the coriander and mix well.
5. Pour over the cream and stir well. Bring just to the boil. Serve garnished with the remaining chopped coriander.
6. Serve with boiled rice.

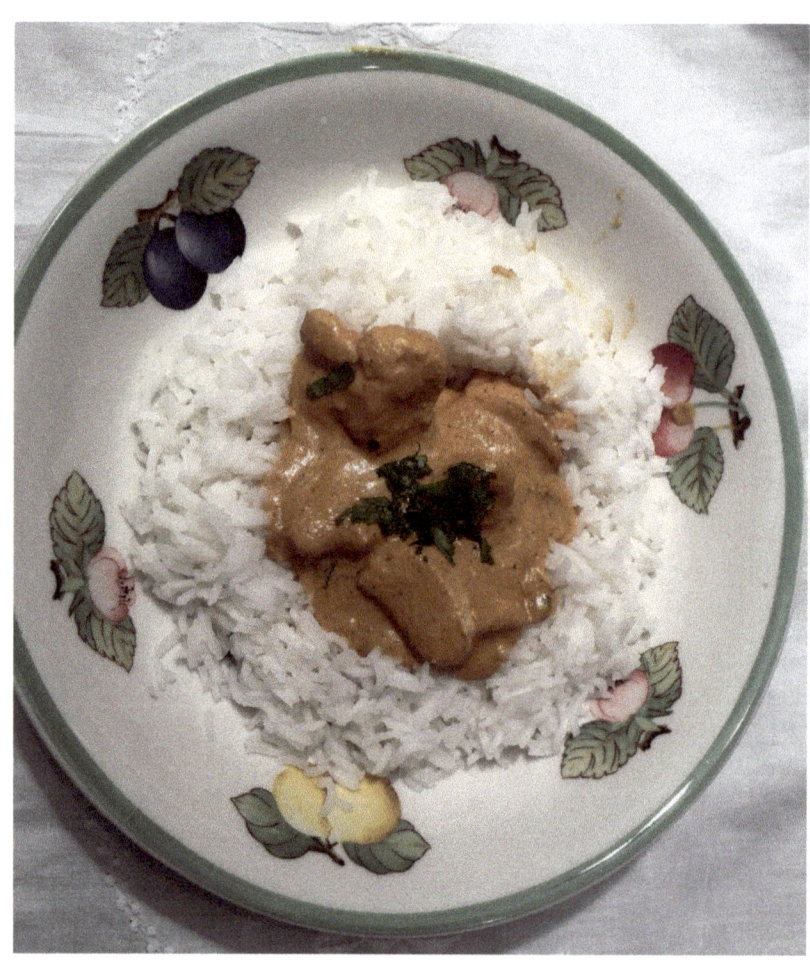

A Whisper of the East

Through ancient spice and scented air,
A dish so rich, so soft, so fair.
With almonds ground and saffron bright,
It fills the soul with golden light.

A simmered taste, a tender glow,
A warmth that lingers soft and slow.
With rice beside and herbs so fine,
A meal to share, a gift divine.

—*Inspired by John Buchan*

Balti Chicken Pasanda

Serves 4

Ingredients

- 4 Tbsp Greek yogurt
- ½ tsp black cumin seeds
- 4 cardamom pods (crushed)
- 6 whole black peppercorns
- 2 tsp garam masala
- 5 m cinnamon stick
- 2 Tbsp ground almonds
- 3 cloves garlic, finely chopped
- 20 g fresh ginger finely chopped
- ½–1 tsp chilli powder
- 1 tsp salt
- 4–6 chicken breasts, chopped into bit size pieces
- 5 Tbsp olive oil
- 2 medium onions, finely sliced
- 2 fresh green chillies pips removed and finely chopped (optional – the pips make the curry hot)
- 2 Tbsp coriander, chopped
- 120 ml single cream
- Steamed rice

Method

1. Mix the yoghurt, cumin seeds, cardamom, peppercorns, garam masala, cinnamon stick, ground almonds, garlic, ginger, chilli powder and salt in a medium mixing bowl. Add the chicken pieces and leave to marinate for at least 2 hours.

2. Heat the oil in a large frying pan. Fry the onions until soft. Pour in the chicken mixture and stir until it is well blended with the onions.

3. Cook over medium heat for 12–15 minutes or until the chicken is cooked and the sauce has thickened.

4. Add the green chillies and fresh coriander (reserve a little for decoration when serving). Pour in the cream. Bring to the boil and serve with steamed rice.

Chicken

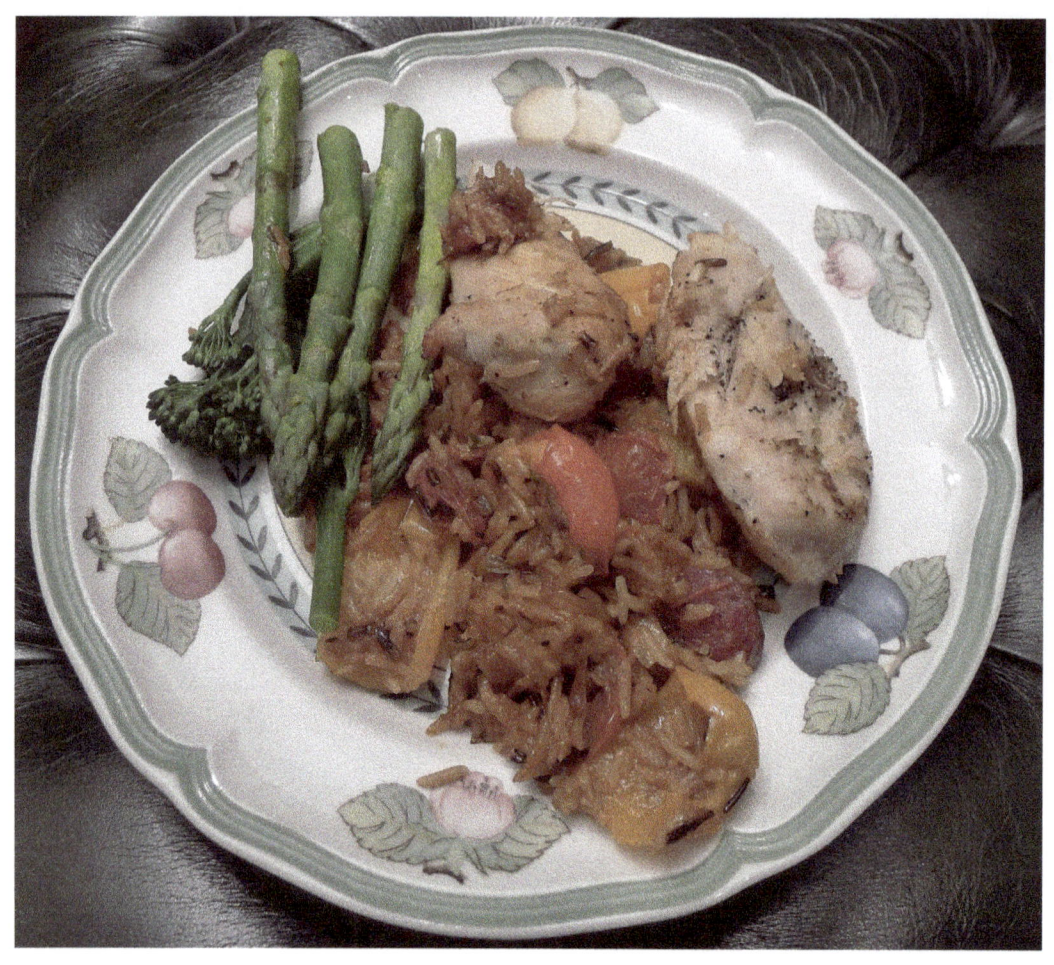

88

A Feast of Sun and Fire

The peppers blaze, the chorizo sings,
A dish of heat, where summer clings.
The orange glows, the olives bright,
A golden plate, a bold delight.

The rice drinks deep, the wine flows free,
A taste of land and rolling sea.
With thyme and fire, with love and cheer,
A Basque-born meal to bring you near.

—*Inspired by Robert Burns*

Chicken Basque

Serves 4

Ingredients

- 6 chicken breasts
- 2 large red peppers
- 2 medium onions
- 2-3 Tbsp olive oil
- 150 g chorizo sausage, skinned and cut into slices (more if desired)
- 285 g jar sun-dried cherry tomatoes
- 4 large garlic cloves, chopped
- 2 Tbsp double concentrate tomato puree
- ½ level tsp paprika
- Brown or white rice measured to the 225 ml (8 oz) level in a glass measuring jug
- 275 ml (10 oz) chicken stock (or stock cube)
- 170 ml (6oz) dry white wine
- 1 orange, cut into slices
- 2 tsp chopped thyme
- 100 g black pitted olives
- Salt and freshly milled black pepper

Method

1. Start by seasoning the chicken joints well with salt and pepper. Next, cut the red peppers in half, remove the seeds and pith, and cut each half into 6 pieces. Then, peel the onions and cut them into pieces. Then, drain the sun-dried tomatoes and wipe them dry with kitchen paper.

2. Now heat 2 Tbsp of olive oil in a large frying pan on medium heat. Add the chicken pieces at a time, and brown them to a nutty golden brown colour on both sides. Put to one side.

3. Next, add more oil to the frying pan and increase the heat. As soon as the oil is hot, add the onion and peppers and allow them to brown at the edges, moving them around for about 5 minutes.

4. Add the chorizo, sun-dried tomatoes, and garlic and toss for a minute or two until the garlic is pale golden and the chorizo has taken on some colour. Next, stir in the rice, and when the grains have a good oil coating, add the tomato paste, paprika, and chopped thyme. Pour in the stock and wine, add some seasoning, and bring to a simmering point.

5. Then, transfer to a wide, shallow casserole dish (with a tight-fitting lid). Add more seasoning, then place the sliced orange on top and scatter with olives. Cover with the chicken.

6. Cover with a tight-fitting lid and cook for one hour in the oven at 180* C. Remove the lid halfway through cooking to see if any more liquid needs to be added

7. Serve with a green vegetable, broccoli or mange tout.

Chicken

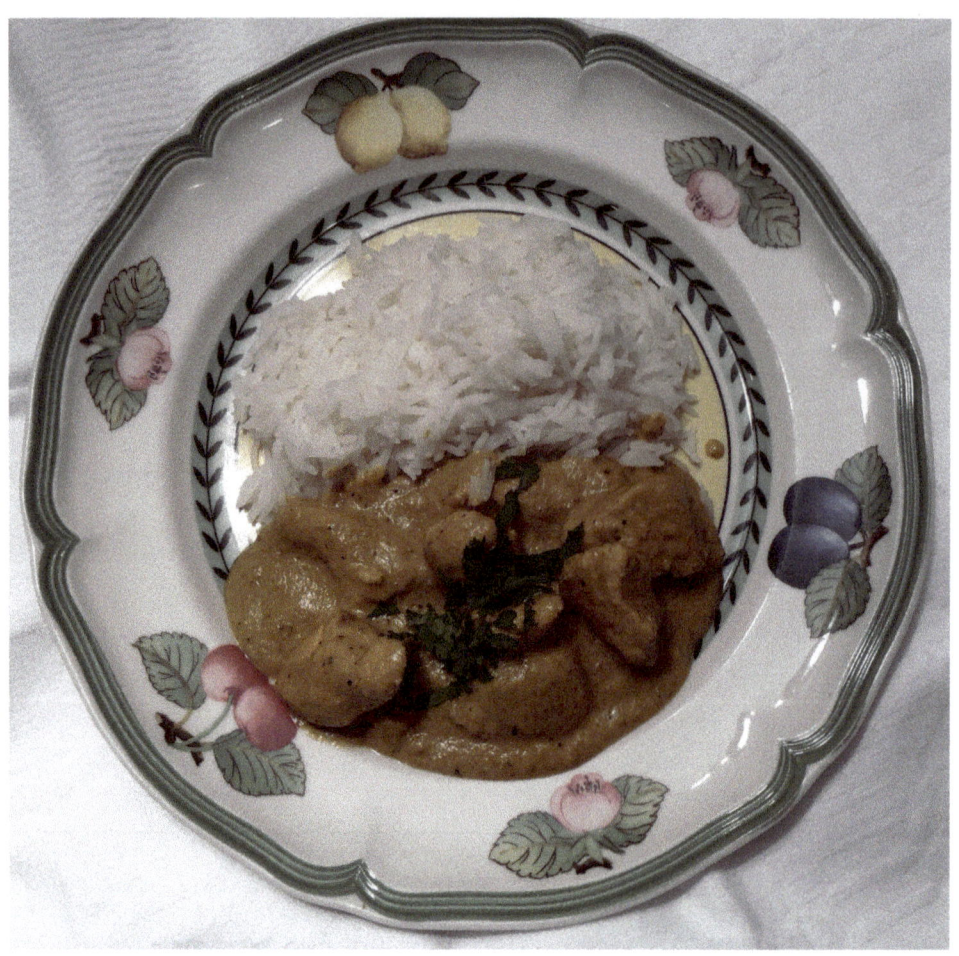

A Bowl of Gentle Gold

A whisper soft, a spice so mild,
A dish that soothes both heart and child.
With almonds kissed and saffron sweet,
A fragrant tale, a dream complete.

The cream swirls in, the warmth unfolds,
A story steeped in hues of gold.
So take a sip, let comfort stay,
A dish to chase the chill away.

—*Inspired by Contemporary Scottish Poets*

Chicken Korma

Serves 4

Ingredients

- 3 Tbsp butter
- 1 Tbsp sunflower oil
- 2 medium onions, chopped
- 10 g chunk of fresh root ginger, peeled and finely grated
- 4 garlic cloves, sliced
- ½ tsp ground cardamom
- 1 Tbsp ground cumin
- 1 Tbsp ground coriander
- 1 Tbsp garam masala
- ½ tsp ground turmeric
- ¼ tsp hot chilli powder (optional)
- 1 bay leaf
- 4 cloves
- Small pinch of saffron (optional)
- 3 Tbsp ground almonds
- 1 Tbsp caster sugar
- 1½ tsp flaked sea salt, plus extra to season
- 300 ml cold water
- 2 Tbsp sunflower oil
- 4 boneless, skinless chicken breasts
- 100 ml double cream
- Freshly ground black pepper

Method

1. Melt the butter and oil in a large nonstick saucepan and add the onions, ginger, and garlic. Cover the pan and cook over medium heat for 10 minutes, then stir in the cardamom, cumin, coriander, garam masala, turmeric, chilli powder, and bay leaf. Pinch the ends off the cloves and add them to the pan; throw away the stalks. Cook for 5 minutes more without covering the pan until the onions are very soft, stirring optionally.

2. Stir in the saffron, almonds, sugar, salt, and water into the pan and gently simmer. Cook for 5 minutes, stirring regularly, then remove the pan from the heat and set aside. Remove the bay leaf.

3. Cut each chicken breast into 7-8 bite-sized pieces and season with salt and freshly ground black pepper. Heat the sunflower oil in a large, nonstick frying pan. Fry the chicken over medium heat for 3-4 minutes until lightly coloured on all sides, turning regularly. While the chicken is cooking, blitz the onion mixture with a stick blender or in a food processor until it is as smooth as possible.

4. Tip the spiced onions puree into the pan with the chicken. Bring it to a simmer and cook for 5-6 minutes, stirring occasionally, until the chicken is tender and just cooked through. Stir in the double cream, then gently simmer, stirring constantly. Serve with rice.

Chicken

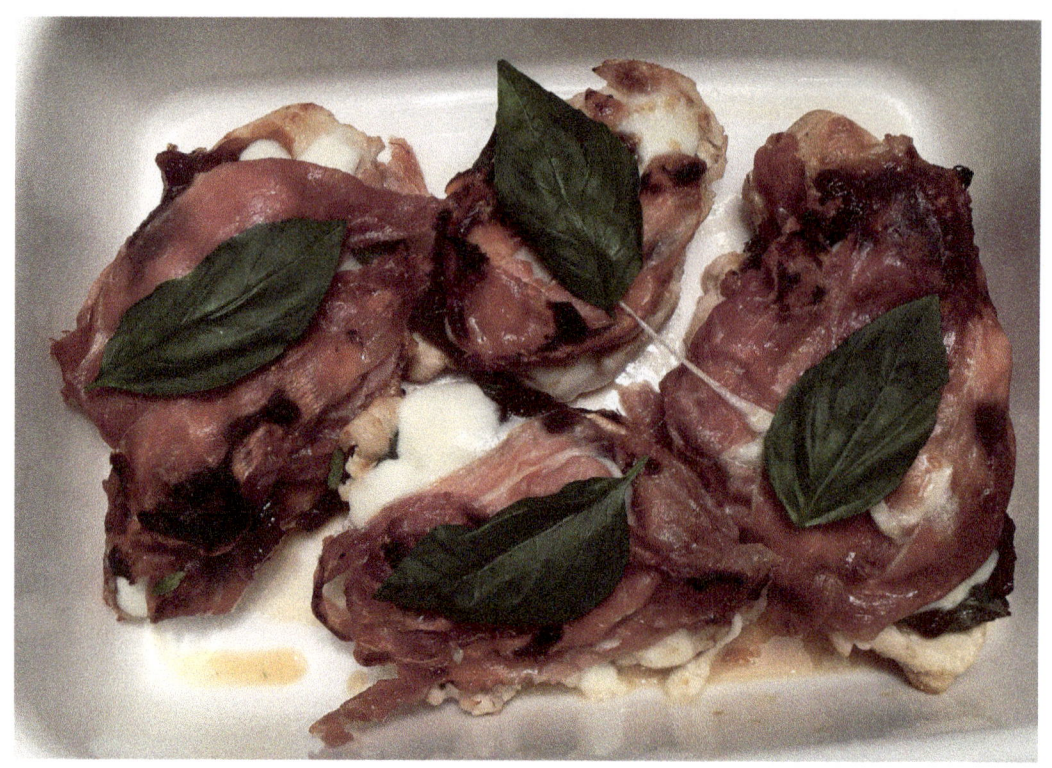

A Rich Embrace

A fold of silk, a warming breeze,
Where prosciutto wraps with tender ease.
With sage so bold and cheese so light,
A meal to charm, a pure delight.

A flicker crisp, a bubbling glaze,
A taste that sets the soul ablaze.
So carve, so share, so lift the glass,
A dish of joy, let none surpass.

—*Inspired by Robert Louis Stevenson*

Chicken with Mozzarella, Prosciutto, and Sage

Serves 4

Ingredients

4 large boneless chicken breasts

4 Tbsp olive oil, plus extra for drizzling

12 sage leaves

8 Tbsp plum chutney (or onion chutney)

2 balls of buffalo mozzarella cheese, about 150 g each

8 slices prosciutto

8 sprigs fresh basil

Sea salt and freshly ground black pepper

Method

1. Cut the chicken breasts in half, but not all the way through enough to open them out flat (called butterflying). Season the chicken well and cook in a hot sauté pan in olive oil, colouring both sides well for about 8-10 minutes.

2. Place 3 sage leaves and 2 Tbsp of chutney on each breast when the chicken is cooked.

3. Remove the mozzarella from the packets and drain. Chop into small pieces and place onto one-half of each butterflied chicken. Finish by wrapping 2 slices of prosciutto ham around each chicken. Drizzle with olive oil and season generously.

4. Place under a preheated grill to crisp the bacon. This will only take a short time and will also melt the cheese.

5. Place the chicken on plates, and pour the remaining pan juices over the top. Garnish with fresh basil.

6. Serve with vegetables, mashed potatoes or salad.

Chicken

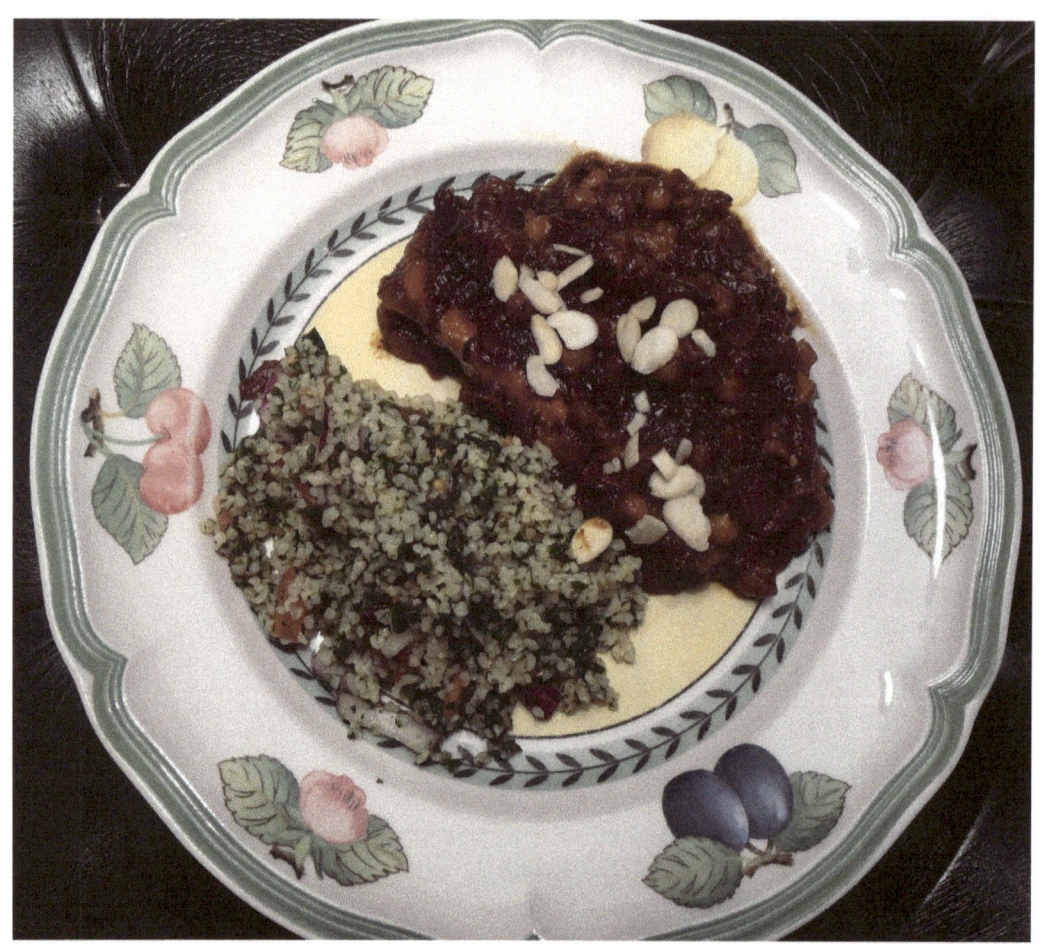

A Song of Spice and Sweet Delight

The cinnamon hums, the saffron glows,
A dish where desert fragrance flows.
With honey's kiss and dates so deep,
A meal to stir the soul from sleep.

The apricots dance, the chickpeas twine,
A touch of mint, a sip of wine.
A meal of warmth, a spice-wrapped dream,
A tale of lands by fire's gleam.

—*Inspired by Sir Walter Scott*

Chicken Tagine

Serves 4-6

Ingredients

- 50 g butter
- 1 medium chicken, cut into 10 pieces or 6 large chicken breasts
- 1 Tbsp sunflower oil plus 25 g butter to pan fry the chicken
- 2 onions, finely chopped
- 3 garlic cloves finely chopped
- 5 cm (2 in) piece of root ginger, grated
- 2 cinnamon sticks
- 2 tsp Ras-el-Hanout (North African spice blend)
- 1½ tsp salt
- 1 tsp freshly ground black pepper
- 1 tsp ground turmeric
- 1 tsp ground cinnamon
- 1 preserved lemon, roughly chopped
- 3 Tbsp honey
- 750 ml chicken stock
- 150 g dates, stones removed, halved
- 150 g soft apricots, chopped
- Salt and freshly ground black pepper
- 2 Tbsp chopped fresh parsley
- 400 g chickpeas (soak overnight to soften before using)
- 400 g chopped tomatoes
- 2 Tbsp fresh mint
- 75 g flaked almonds

Method

1. Heat the 50 g butter in a frying pan. Add the onions, garlic, ginger, and fry for 2-3 minutes or until softened. Stir in the spices and cook for one minute.
2. Add the preserved lemons, honey, chickpeas, tin tomatoes, dates, apricots, and stock and bring the mixture to a boil.
3. Reduce the heat until simmering, cover with a lid, and cook for 1 hour. The flavours develop more if left overnight.
4. The following day, reheat.
5. Then, fry the chicken, a few pieces at a time, in the butter and oil in a large frying pan for 2-3 minutes on each side or until golden brown. Replace the chicken in the tagine and cook slowly until thoroughly cooked.
6. Season to taste with salt and freshly ground pepper, then stir in the parsley and mint. Decorate with flaked almonds.
7. Serve with herby tabbouleh (see recipe).

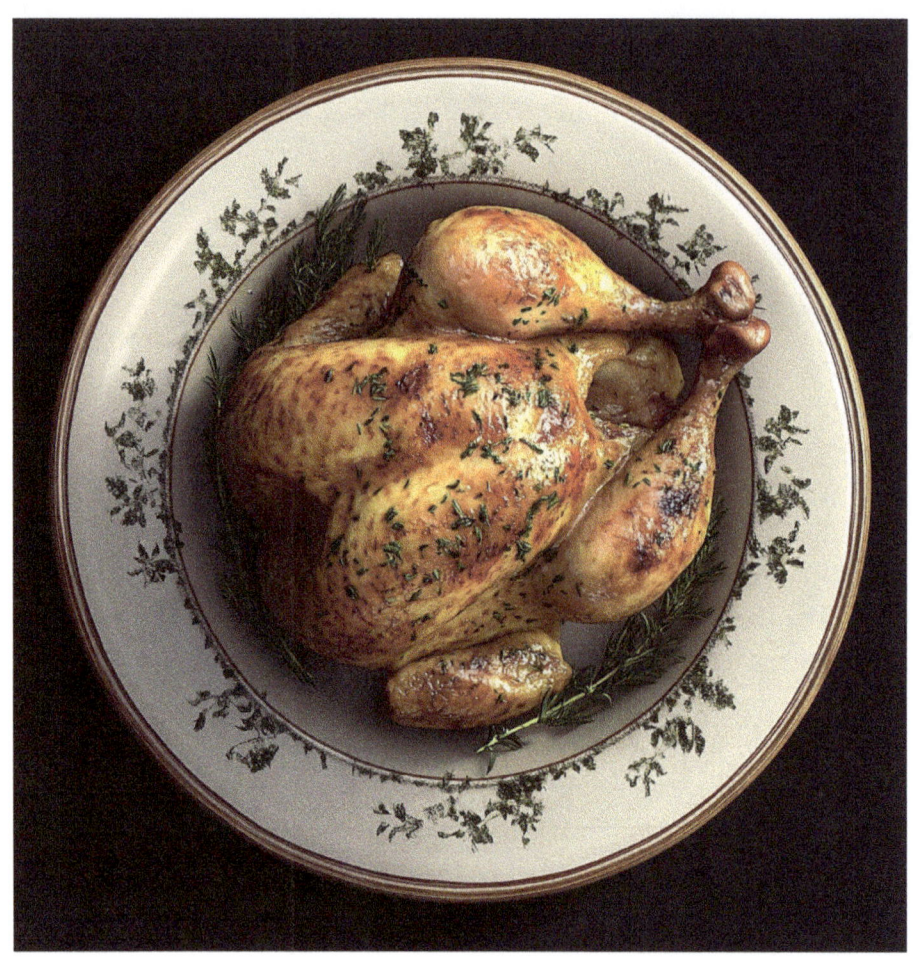

A Herb's Soft Whisper

A garden's breath, a summer's taste,
With tarragon both bold and chaste.
A tender sip, a creamy dream,
Where mushrooms waltz in velvet stream.

A dish of ease, yet fine and bright,
A golden plate, a touch so light.
With wine and warmth, a poet's cheer,
A meal to keep the heart sincere.

—Inspired by Contemporary Scottish Poets

Chicken with Tarragon

Serves 4

Ingredients

- 4 chicken breast fillets, skinless
- 1 Tbsp olive oil
- 50 g unsalted butter
- 2 medium onion, thinly sliced
- 120 g button mushrooms, thinly sliced
- 2 garlic cloves, crushed
- 150 ml white wine
- 300 ml chicken stock (or a chicken stock cube made up as per instructions)
- 150 ml double cream
- 2 Tbsp plain flour
- 15 g tarragon leaves (8 for decoration)
- Maldon salt
- Fresh ground white pepper
- Lemon juice

Method

1. Heat the oil and 25 g of butter in a large frying pan until hot. Lightly bash the chicken breast between 2 sheets of cling film until even in thickness, season well with salt and pepper.

2. Add the chicken breast one at a time to the pan and cook for two to three minutes on each side until browned. Put to one side and cover to keep warm.

3. Add the onions. Once they have started to soften, add the garlic and mushrooms. Cook for a few minutes, and then add the flour. Continue to cook for a few minutes, then add the wine and stock. Bring to the boil, then lower the heat.

4. Return the chicken breast to the pan, and cook slowly until cooked, turning a couple of times to ensure the chicken is cooked evenly.

5. When the sauce has become thick, add the cream and tarragon to the pan. Check the seasoning and add a few drops of lemon juice.

6. Keep warm until you are ready to serve. (If you are keeping it for any length of time, do not add the tarragon. Cover the surface of the mixture with a buttered wrapper to prevent the skin from forming. Leave it to cool. When reheating, add two Tbsp of water and the tarragon.)

7. To serve, lay out four warm plates, placing a chicken breast on each one and spooning over the sauce.

8. Serve with asparagus and rice. Decorate with a couple of tarragon leaves.

Chicken

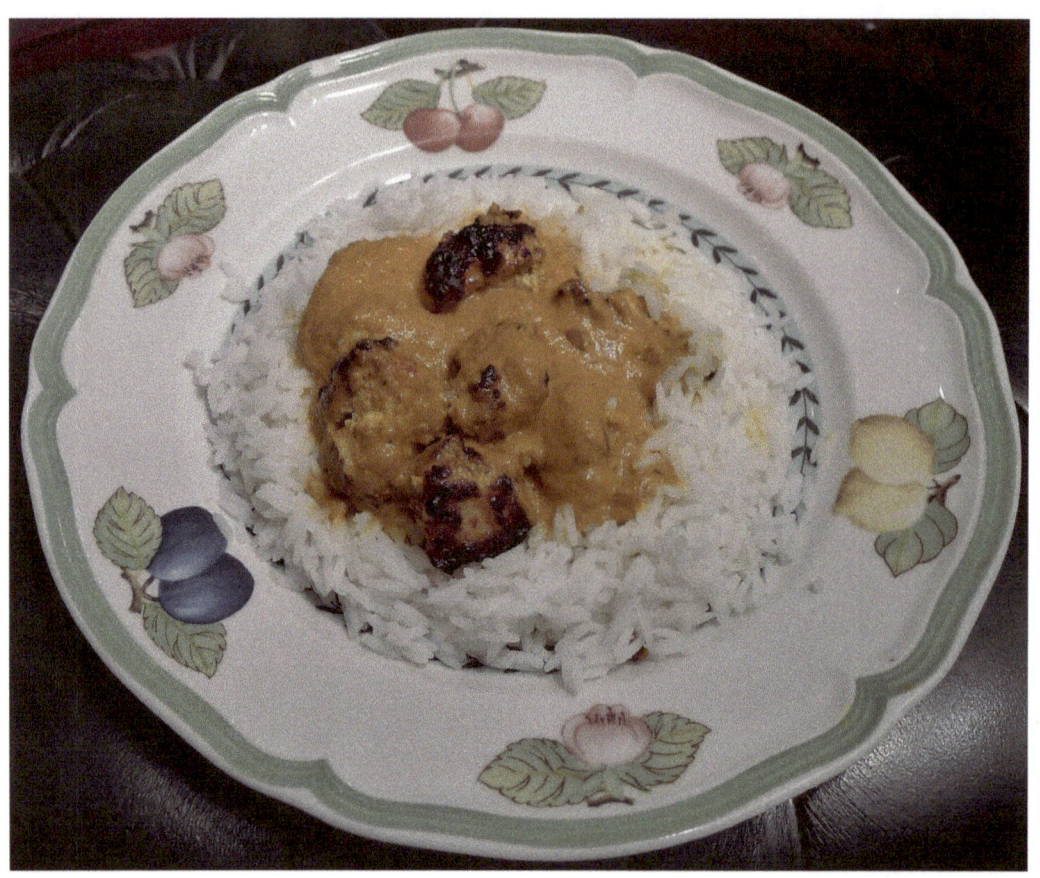

A Fire and Feast

The embers glow, the skewers char,
A dish that sings from lands afar.
With spice so bold and yoghurt sweet,
A taste where fire and silk do meet.

The masala swirls, the sauce runs deep,
A dish where golden secrets keep.
With every bite, the warmth expands,
A tale now shared in distant lands.

—*Inspired by Robert Louis Stevenson*

Chicken Tikka Masala

Serves 4

Ingredients

2 Tbsp cumin seeds
2 Tbsp coriander seeds
2 whole cloves
1 tsp black peppercorns
Small piece of cinnamon stick
½ tsp ground fenugreek
1½ tsp ground turmeric
2 tsp ground paprika
¼–½ tsp chilli powder
1 tsp flaked sea salt
2 garlic cloves, crushed
20 g chunk of fresh root ginger, peeled and grated
4 heaped Tbsp plain yoghurt
4 large boneless chicken breasts cut into 7–8 pieces

Sunflower oil, for greasing skewers

For the Masala sauce

2 Tbsp softened butter
2 Tbsp sunflower oil
3 medium onions, chopped
4 garlic cloves, crushed
25 g chunk of fresh ginger, peeled and finely grated
½ tsp ground turmeric
3 Tbsp tomato purée
2 tsp caster sugar
1 tsp flaked sea salt
400 ml cold water
2 Tbsp double cream

Method

1. Put the cumin and coriander seeds, cloves, peppercorns, and cinnamon stick in a dry frying pan over medium heat. Cook for 1–2 minutes, stirring regularly, until lightly toasted—you know they are ready when you can smell the wonderful spicy aroma. Now, allow the spices to cool.
2. Tip everything into a pestle and mortar or electric spice grinder. Add the fenugreek, turmeric, paprika, chilli powder and salt and grind everything to a fine powder.
3. Spoon 3 Tbsp of this spice mixture into a mixing bowl and stir in the garlic, ginger, and yoghurt. Mix thoroughly and set aside.
4. Stir the chicken pieces into the spiced yoghurt, cover with cling film, and refrigerate for at least 4 hours, ideally overnight.
5. To make the masala sauce, heat the butter and sunflower oil in a large nonstick pan. Add the onions, garlic, and ginger. Cover and cook over low heat for 10 minutes, stirring occasionally.
6. Remove the lid, increase the heat slightly and stir in the rest of the powdered spices, plus ½ tsp of turmeric. Fry for 3 minutes, stirring regularly.
7. Stir in the tomato purée, sugar, salt, and fry for 2–3 minutes, stirring constantly. Add the water to a gentle simmer and cook for 5 minutes more, adding the cream for the last 30 seconds of the cooking time.

8. Remove from the heat and blitz with a stick blender until the sauce is as smooth as possible. Pour this into a heat-proof bowl, cover with cling film, cool, and chill until you are ready to cook the chicken. Remove the chicken pieces from the marinade.
9. Remove the chicken from the marinade. Thread the chicken pieces onto lightly greased, long metal skewers. You should be able to fit about 6 chunks of chicken on each skewer, leaving 1-2 cm between each piece. Save the leftover marinade.
10. Preheat the grill to its hottest setting, and place the skewers on a rack over a grill pan lined with foil. Slide the pan onto a shelf, put it as close to the heat as possible, and cook the chicken for 5 minutes.
11. Turn each skewer, holding it with an oven cloth, and cook on the other side for another 4-5 minutes or until the chicken is cooked through and lightly charred.
12. While the chicken grills, tip the masala sauce and the remaining marinade into a large nonstick frying pan. Bring to a gentle simmer and cook for 2-3 minutes, stirring regularly.
13. Take the chicken skewers from under the grill and slide a fork down the length of each skewer to plop the pieces into the hot sauce. Stir well and bubble for a few seconds more. Serve hot with rice.

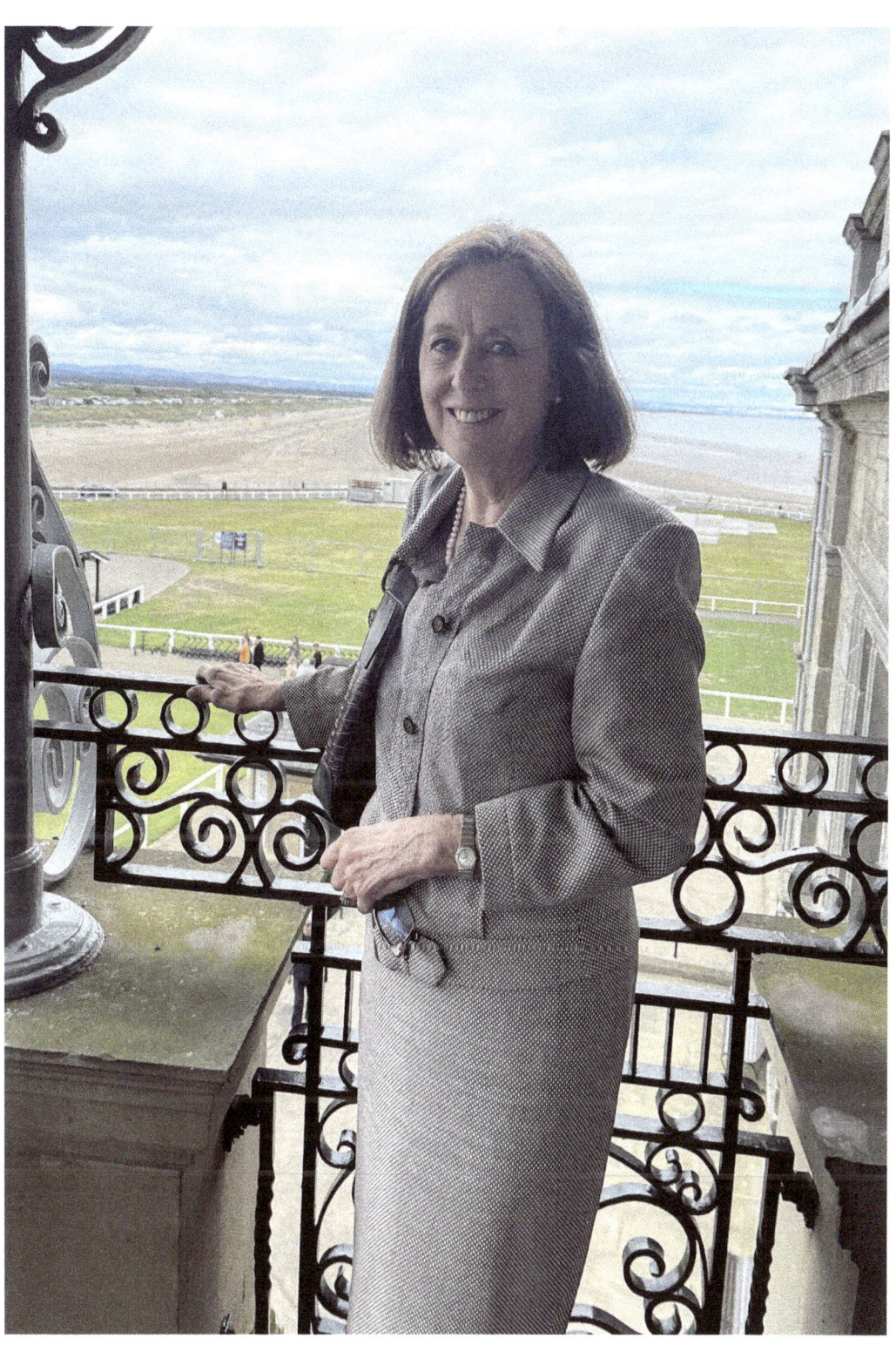

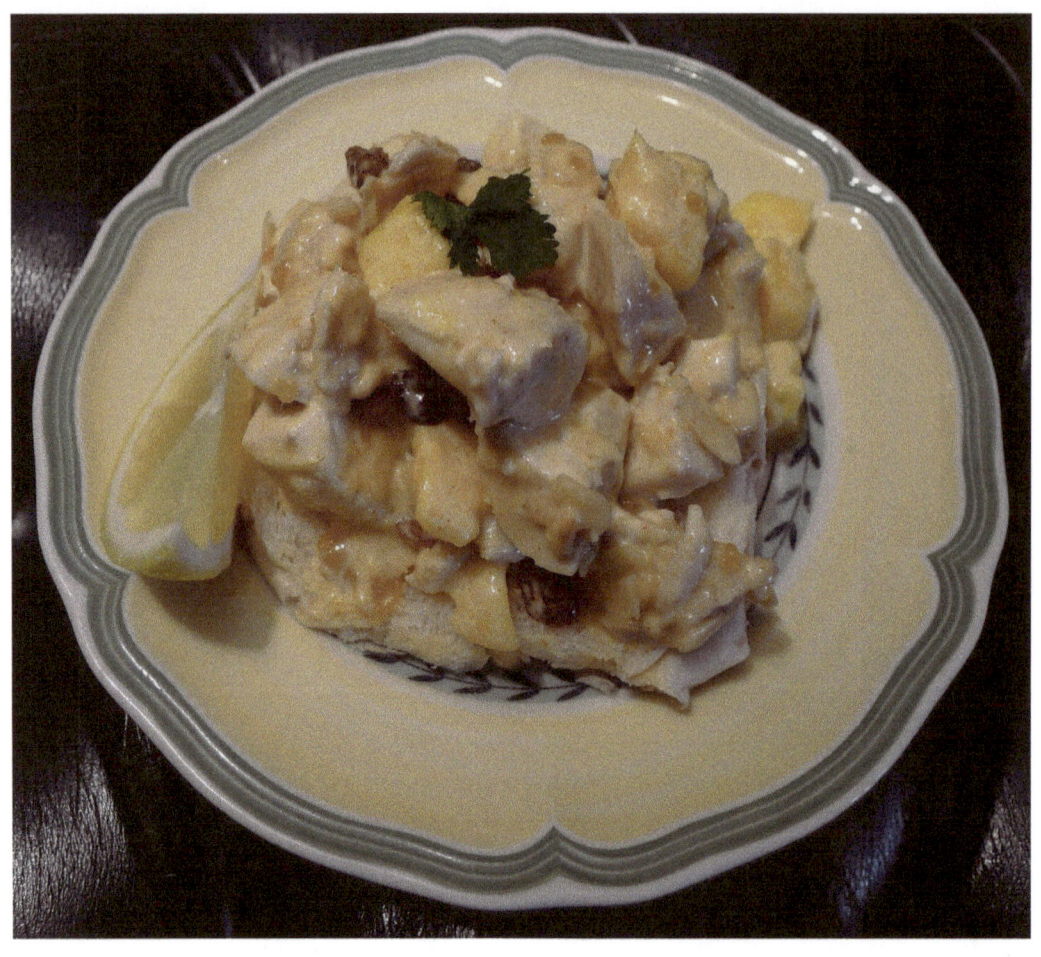

A Royal Fare*

A dish once served with golden cheer,
A taste of spice, both bright and clear.
With mango sweet and cashew's bite,
A meal both rich and feather-light.

A toast is raised, a table set,
A feast of past, remembered yet.
A touch of charm, a regal grace,
A dish that time shall not erase.

—*Inspired by John Buchan*

Coronation Chicken

Serves 4-6

Ingredients

1 large firm, ripe mango

50 g sultanas

1 kg chicken breast cooked and skinned and cut into 12mm strips

150 ml mayonnaise

1½ tsp mild curry powder

1 Tbsp mango chutney

1 tsp lemon juice

Salt and pepper

100 g cashew nuts

Method

1. Remove the skin from the mango. Chop the flesh off either side of the stone and slice it into mango strips.
2. Put three quarters off the mango strips, sultanas and the chicken in a large bowl.
3. Mix the mayonnaise with the curry powder, chutney and lemon juice, and season. Pour over the chicken mixture and toss gently. Add half the nuts and mix in well.
4. Transfer to a serving dish and garnish with the remaining mango strips and cashew nuts.
5. Serve with a rice salad on a bed of crispy green salad.

If you chop the nuts, mango, and chicken into smaller pieces, this makes a delicious, moist sandwich filling.

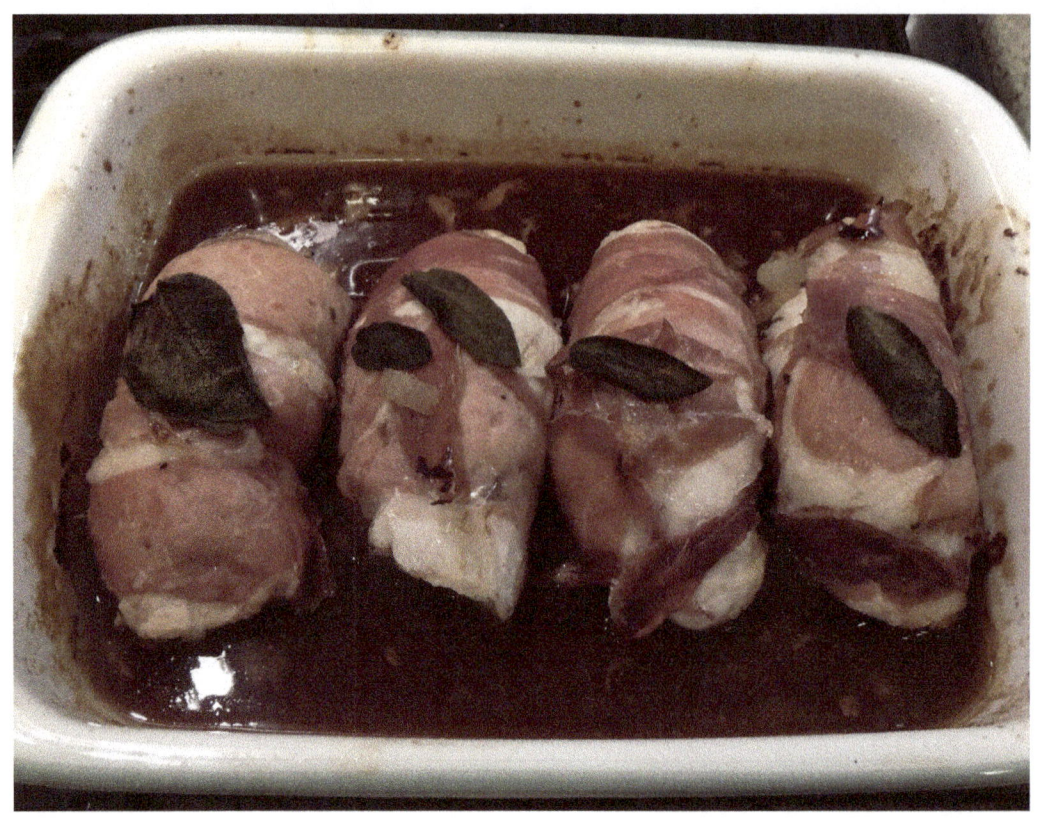

A Feast of Hearth and Home

A wrap of warmth, a sage's grace,
A dish that holds the hearth's embrace.
With chestnuts deep and ham so fine,
A taste of autumn's sweetest wine.

The sauce runs rich, the plates are filled,
A meal where love and hands have skilled.
A fork is raised, the candle's gleam,
A feast of warmth, a winter dream.

—Inspired by Robert Burns

Ham-wrapped Chicken with Chestnut Stuffing

Serves 4

Ingredients

7 g dried mushrooms

Chestnut stuffing see recipe

4 skinless free-range chicken breasts

12 fresh sage leaves

8 slices of dry-cured ham

For the Madeira sauce

600 ml of fresh chicken stock

150 ml Madeira

1 tsp balsamic vinegar

You will need

4 wooden cocktail sticks

Shallow oven-proof dish

Method

1. Tip the mushrooms into a food processor and blend until they are almost powdered.

2. Place the chicken breasts in between 2 sheets of cling film and lightly beat with a rolling pin until they are an even thickness.

3. Place the parma ham on top of the chicken breast, turn over and then scatter each one with some of the mushroom powder and divide the chestnut stuffing between the breasts. Place 2 sage leaves on each breast, then roll in a slice of ham like a Swiss roll. Secure with a cocktail stick, and chill until ready to serve.

4. To make the sauce, tip the stock into the pan with the Madeira and vinegar and leave to bubble over high heat until the liquid has reduced by half. Cool, and then chill.

5. When ready to eat, preheat the oven to 200°C. Arrange the chicken in the dish and pour over the Madeira sauce. Cover with foil, then place in the oven for 20 minutes until the chicken is cooked. Leave to stand for 5 minutes, then remove the cocktail sticks and slice at an angle.

6. Serve with bubble and squeak cakes and green beans. Spoon the sauce around the chicken. Garnish with sage sprigs.

Chicken

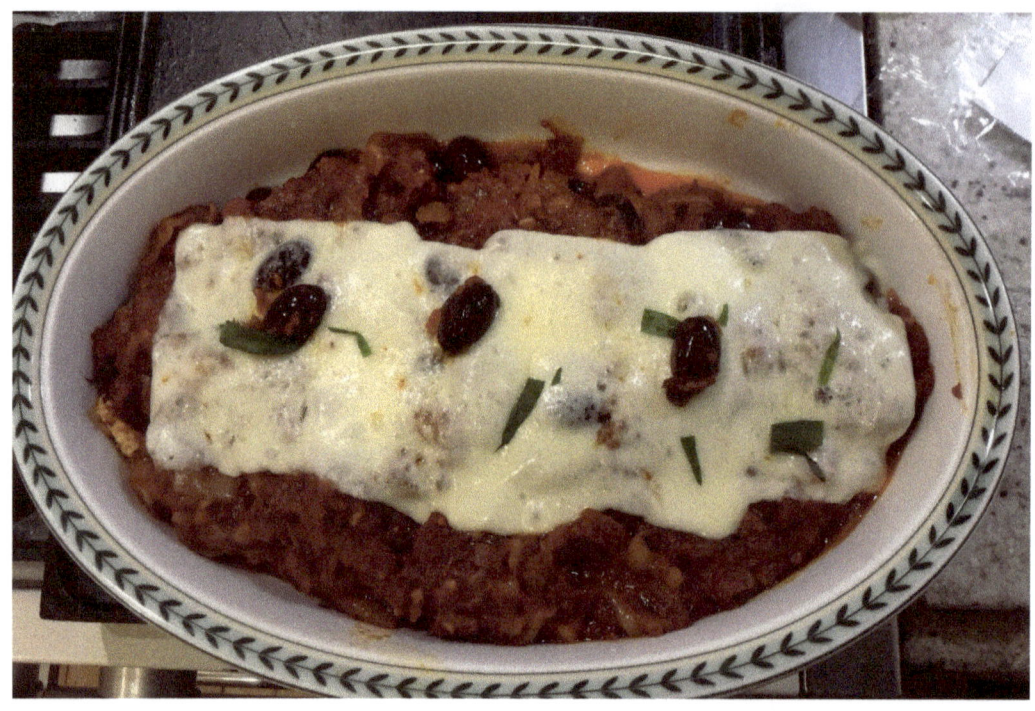

A Tale of Vine and Hearth

The olives dance, the garlic sings,
A meal where joy and comfort clings.
With tomatoes bright and cheese so bold,
A tale of love in plates retold.

A touch of thyme, a sip of red,
A dish where every heart is fed.
A song of home, a southern breeze,
A taste of life, of art, of ease.

—*Inspired by Robert Louis Stevenson*

Italian Style Chicken

Serves 4

Ingredients

4 large chicken breasts, skinned
2 cloves of garlic, crushed
2 Tbsp chopped tarragon
Salt and pepper
15 g butter
3 Tbsp oil
1 onion, finely chopped
2 shallots, finely chopped
400 g chopped tomatoes
2 Tbsp tomato puree
2 tsp sugar
1 tsp oregano
150 ml chicken stock
150 g mozzarella cheese, sliced
100 g Black olives
Mint to garnish

Method

1. Season the chicken breasts with garlic, tarragon, salt, and pepper. Melt the butter and 1 Tbsp oil in a frying pan, and gently fry the chicken for 3 minutes on each side. Transfer to a flameproof dish.

2. Heat the remaining oil in a saucepan. Add the onion and shallots and fry for 5 minutes.

3. Add the tomatoes, tomato puree, sugar, oregano, and chicken stock. Season to taste with salt and pepper and cook for 30 minutes over low heat. Add pitted olives.

4. Preheat the oven to 180°C.

5. Spoon the tomato sauce over the chicken breasts, cover with foil and place in the oven. Cook for 25 minutes.

6. Set the grill to high. Remove the chicken from the oven and cover it with mozzarella cheese. Place under the grill for 3-5 minutes or until the cheese has melted.

7. Garnish with mint leaves and serve

Chicken

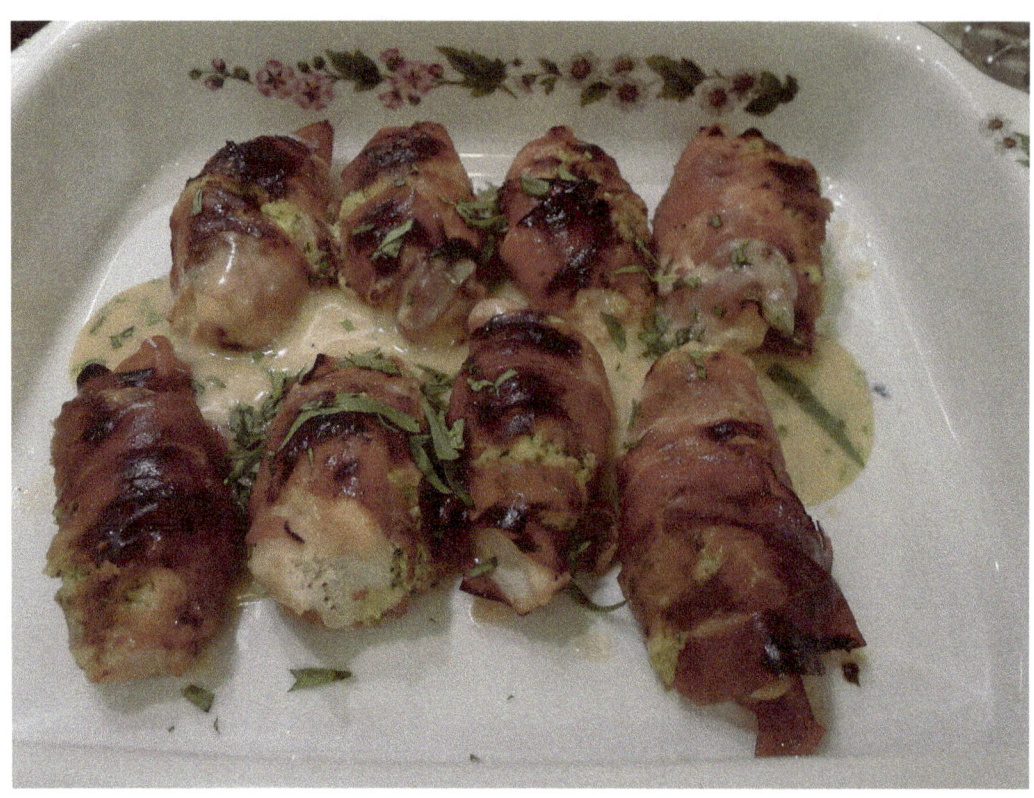

A Feast of Layers Deep

A cream of spice, a pepper's glow,
A dish of depth, a warmth to show.
With ham wrapped tight and tarragon bright,
A bite of boldness, rich yet light.

A honeyed glaze, a sauce so free,
A taste of land and rolling sea.
A meal of skill, of hands that know,
A dish where time moves soft and slow.

—*Inspired by Sir Walter Scott*

Peppered Chicken with Tarragon and Parma Ham

Serves 6

Ingredients

6 skinless, boned chicken breasts

150 g pack black-pepper full-fat cream cheese (Boursin)

3 Tbsp chopped tarragon, plus extra leaves, to decorate

12 slices of Parma ham

A knob of butter

3 Tbsp clear honey

200 g full-fat crème fraîche

Small squeeze of lemon

Salt and freshly ground black pepper

1 heaped tsp of cornflour mixed with a small amount of cold water

Method

1. Preheat the oven to 180°C

2. Put the chicken breasts on a board. Using a sharp knife, make a pocket in the side of each breast, cutting through to the middle.

3. Mix the cream cheese with 2 Tbsp of the tarragon and season well. Divide the mixture between the chicken breast pockets, pushing it into each one. Wrap each breast in two slices of Parma ham so the chicken is completely covered.

4. Grease a small roasting tin with butter, then arrange the chicken inside. Drizzle over 2 Tbsp of honey, then roast for about 25–30 minutes or until the chicken is golden brown and no longer pink in the centre. Remove the chicken breasts from the tin and leave to rest for 5 minutes while making the sauce.

5. Add the crème fraîche, the remaining tablespoon of honey, and cornflour mixed with water and lemon to the roasting tin. Put the tin on the hob and bring gently to a boil, incorporating the chicken juices with a wooden spoon to release the chicken juices (be careful not to scrape the base where it has burnt, or it will become bitter).

6. Add the remaining chopped tarragon and season.

7. Serve the chicken sprinkled with a few tarragon leaves and with the sauce alongside for everyone to help themselves.

Chicken

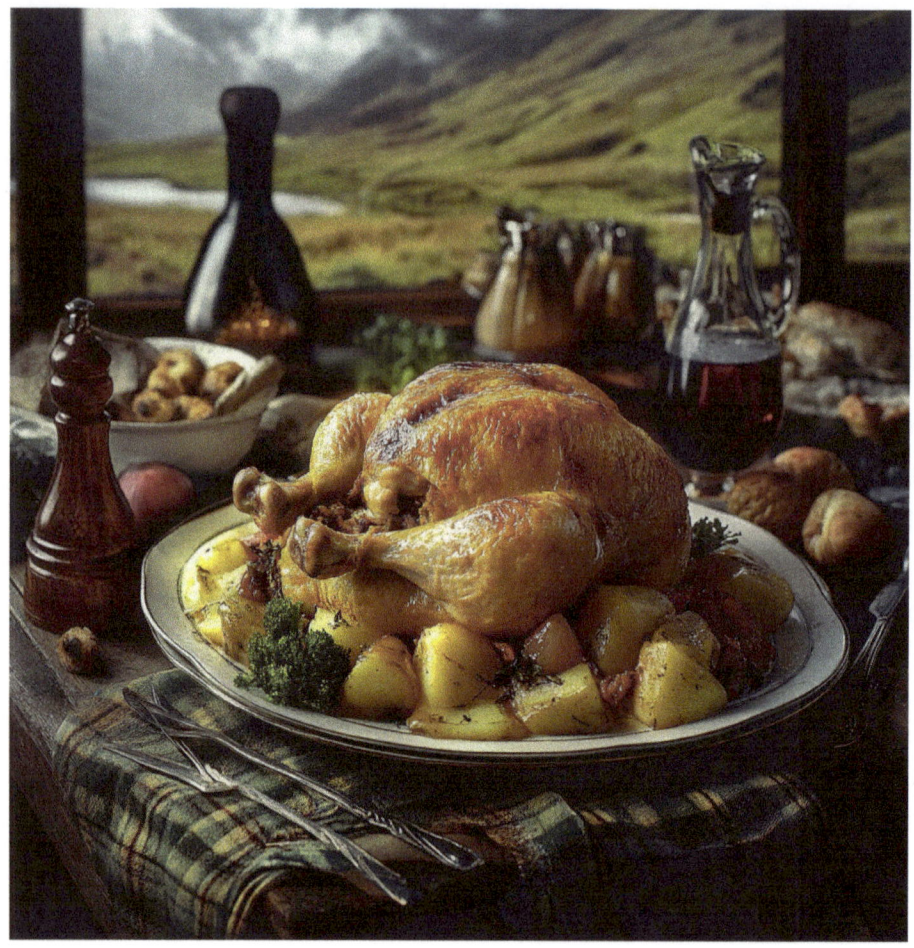

A Sunday's Grace

*The oven hums, the table's set,
A feast that none shall e'er forget.
With golden skin and stuffing deep,
A meal that love and hands do keep.*

*The gravy flows, the plates are passed,
A taste of home that's built to last.
A simple dish, yet rich in lore,
A Sunday's gift forevermore.*

—*Inspired by Robert Burns*

Roast Chicken Dinner

Many of these recipes are suitable to use with turkey.

Serves 4

Ingredients

One chicken

Half a lemon

Stuffing

Salt and pepper

100 g smoked back bacon or streaky bacon

Olive oil/butter

12 chipolata sausages

Method

1. Preheat the oven to 180°C

2. Remove the wishbone; this will make carving easier. Place softened butter under the skin of the bird. (Basting) Rub with olive oil all over the bird. Liberally sprinkle with salt and pepper. Place half a lemon in the cavity. Stuff the bird at the neck end with one of the stuffings.

3. Stuffing recipes are shown below. Place the bird in the oven for one hour. During this time, baste the chicken with the juice that escapes from the bird.

4. After one hour in the oven, remove the chicken and place the bacon on it. Place the sausages around the bird. You can also put the potatoes, which will be roasted, in the pan; see below. Coat the carrots with olive oil to stop them drying out.

5. Cook the chicken for a further 50 minutes turning the sausages and carrots periodically to ensure even cooking.

6. To test the chicken is fully cooked, insert a sharp knife into the leg of the chicken and the juices should run clear.

7. Remove the chicken from the oven, cover with foil, and allow the bird to rest before carving. This gives you time to make the gravy!

Bread Sauce

Serves 6

Bread sauce can be made several weeks in advance and frozen. You will need a dish that is freezer and oven-proof. Butter the dish well, pour the finished bread sauce into it, put dabs of butter over the surface, cover, and freeze. When needed, thaw and reheat to serve. The amount of cloves is of personal preference. It must be made from a good unsliced loaf, or it will be gluey.

Ingredients

1 large onion, stuck with cloves

850 ml (1½ pints) milk

250 g (8 oz) of stale breadcrumbs, vary the quantity depending on how thick you want the sauce

50 g (2 oz) butter

Salt and freshly ground black pepper

Method

1. Put the clove-stuck onion in the milk in a saucepan and cook on low heat for 20 minutes to infuse the milk with the onion and cloves' flavour.
2. Remove from the heat, cover and leave for 2 hours.
3. Stir in the breadcrumbs; cook gently for a few minutes, then stir in the butter and seasoning.
4. When the butter has thoroughly melted, remove the onion and pour the bread sauce into a buttered serving dish.
5. Cool thoroughly, cover and freeze.

Carrots

1. Carrots are peeled and diced; place in hot, salted water with a little sugar added to the water, bring back to the boil, turn down the heat, and simmer for 8 minutes.

Chestnut Stuffing

Enough stuffing for a turkey for 8 people /half this amount for a chicken

Ingredients

200 g smoked streaky bacon, rind removed and chopped

40 g butter

Turkey liver chopped (optional)

1 onion chopped

1 stick of celery

500 g chestnuts vacuum packed or canned, chopped

50 g fresh bread crumbs

2 tsp grated lemon rind

Salt

Freshly ground pepper

Juice of 2 lemons

Method

1. Cook the bacon gently until all the fat runs out. Add the butter and fry the liver, onion and celery until slightly coloured.

2. Stir in the chopped chestnuts or puree into the pan. Add the breadcrumbs, lemon juice, and rind and mix well. Season to taste with salt and pepper.

Cranberry and Orange Relish

Serves 8

Ingredients

600 g fresh cranberries

The rind and juice of one orange

4 cm piece of cinnamon stick

4 cloves (wrapped in muslin)

1 heaped tsp of freshly grated root ginger or ½ tsp of ground ginger

100 g castor sugar

2-3 Tbsp of port

Method

1. Pulse the cranberries in a food processor for 3 seconds.

2. Grate the rind and squeeze the juice from the orange.

3. Place the cranberries, rind, juice, ginger, sugar and spices in a pan. Bring it to a boil, turn down the heat and let it simmer gently for 10 minutes with the pan lid on.

4. Then, remove the pan from the heat. When it is cold, stir in the port and pour into a serving dish. Cover with cling film and keep in the fridge until needed. Don't forget to remove the cloves and cinnamon before serving.

Gravy

Makes 1 litre

Ingredients

1 Tbsp flour
Chicken or vegetable stock

Method

1. After taking the cooked chicken out of the oven, remove it from the pan, place it on a dish, cover it, and keep it in a warm place to allow it to rest.

2. Tip the pan in which the chicken was cooked to one side. This will enable you to spoon off the excess fat into a bowl (it will visibly separate from the meat juices), leaving behind 1-1½ Tbsp of fat.

3. Place the pan over a low heat.

4. Add 1 heaped Tbsp of plain flour to the pan, and mix well with a wooden spoon to blend the fat into the flour until you get a smooth paste, scraping the base and sides of the tin to incorporate any crusty residue.

5. Then gradually whisk in the stock (about 1 and a 1/2 pints of chicken/vegetable stock). Sieve into a clean saucepan, whilst stirring bring to the boil to thicken. Turn down the heat Add some gravy browning if necessary and season to taste.

Get Ahead Gravy

Prepare in advance

Ingredients

2 celery sticks, trimmed and roughly chopped
2 carrots, roughly sliced
2 onions, peeled and quartered
5 fresh bay leaves
5 fresh sage leaves
4 sprigs of fresh rosemary
2 star anise
2 rashers of smoked streaky bacon

8 chicken wings
Olive oil
Sea salt
Freshly ground black pepper
4 Tbsp plain flour
60 ml sherry or port (optional)
2 heaped dessert spoons of cranberry sauce for finishing

Method

1. Preheat the oven to 200°C.

2. Put the vegetables, herbs and star anise into a sturdy-bottomed roasting tray. Scatter the bacon on top. Break the chicken wings open, put them onto a board and bash the bones with a rolling pin, releasing more of their flavour.

3. Put them in the pan, drizzle with olive oil, sprinkle over a few pinches of salt and pepper, then toss everything together and put the tray in the oven to cook for 1 hour, or until the meat is tender and falling off the bones.

4. Take the pan out of the oven, put it on the hob over low heat, and use a potato masher to grind and mash everything. Scrape all the goodness from the pan as you go. The longer you let everything fry, the darker your gravy will be.

5. Gradually mix in the flour to thicken the mixture. When the flour is combined, pour in 2 litres of hot water, turn the heat up, and bring it to a boil for 10 minutes till thickened. Then, turn down the heat and simmer for about 25 minutes, stirring occasionally. If you want to add 60 ml sherry or port for flavour, do that now.

6. When it reaches the consistency you're looking for, check the seasoning and push it through a sieve into a large bowl. Discard anything left behind. Once it has cooled to room temperature, put it into containers or freezer bags and pop them in the freezer.

7. To finish the gravy, remove it from the freezer and defrost it. You can add any essence from the turkey (spoon off the fat first). Bring to a boil over the hob. Add cranberry sauce if you want. Heat the gravy until piping hot, strain through a sieve, and pour into another pan. Skim off any fat. Leave on a low heat until ready to serve.

Lemon and Thyme Stuffing

Ingredients

6 slices white bread

¾ onion

1 lemon

Salt and freshly ground pepper

3 heaped tsp mixed herbs (thyme & oregano)

Method

1. Remove crust from white bread and place in food processor for 1 minute to make bread crumbs

2. Put onion in food processor and pulse for 10 seconds.

3. Juice and grate lemon. Mix all together, add more lemon juice if needed.

Mashed Potatoes

Serves 4

Ingredients

500 g potato peeled weight and cut into cubes
70 g butter
60 ml milk
1 tsp of salt
Freshly ground pepper

Method

1. Put the potatoes in a large pan, cover with cold water, add salt, and bring to a boil. Turn down to medium heat and cook until tender, about 15-20 minutes. Drain and replace into the pan, leaving the lid on for 2 minutes.

2. Put the potato through a potato ricer or use a masher. Add the butter and milk, mix well, and season with salt and pepper.

Roast Potatoes

Ingredients

1 large potato for each person
4 Tbsp duck fat
4 Tbsp vegetable oil

Using floury potatoes such as King Edwards, Desiree, or Maris Piper is essential.

Method

1. Cut each potato into 2 or 3 pieces, place in cold salted water, bring to a boil, turn down the heat, and simmer for about 6 minutes or until soft around the edges. Drain the potatoes, replace them back in the pan, cover with a lid, and let them steam for a few minutes to dry.

2. To ensure the edges are fluffy, toss them in the pan with the lid on to roughen them up slightly.

3. It is essential to get the fat smoking hot before adding the potatoes. A mixture of vegetable oil with a high flame point and goose fat, which gives a delicious flavour, will enable you to reach a very high temperature without burning.

4. Do not overcrowd the tin when roasting them. Depending on appetites, allow 2-4 chunks of potato per person.

5. Roast potatoes must be cooked at high temperature (200°C) and turned once or twice until golden.

Sausage Meat Stuffing with Onion & Sage

450 g pork sausage meat

1 medium onion, peeled and finely chopped

1 Tbsp finely chopped parsley

1 tsp dried mixed herbs

12 sage leaves, chopped

50 g fresh breadcrumbs

Salt

Freshly ground black pepper

Method

1. Break up the sausage meat with a fork. Add the other ingredients, salt and pepper to taste, and mix thoroughly. Use half this amount for a small chicken.

Skirlie

Ingredients

4 Tbsp sunflower oil

One small onion

150 g fine oatmeal

Good pinch of salt

Method

1. Finely chop a small onion.

2. Heat 4 Tbsp of sunflower oil in a small frying pan and fry the onions over medium heat until soft and transparent.

3. Add the oatmeal and stir until it soaks up all the oil. Finally add the salt.

For extra flavour, add some of the essence from the cooked chicken.

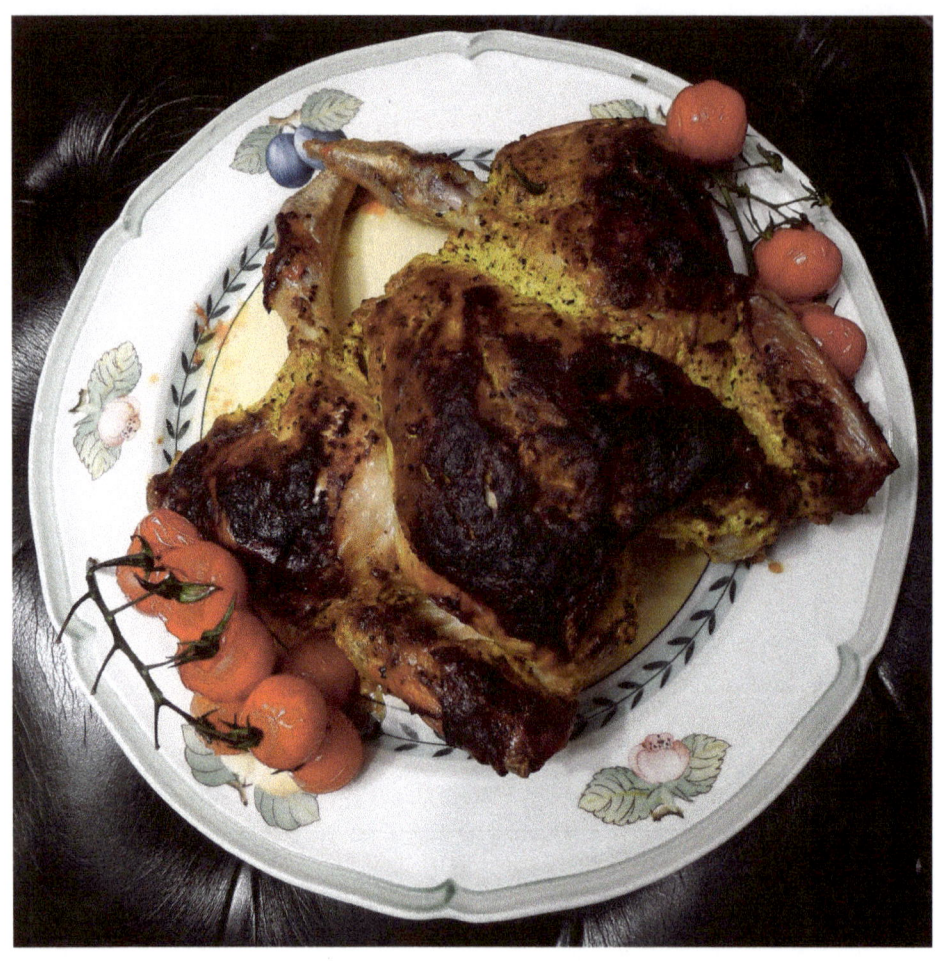

A Flame-Kissed Feast

*A crackling fire, a summer's glow,
A feast of spice, of seeds that sow.
The fennel hums, the lemon sings,
A taste where joy and ember clings.*

*The skin turns crisp, the juices run,
A meal that glows beneath the sun.
With hands that carve, with plates held high,
A dish of warmth beneath the sky.*

—*Inspired by Robert Louis Stevenson*

Spatchcock Chicken

Chicken breasts with Greek yoghurt and Indian Spices

Serves 4

Ingredients

- 1 spatchcocked whole chicken, approx 2 kg, skin on
- Or 4 large chicken breasts, skin on
- 300 g cherry tomatoes
- For the marinade
- 1 tsp fennel seeds
- 1 tsp fenugreek seeds
- 2 tsp black onion seeds
- 1 tsp ground turmeric
- 2 tsp dried oregano
- 2 tsp sesame oil
- 2 tsp garlic, peeled and finely chopped
- 2 Tbsp root ginger, peeled and finely chopped
- 250 ml plain Greek yoghurt, whisked until smooth
- 4 Tbsp lime or lemon juice
- Salt and pepper
- 1 Tbsp water

Method

1. To make the marinade, grind all the seeds for 1 minute in a spice grinder or using a pestle and mortar, then mix with the remaining ingredients. Adding water will loosen the mixture.
2. Spread the marinade all over the chicken and under the skin, then place it on a plate or baking tray, cover it with cling film, and refrigerate it for at least 2 hours or up to 24 hours.
3. When ready to cook, preheat the oven to 200°C
4. Remove the chicken from the fridge and place it in a roasting tin. Cover with foil and bake for 25 minutes. Add the cherry tomatoes to the tin and continue cooking for a further 15 minutes. Remove from the oven, carve the chicken into slices and serve with the tomatoes and some boiled rice or dressed salad.

To spatchcock a chicken, turn the bird's breast side down on a board and use scissors to cut through the flesh and bone along both sides of the backbone at a 5 cm width. Cut from the tail to the head end, completely removing the backbone. Turn the bird back over and press lightly down until the bird is flattened.

If using chicken breasts, cut down on the cooking time.

Chicken

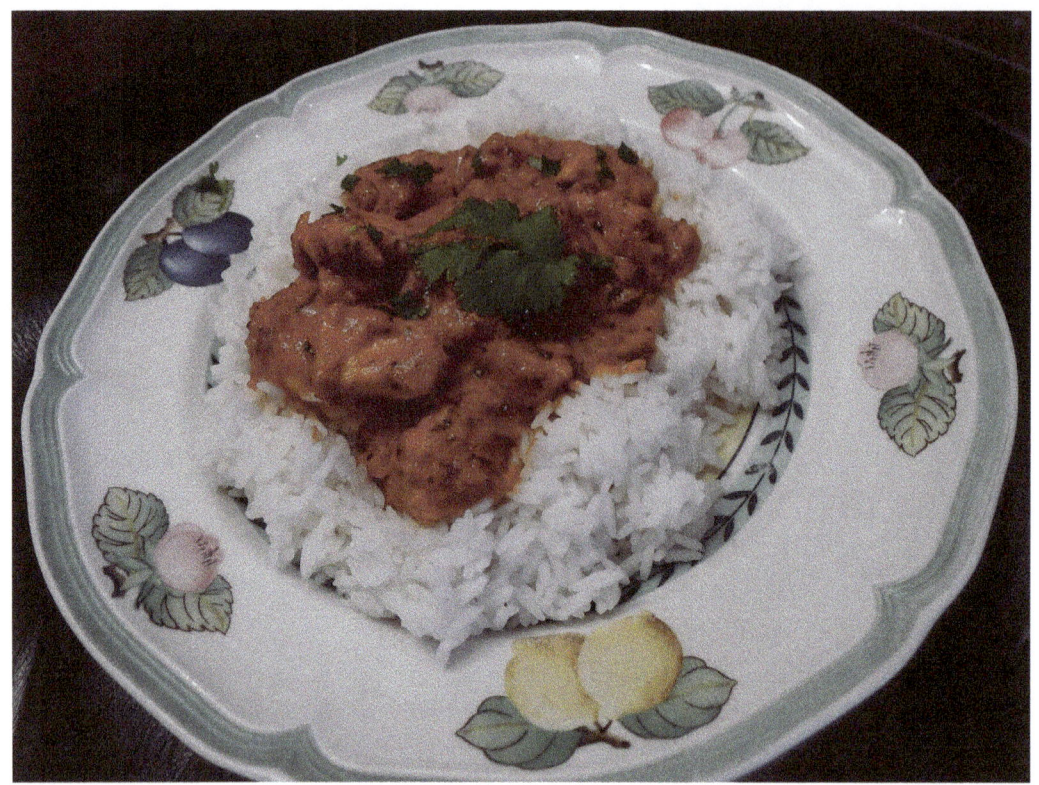

A Balance Bold and Bright

*A dish of spice, yet touched with sweet,
Where tang and warmth in contrast meet.
The mango sways, the chutney glows,
A plate where spice and sugar flows.*

*A balance struck, both rich and wise,
A feast to set the soul to rise.
With rice so light and sauce so deep,
A taste that lingers, bold to keep.*

—Inspired by Contemporary Scottish Poets

Sweet and Sour Balti Chicken

Serves 4

Ingredients

- 3 heaped Tbsp tomato puree
- 250 g Greek yogurt
- 1½ tsp garam masala
- 1 tsp chilli powder
- 2 chopped garlic cloves
- 1 onion, finely sliced
- 2 shallots, finely sliced
- 2 Tbsp mango chutney
- 1 tsp salt
- ½ tsp sugar
- 2 Tbsp sunflower oil
- 675 g chicken breasts, skinned, boned and cubed
- 200 ml water
- 2 Tbsp fresh coriander, chopped (reserve some for decoration)
- 2 Tbsp of single cream (optional)

Method

1. Blend together the tomato puree, yoghurt, garam masala, chilli powder, mango chutney, salt and sugar in a medium mixing bowl
2. Add the chicken breasts and marinate for 2 hours.
3. Heat the oil and gently fry the onions and shallots. Then add the garlic and cook for a further 3 minutes. Pour in the chicken mixture and bring to the boil. Turn down the heat and cook for a further 15 minutes until the chicken is fully cooked. Add the water to thin the sauce slightly as the chicken mixture cooks.
4. Finally, add the fresh coriander and cream, cook for 2 minutes, decorate with a sprinkling of coriander, and serve with plain rice.

Chicken

Flint Family Cookbook

Ham

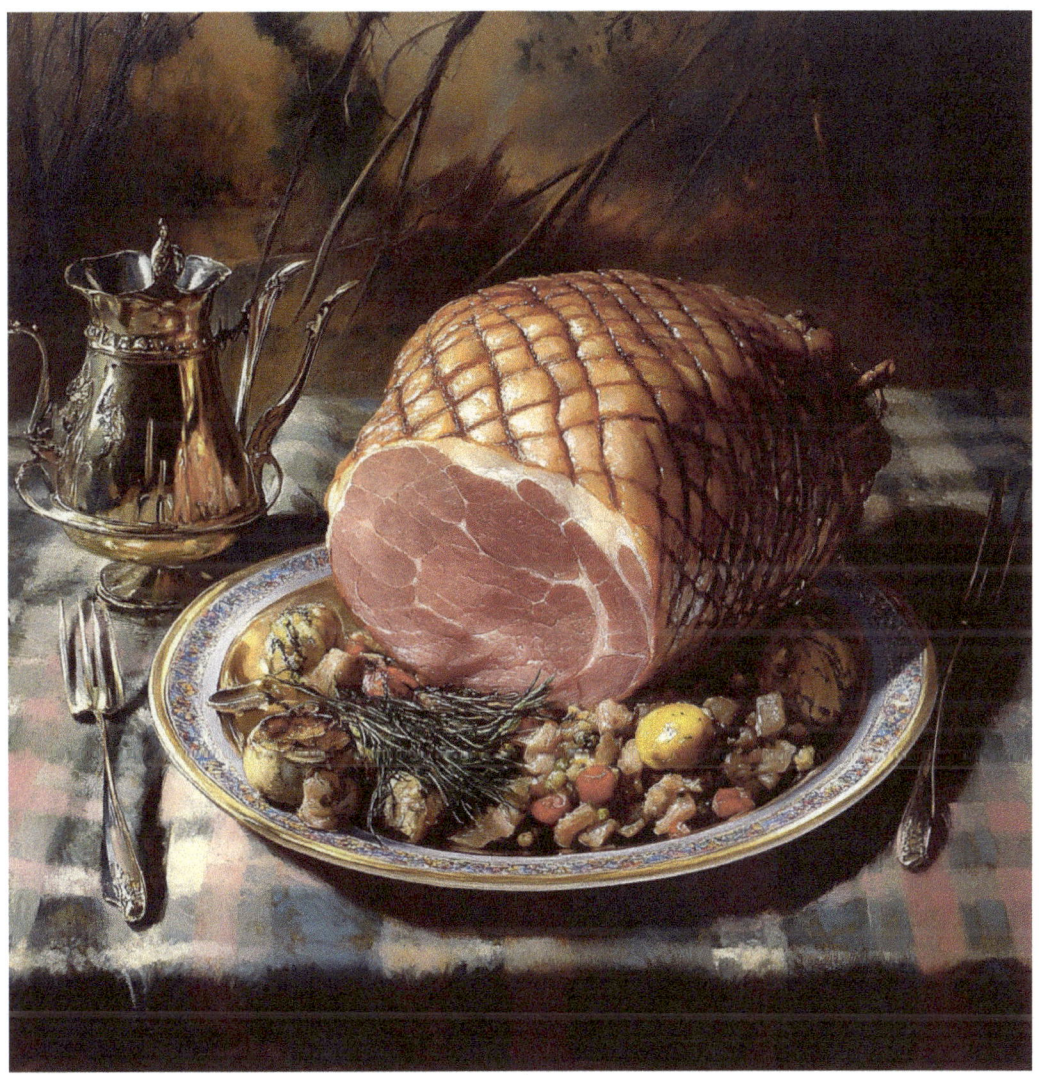

Ham

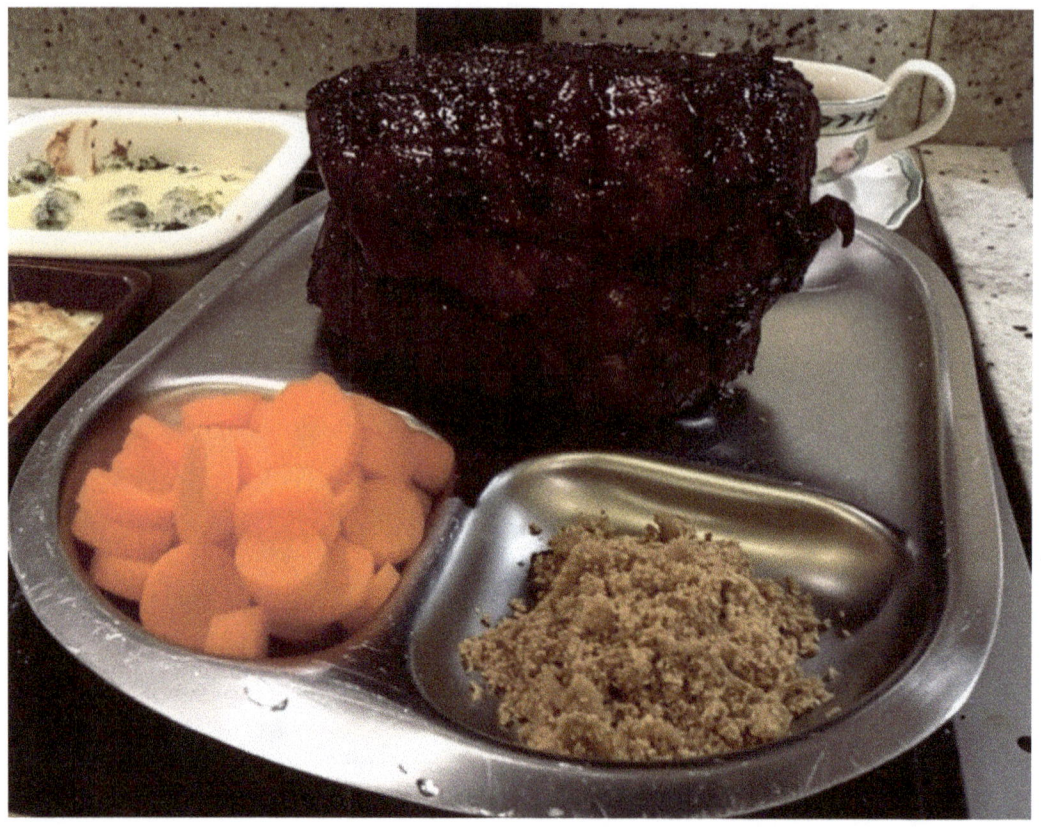

A Feast for the Table

The firelight hums, the table set,
A feast of gold, a joy well met.
The gammon simmers, rich and deep,
A secret stock the pot shall keep.

With honey brushed and treacle bright,
The oven's glow brings pure delight.
A glaze of spice, a touch of cheer,
A meal to mark the festive year.

—Inspired by Robert Burns

Honey Glazed Ham - Boiled and Roasted

Boiled gammon with treacle glaze, finish off by roasting

Serve 10-12

Ingredients

4 kg smoked gammon

4 bay leaves

8 cloves

12 black peppercorns

1 large onion, peeled and cut in half

4 cartons of apple juice concentrate (or 1 large bottle of cider)

100 g Demerara sugar

For the glaze

225 g clear honey or treacle

30 cloves

6 Tbsp Demerara sugar

Method

1. Place the ham in a large saucepan. Add the bay leaves, cloves, black peppercorns, sugar, and all the apple juice. Pour in enough cold water to cover the ham.

2. Bring the water to the boil over medium heat, skimming if necessary. Cover the pan and simmer for about 4 ½ hours. (20 minutes for each 450 g).

3. Remove the ham from the stock. (Reserve the stock to make soup.) Carefully cut away the rind when the ham is cool enough to handle. Score the fat in a diamond pattern.

4. Brush all over the surface of the ham with honey or treacle. Stick the cloves into the fat to make a lattice pattern. Sprinkle the sugar all over the ham.

5. Place the ham into a roasting tin and bake in a preheated oven at 180°C for 20 minutes.

6. Either transfer the ham to a dish to cool, wrap it in foil, and chill it overnight. Remove the ham from the refrigerator and leave it at room temperature for 4-5 hours before serving. Alternatively, serve it hot straight from the oven.

Ham

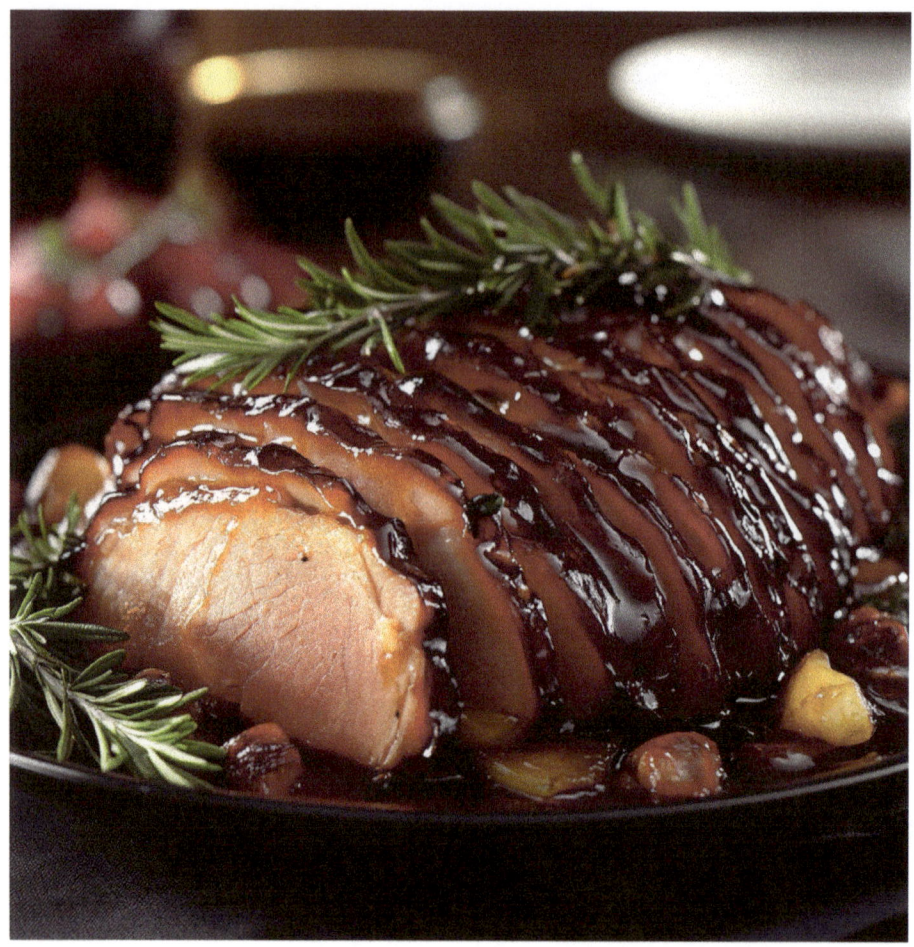

A Patience Well Rewarded

The embers fade, the night grows still,
Yet in the oven, warmth does thrill.
A simmered prize, both bold and sweet,
A scent that calls the hands to meet.

The cloves pressed in, the fat scored neat,
A dish where time and flavour meet.
A waiting hand, a resting grace,
A meal to bring a smile in place.

—*Inspired by John Buchan*

Honey Glazed Ham – Slow Cooked

Slow oven-cooked gammon 12-15 hours

Serves 10-12

Ingredients

4 kg smoked gammon rinds on

75 g black treacle

75 g runny honey

For the glaze

15 ml Tbsp whole cloves

4 15 ml Tbsp black treacle

4 15 ml Tbsp Demerara sugar

15 ml tablespoon Dijon mustard

Or

4 Tbsp runny honey

4 Tbsp English mustard

1 Tbsp whole cloves

Method

1. Preheat the oven to 200°C, and let your gammon come to room temperature.

2. Line a large roasting tin with two pieces of foil overlapping the sides (these will be brought together to wrap around the gammon). Lay one vertically and the other horizontally (shaped in a cross), then sit a wire rack on this foil. Place the gammon on the rack in the middle and pour the black treacle all over it.

3. Wrap the gammon in the foil, trying to create a good seal around the gammon.

4. Put it into the oven for 30 minutes on high, then turn down the heat to 110°C and leave it for 12-15 hours.

5. Remove the gammon from the oven. Turn up the oven to 200°C. Open up the foil. Remove the gammon to another baking dish (Be careful not to burn yourself from the hot liquid.)

6. Remove the skin from the gammon, leaving as much fat as you can. Using a sharp knife, cut a diamond pattern in the fat layer, drawing the lines one way and then the opposite way about 2 cm apart.

7. Stud the centre of each diamond with a clove. Mix the treacle with the Demerara sugar and the Dijon mustard in a small bowl and spread over the gammon.

8. Pop the gammon back in the hot oven for 20 minutes. Remove from the oven, place the gammon on a flat dish or wooden board, cover with tin foil, and allow to rest before carving.

Flint Family Cookbook

Veal

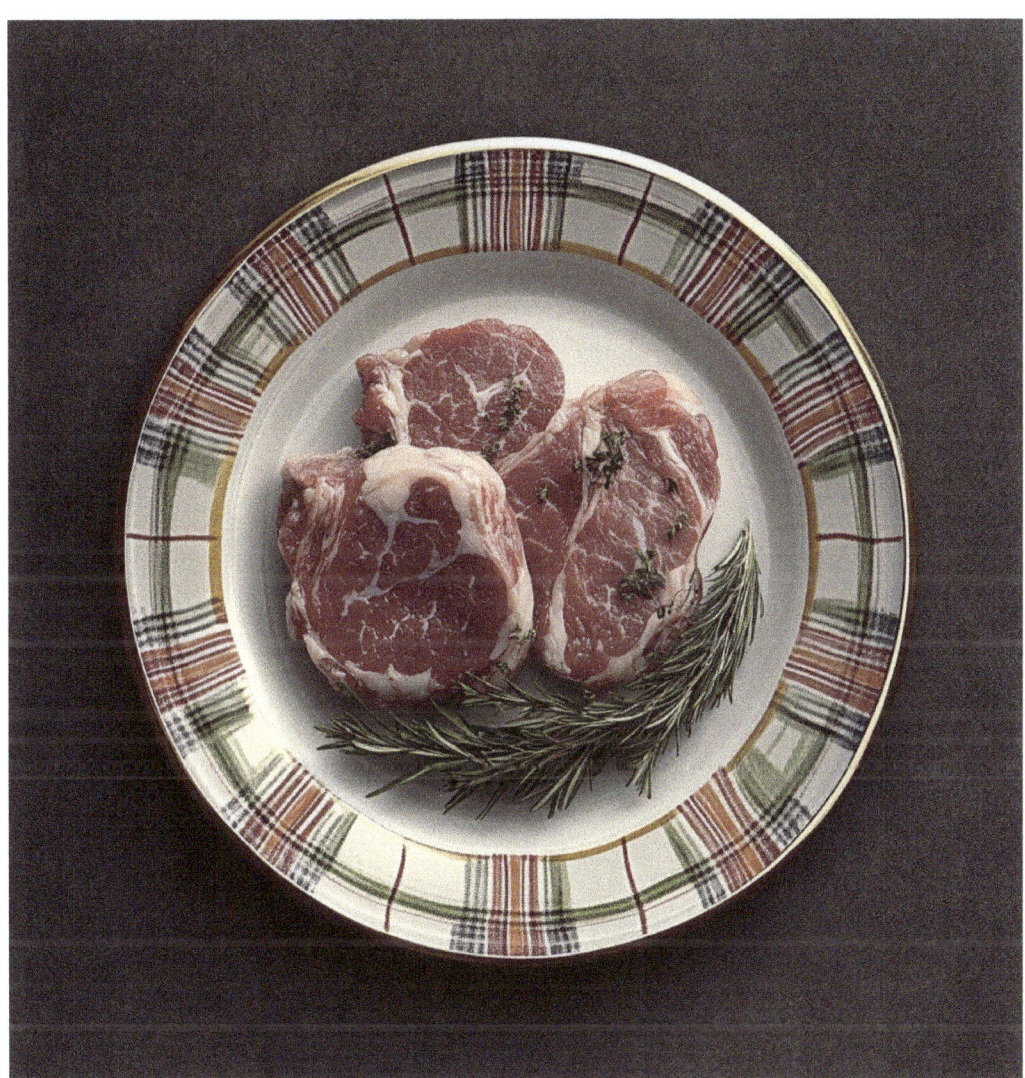

Veal

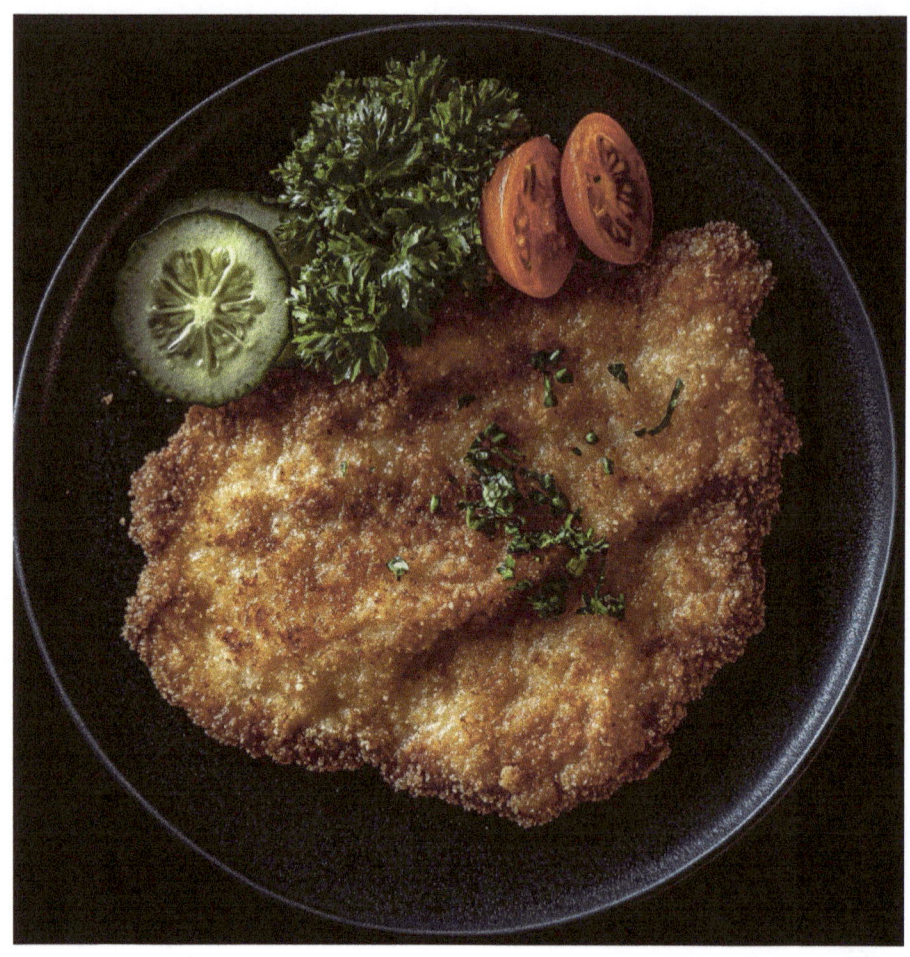

A Crisp and Golden Bite

A golden crust, so light, so fine,
A tender cut, a touch divine.
With butter's kiss and crumbs pressed tight,
A meal that glows in golden light.

A squeeze of lemon, sharp and bright,
A dish to bring the heart delight.
With capers bold and anchovies near,
A taste of warmth, of joy, of cheer.

—Inspired by Robert Louis Stevenson

Wiener Schnitzel

Serves 4

Ingredients

4 veal escalopes weighing about 480 g

Salt and pepper

4 Tbsp plain flour

1 egg, beaten

150 g fresh breadcrumbs

75 g butter

2 Tbsp vegetable oil

8 anchovy fillets, drained and cut in half (optional)

1 egg hard-boiled and the yolk and white chopped separately (optional)

Lemon slices, halved cherry tomatoes, cucumber and parsely to garnish

Method

1. Flatten each escalope thinly between two sheets of damp greaseproof paper.
2. Season the meat, then coat it in plain flour (shake off any excess), beaten egg, and breadcrumbs, pressing the crumbs on well.
3. Heat the butter and oil in a large frying pan. Fry the escalopes, two at a time, for 3-5 minutes on each side until golden. Drain on absorbent kitchen paper and keep warm while cooking the remaining escalopes.
4. Serve with anchovy fillets, chopped egg, lemon slices, cherry tomatoes, cucumber, parsley and chips!

Flint Family Cookbook

Beef

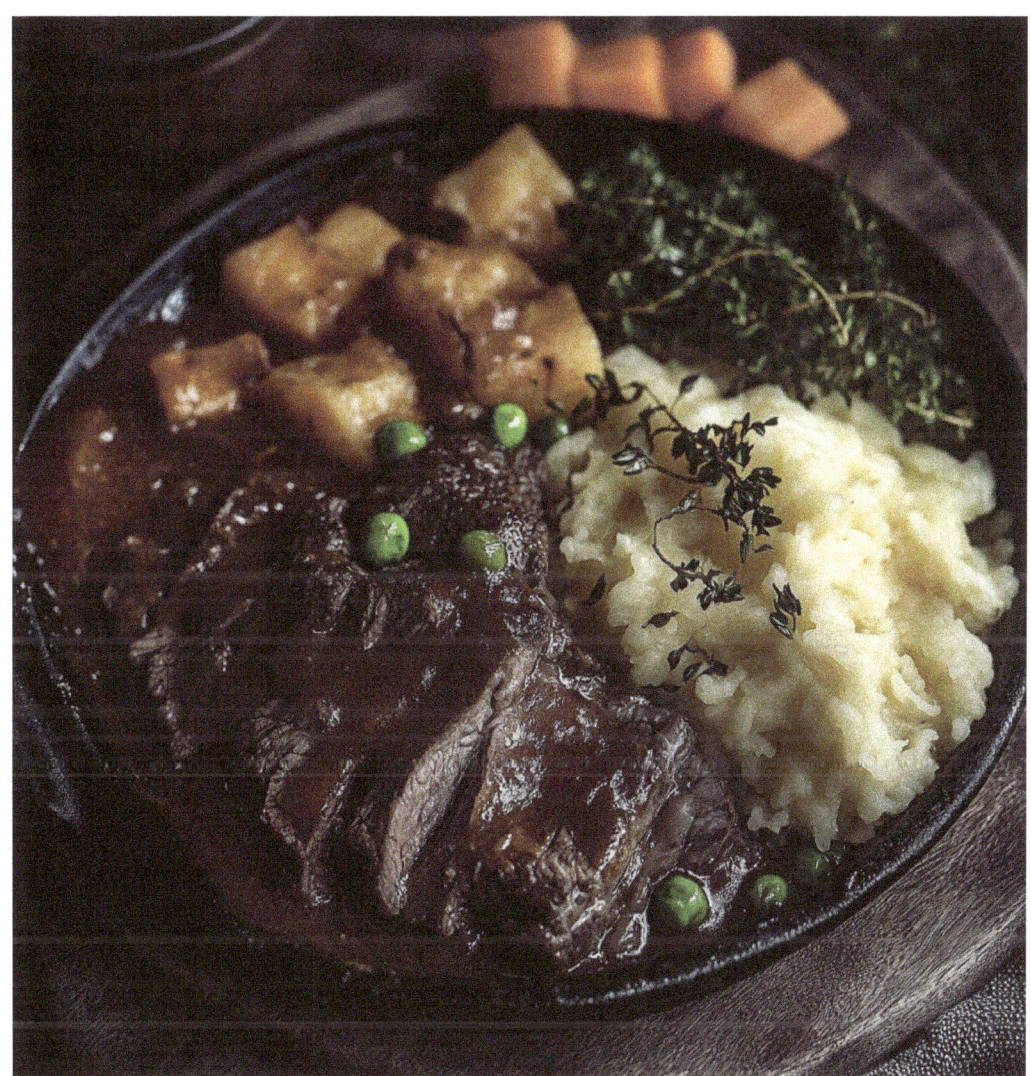

133

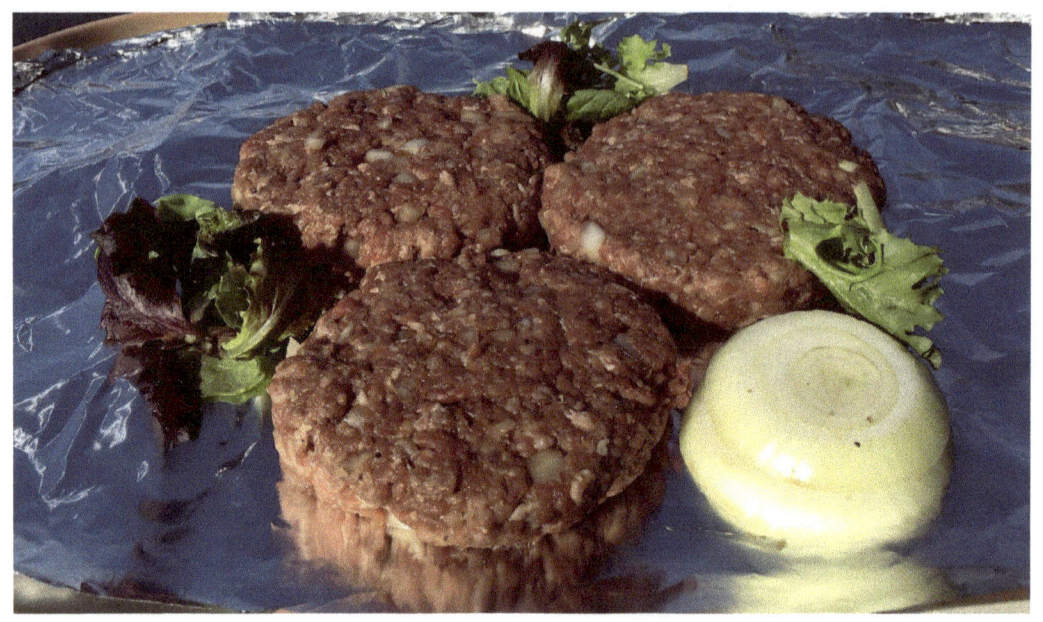

A Feast by the Fire

The grill does roar, the coals burn bright,
A patty pressed, a pure delight.
With onion's bite and nutmeg's grace,
A meal to share in open space.

The bread roll waits, the cheese melts near,
A taste of summer, bold and clear.
With hands held high, the plates are filled,
A feast of fire, a hunger stilled.

—Inspired by Robert Burns

Beef Burgers

Serves 3

Ingredients

450 g 10% fat ground Aberdeen Angus mince

1 small onion finely chopped

1½ Tbsp of soya sauce

1 Tbsp of Lea and Perrins

½ tsp of grated nutmeg

½ tsp of freshly ground pepper

1 tsp of salt

3 large bread rolls

Optional

Sliced raw onion & cheddar cheese 40 g.

Method

1. Chop the mince, place into a bowl with the rest of the ingredients. Give it a good mixing, this is easier by hand.
2. Divide the mixture into three, squeeze together and roll into a ball, place on a flat surface and pat into a round shape about 2 cm thick (it tends to shrink when cooked and is therefore better to be made large in size)
3. Cook on the BBQ for 4 minutes per side.
4. Grate cheddar cheese on top for the last 2 minutes; with a slice of raw onion on top, serve in a roll.
5. Serve with a green salad, cherry tomatoes, coleslaw, and potato salad.

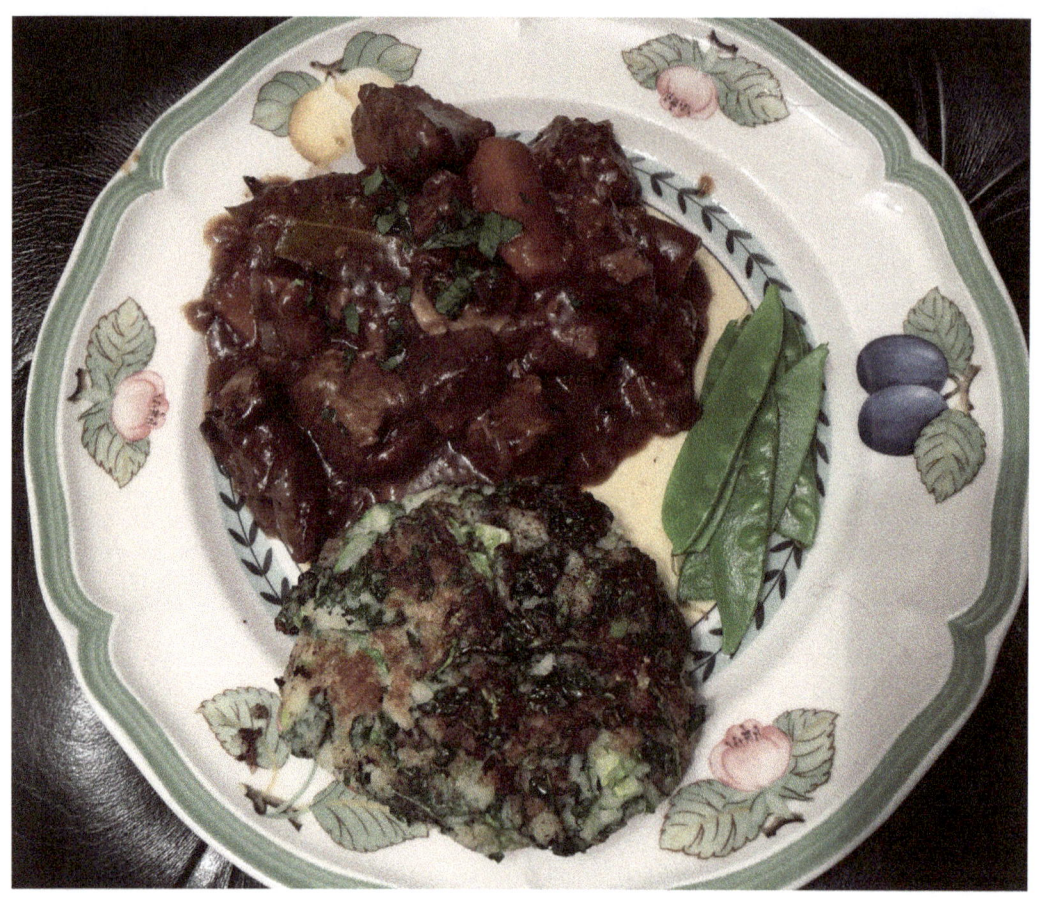

A Slow and Sturdy Brew

A stew of strength, both dark and deep,
Where onions waltz and spices steep.
The ale flows in, the bay leaf sways,
A meal to warm the winter's haze.

The beef grows tender, rich and bold,
A tale of warmth, of hearths of old.
With mash and greens, the plate is laid,
A feast where simple joys are made.

—Inspired by John Buchan

Beef Carbonnade

Serves 4

Ingredients

- 750 g braising steak cut into 4 cm cubes
- 3 Tbsp plain flour
- 1 tsp salt
- Freshly ground black pepper
- 4 Tbsp oil
- 2 large onions, peeled and thinly sliced
- 1-2 garlic cloves, peeled and crushed
- 300 ml brown ale
- 300 ml beef stock°
- 2 Tbsp tomato ketchup or 1 Tbsp tomato puree
- Pinch of ground mace or nutmeg
- 1 bay leaf
- 2 tsp brown sugar
- 2 tsp vinegar
- 1½ tsp French mustard
- 3-4 carrots, peeled and cut into sticks
- 100 g button mushrooms, trimmed and sliced
- Chopped fresh parsley, to garnish (optional)

Method

1. Preheat oven to 160°C
2. Coat the meat with flour seasoned with salt and pepper. Heat 3 Tbsp of the oil in a pan and fry the meat in batches until browned. Transfer to a casserole.
3. Fry the onions and garlic in the same pan with the remaining oil added, until lightly coloured, then stir in the remaining seasoned flour and cook for 1 minute.
4. Gradually add the brown ale and stock and bring to the boil. Add the ketchup, nutmeg, plenty of salt and pepper, bay leaf, sugar, vinegar and mustard and pour over the beef.
5. Add the carrots to the, casserole, mix well, cover tightly and cook in a preheated oven for 1 ¼ hours.
6. Taste and adjust the seasoning, add the mushrooms and return to the oven for 25-30 minutes until quite tender. Discard the bay leaf and serve sprinkled with chopped parsley.
7. Serve with mashed potatoes and mange tout.

Beef

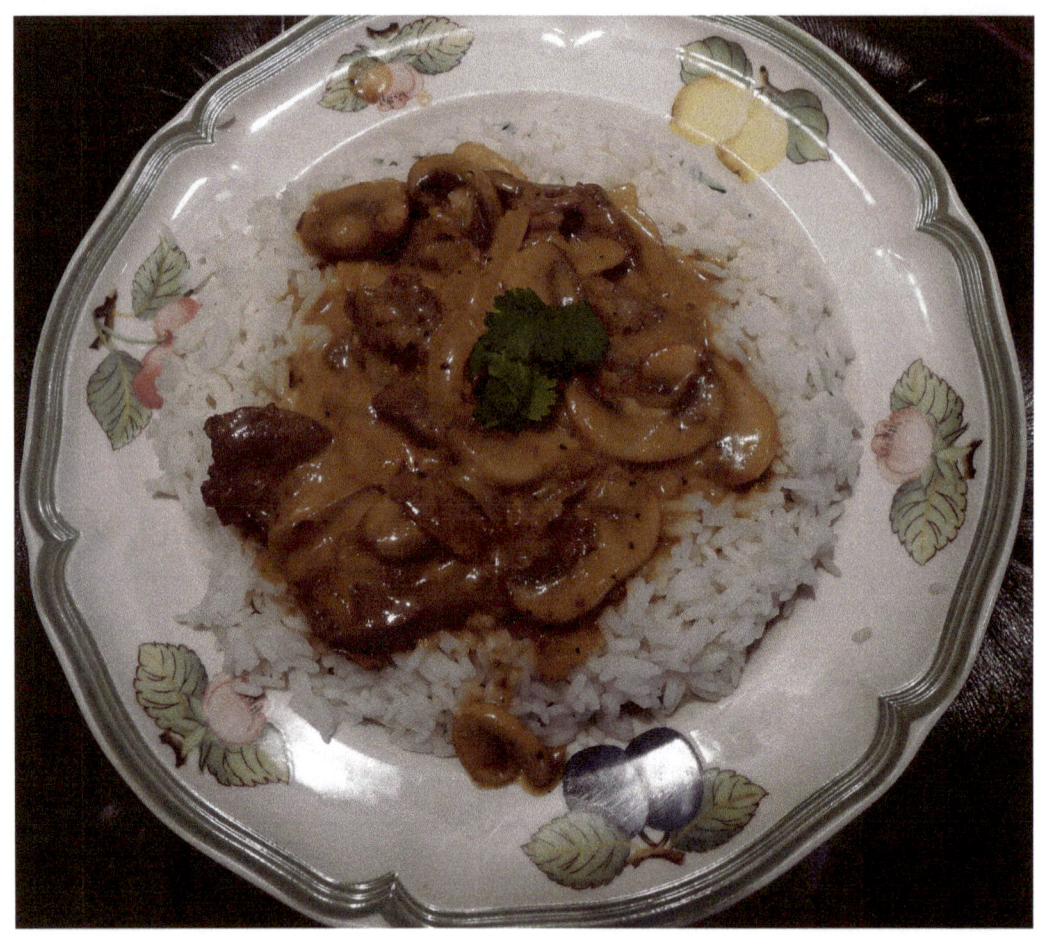

A Dance of Cream and Fire

A flick of flame, a pan's embrace,
The fillet turns with nimble grace.
The brandy leaps, the mushrooms glow,
A dish where velvet flavours flow.

A swirl of cream, a final cheer,
A meal to bring the heart sincere.
With rice or bread, so light, so free,
A taste of joy in luxury.

—*Inspired by Robert Louis Stevenson*

Beef Stroganoff

Serves 4

Ingredients

1½ lb fillet steak

2 medium onions

225 g mushrooms

2 Tbsp of butter

300 ml beef stock

Salt

Spicy pepper

1 Tbsp of plain flour

1 tsp English mustard

¼ pt sour cream

Parsley

Olive oil

1 Tbsp of brandy

Method

1. Cut the meat into thin strips 1" long and ¼" thick and leave them sprinkled with salt, pepper and a little olive oil for 30 minutes.

2. Peel and sliced the onions, and mushroom, fry the onions in the butter until soft, then add the mushrooms, fry together for 5 minutes, stirring frequently.

3. Add the flour cook for a further minute .Now add the mustard and beef stock, bring to the boil. Turn down the heat immediately.

4. In another frying pan fry the meat in a little butter, until brown on the outside and pink in the middle. Add to the onions and mushrooms. Heat the brandy in a ladle. Light it and pour over the meat. Stir in the sour cream.

5. Taste, adjust the seasoning, and reheat.

6. Serve with rice, garlic bread and a green vegetable decorate with parsley.

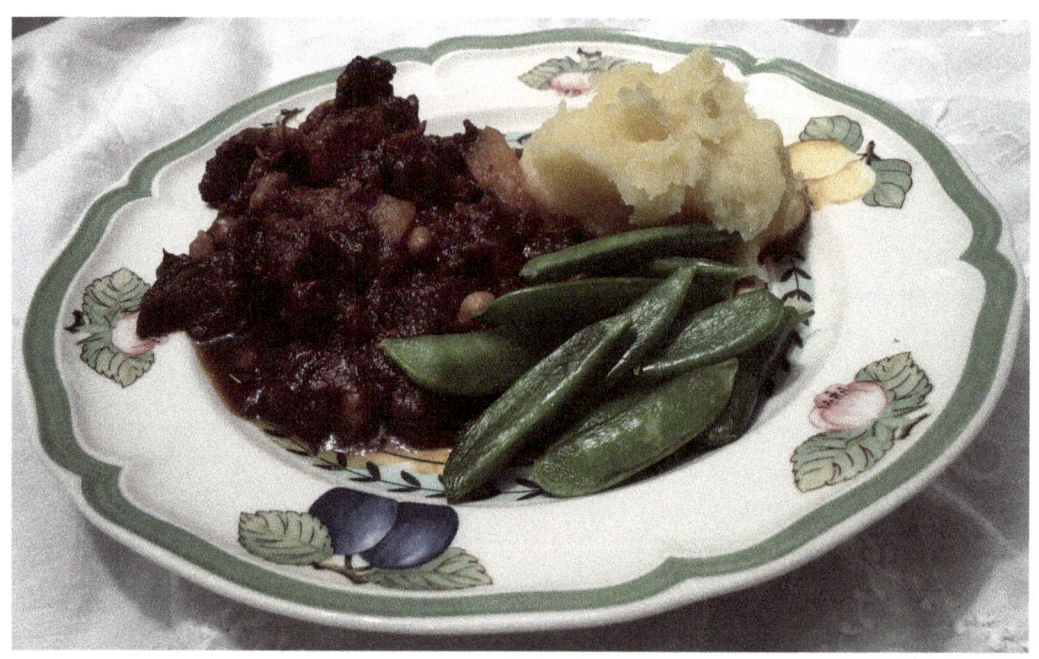

A Song of Spice and Slow Delight

The cumin hums, the saffron sighs,
A dish where desert fragrance lies.
With honey kissed and prunes so deep,
A tale of heat, of time, of sleep.

The beef drinks slow the seasoned air,
A meal both bold and rich with care.
With couscous bright and herbs anew,
A feast of lands both old and true.

—*Inspired by Sir Walter Scott*

Beef Tagine

Serves 6

Ingredients

- 800 g braising steak
- 4 Tbsp sunflower oil
- 2 onions, halved and sliced
- 2 garlic, finely chopped
- 2 tsp ground cumin
- 2 tsp ground coriander
- 1 tsp paprika
- 1 tsp turmeric
- 1 tsp hot chilli powder
- 400 g can chopped tomatoes
- 400 g can chickpeas, drained and rinsed
- 3 Tbsp clear honey
- 1 beef stock cube
- 1 cinnamon stick
- 1 medium sweet potato (around 400 g)
- 25 g bunch fresh coriander
- 250 g no-soak dried soft prunes, chopped
- Flaked sea salt and freshly ground black pepper

Method

1. Trim the beef of any hard fat and cut into roughly 3 cm chunks. Season the meat all over with salt and pepper. Heat one Tbsp of oil in a large in a large frying pan and fry the beef in three/four batches over a high heat until lightly browned on all sides, adding a little more oil to the pan when needed. Transfer each batch to a large casserole/tagine dish once browned.

2. Reduce the heat and add two Tbsp of oil to the frying pan. Fry the onions for five minutes, or until softened and lightly coloured, stirring regularly.

3. Add the garlic and sprinkle with the cumin, coriander, paprika, turmeric and chilli powder cook for 2 minutes, stirring constantly.

4. 5.Stir 250 ml cold water into frying pan and stir vigorously to lift the sediments from the bottom. Tip the onions and spices into the tagine dish.

5. Pour in the tomatoes, chickpeas, prunes and stock cube into the frying pan, bring to the boil, turn down the heat, and then add the honey and cinnamon stick giving a good stir.

6. Pour into the meat and onions. Cover and cook gently for 2 hours. Stir the beef tagine from time to time.

7. Peel the sweet potato and cut into small chunks add to the tagine and continue to cook for 40 minutes, until the beef is tender. Add the chopped coriander reserving some for decoration.

8. Serve with couscous or mashed potato. Sprinkle the remaining coriander over the beef before serving.

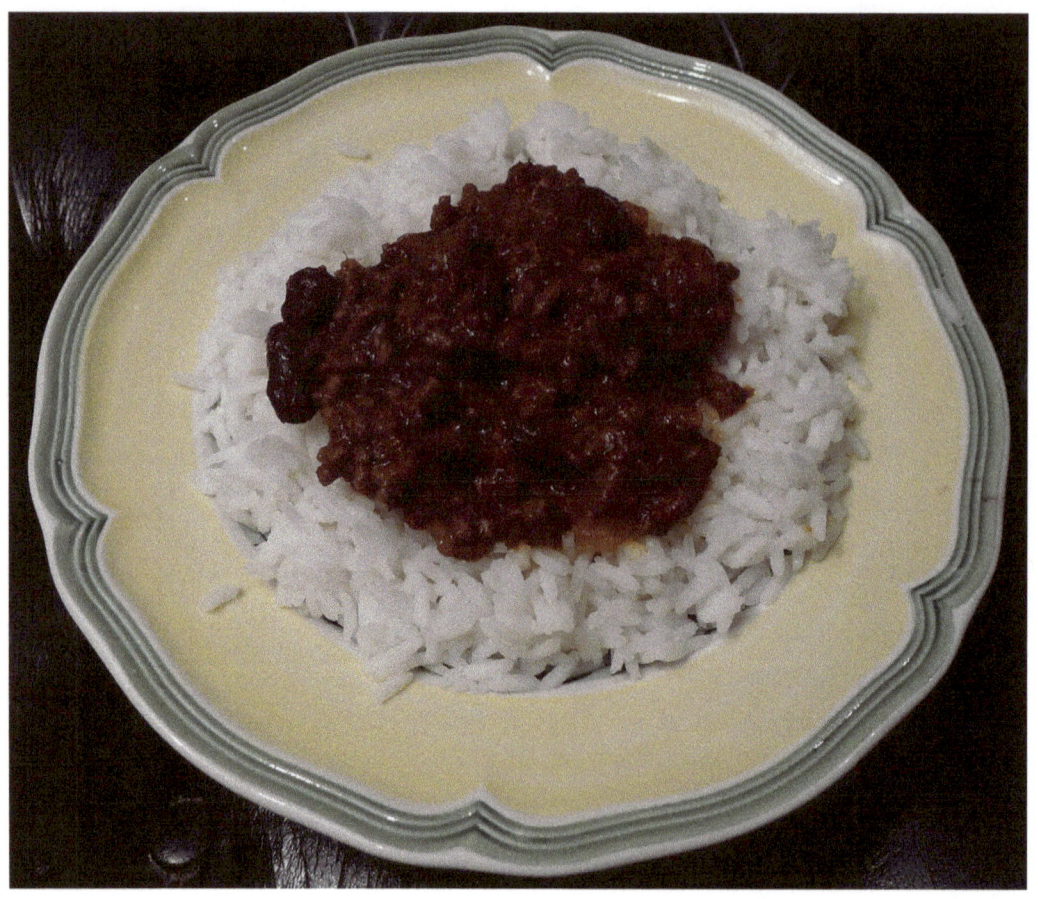

A Flame That Sings

A spark of spice, a simmered glow,
A pot where heat and passion flow.
With cumin bold and peppers bright,
A taste that lingers through the night.

The beans join in, the wine runs deep,
A meal where warmth and fire keep.
With rice beside and bread so fine,
A feast that calls for one more time.

—*Inspired by Contemporary Scottish Poets*

Chilli Con Carne

Serves 6-8

Ingredients

1 kg minced lean beef
2 onions, finely chopped
3-4 cloves of garlic, chopped
2-3 level Tbsp of bacon fat, or sunflower oil
2 425 g tin of Italian chopped tomatoes
300 ml of red wine
½ tsp of chilli powder
1½ heaped Tbsp of plain flour
2 bay leaves
1 tsp of powdered cumin
1 level Tbsp of oregano
4 Tbsp of tomato puree
1 Tbsp of mango chutney
Salt and freshly ground pepper
2 432 g tin of red organic kidney beans
¼ pt water

Method

1. Fry the chopped onions gently in the bacon fat until translucent/golden.
2. Add the garlic and fry for a few minutes.
3. Add the minced beef and fry until completely brown.
4. Add the Italian canned tomatoes water and red wine, bring to the boil. Skim off any residue, cover casserole and simmer very gently for one hour.
5. Blend the chilli powder and flour in a little of the hot pan juices and add to the casserole. At the same time add crumbled bay leaves, cumin, oregano, mango chutney, tomato puree and salt and pepper, to taste. Check seasoning.
6. Add canned red kidney beans and gently heat for a further 30 minutes.
7. Serve with boiled rice, garlic bread and salad.

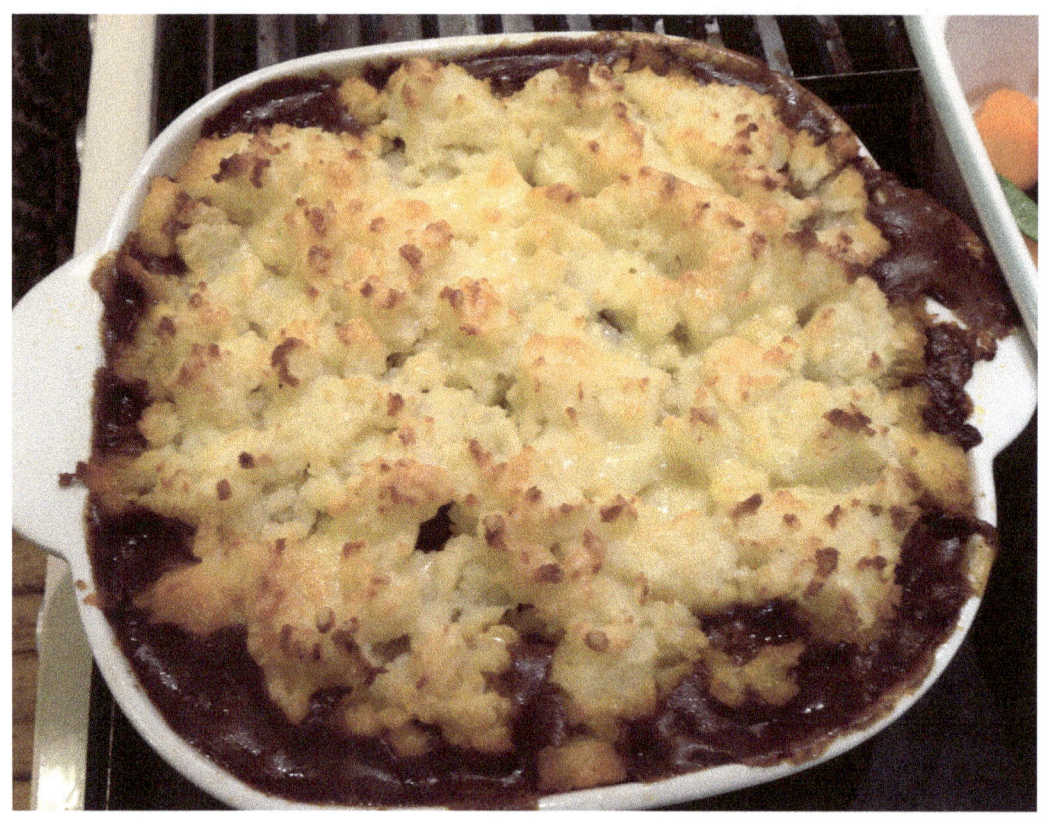

A Hearth's Embrace

A layer rich, a crust so gold,
A tale of warmth from days of old.
The mince stews deep, the flavours blend,
A dish where love and time suspend.

With mash atop and herbs so bright,
It calls us home through fading light.
A bite, a pause, a sigh so free,
A taste of care, of memory.

—*Inspired by Robert Burns*

Cottage Pie

Serves 4-5 generous portions!

Ingredients

800 g potatoes cut into 2 cm cubes

2 Tbsp sunflower

75 ml milk

50 g butter

495 g can of a good oxtail soup

150 ml red wine

1 Knorr beef stock cube

50 g plain flour

600 g of lean mince beef

2 onions, chopped

2 Tbsp fresh or dried thyme

2 Tbsp Worcestershire sauce

2 tsp marjoram

2 Tbsp tomatoes puree

3 Tbsp chopped parsley

Method

1. Steam the potatoes until soft, mash until there are no lumps; add the butter and milk, put to one side.

2. Fry the chopped onions until transparent in the sunflower oil.

3. Add the mince and fry until brown. Add the flour and cook for two minutes.

4. Then add all the rest of the ingredients, season to taste. Bring to the boil, stirring until thickened, check the seasoning. Cover with a lid and simmer gently for 45 minutes until the mince is tender, check the seasoning.

5. Tip the cooked meat into a 3 .5 pt shallow ovenproof dish. Arrange the potato on top of the mince, sprinkle over the cheese if using. Bake in the oven 195°C for 30 minutes until golden brown and bubbling. Serve with cooked carrots and peas.

If the cottage pie is still not tasty enough put another Knorr beef stock cube into the meat mixture.

Beef

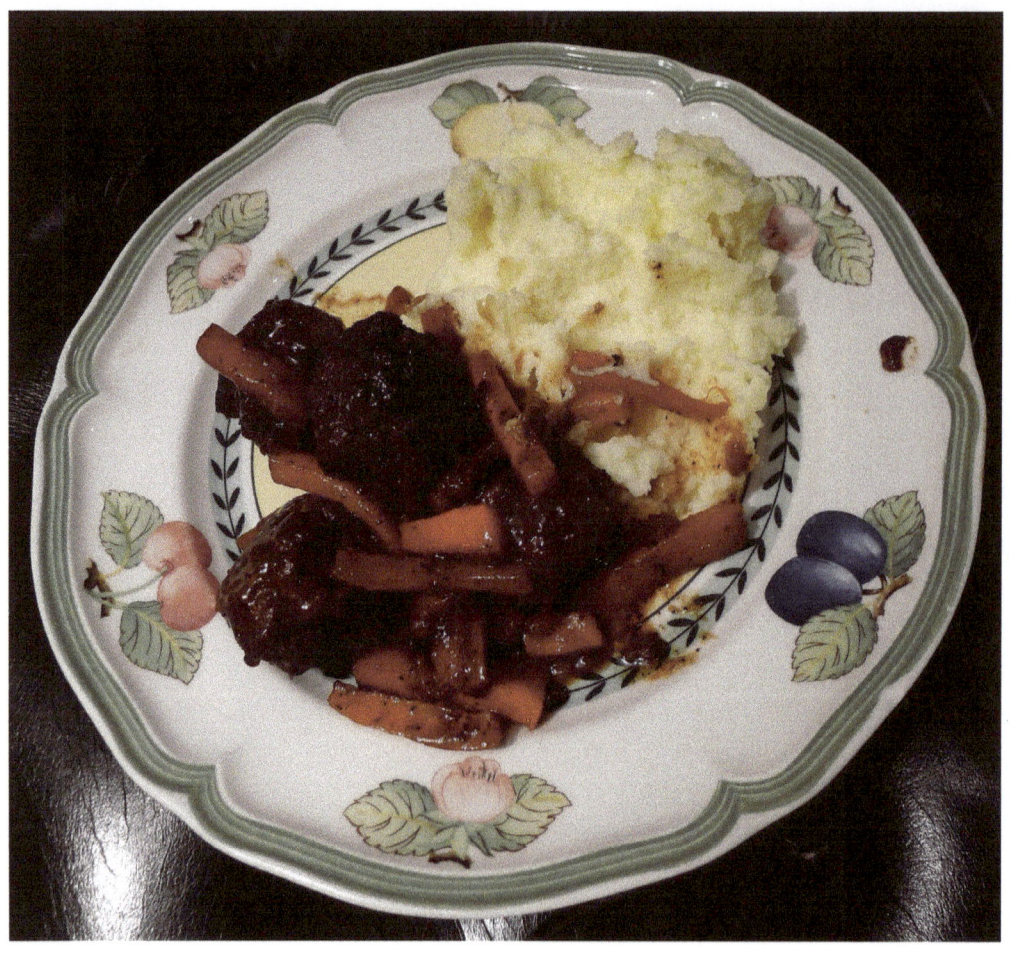

A Bold and Tangy Bite

*The meatballs roll in sauce so fine,
With apple's kiss and mustard's shine.
A tang of spice, a playful cheer,
A taste that lingers, bold and clear.*

*The chutney hums, the Worcestershire sings,
A meal that heat and sweetness brings.
With watercress or mash beside,
A plate where daring flavours bide.*

—*Inspired by Robert Louis Stevenson*

Devilled Meatballs

Serves 4

Ingredients

600 g raw lean mince beef
50 g fresh bread crumbs
1 small onion peeled and finely chopped
1 tsp salt
½ tsp freshly ground black pepper
1 Tbsp Worcestershire sauce
2 Tbsp sunflower oil
225 g carrots, peeled and cut into thin sticks
1 large cooking apple, peeled, cored and diced

For the sauce

1 Tbsp plain flour
1½ tsp English mustard powder
1½ tsp Dijon mustard
1 Tbsp soy sauce
1 Tbsp Worcestershire sauce
1 Tbsp mango chutney
300 ml beef stock
Watercress or parsley to decorate

Method

1. Mix the minced beef thoroughly with the bread crumbs, onion, salt, and pepper and Worcestershire sauce. Divide into 16 and shape into balls

2. Heat the oil in a pan and fry the meat balls gently until browned. Remove from the pan and pour off all but 1 Tbsp of the fat.

3. To make the sauce, stir the flour and dry mustard into the residue in the pan followed by the Dijon mustard, soy sauce, Worcestershire sauce, chutney and stock. Bring to the boil and add plenty of salt and pepper.

4. Lay the carrots and apples in a casserole and arrange the meatballs on top. Pour the sauce over and cover the casserole .Cook in a preheated oven for about 45 minutes.

5. Uncover the casserole, remove any fat from the surface and stir lightly. Garnish with watercress or parsley. Serve with spaghetti or mashed potato.

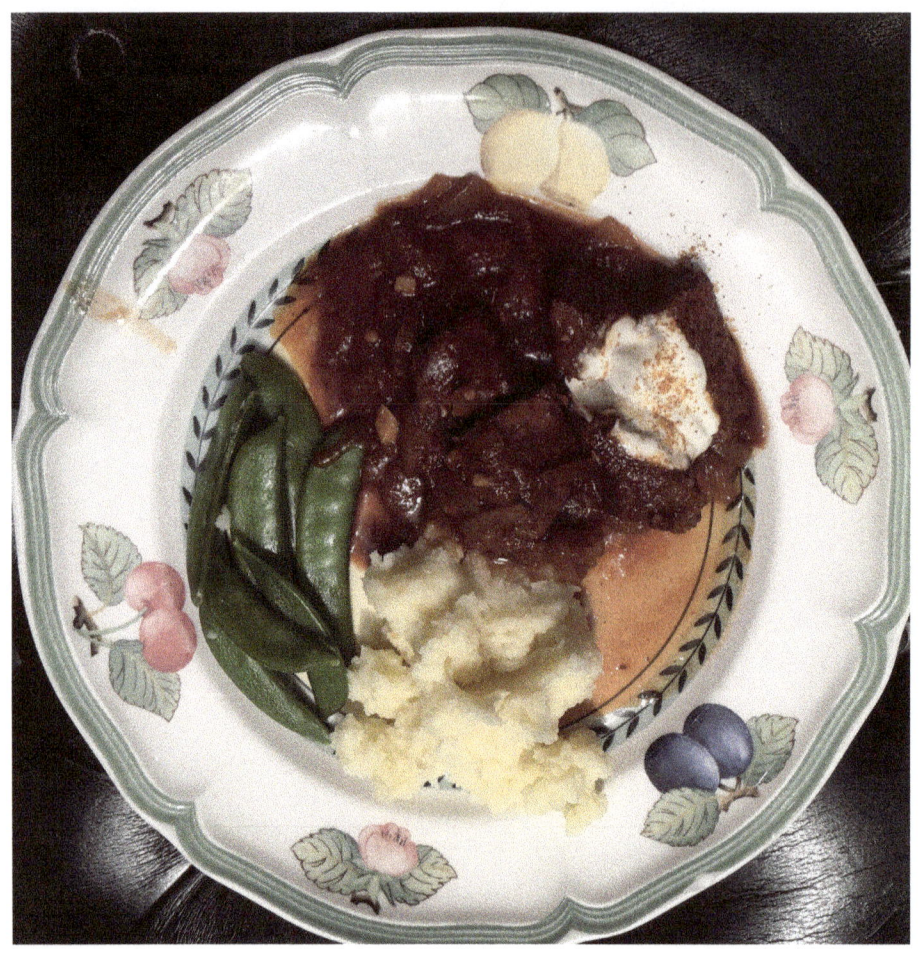

A Stew of Strength

Through spice and smoke, the broth runs deep,
A simmered tale, a dream to keep.
The paprika burns, the onions sigh,
A dish where winter nights pass by.

The beef is rich, the peppers bright,
A meal that brings both strength and light.
With sour cream's swirl and bread so wide,
A taste where comfort does abide.

—*Inspired by Sir Walter Scott*

Goulash

A recipe given to me by our good Swedish friend Attila

Serves 4

Ingredients

750 g braising steak, cut into cubes

4 Tbsp oil

650 g onions, thinly sliced

2 cloves of garlic chopped

2 Tbsp flour mixed with a little stock

800 ml beef stock

Salt and freshly ground pepper

1 tsp marjoram

1 tsp cumin

1 tsp caraway seeds

1 tsp cayenne pepper plus extra for garnish

1 tsp sugar

2 Tbsp sweet paprika powder

2 green peppers, thinly sliced (optional)

5 cherry tomatoes, halved or 1 tin plum tomatoes, quartered

4 Tbsp tomato puree

175 ml red wine

100 ml sour cream for decoration

Method

1. Heat the oil and sear the meat in batches, put to one side.

2. Fry the onions and peppers in the remaining oil in the casserole dish for 5 minutes, add the chopped garlic, add all the herbs and spices and cook for a few minutes. Add the flour cook for a couple of minutes. Turn up the heat add all the tomatoes, stock and red wine, bring to the boil.

3. Cook for 1½ hours until tender in the oven at 160°C

4. Serve with mashed potatoes, and mange tout. Decorate with sour cream and cayenne pepper. Best reheated the following day.

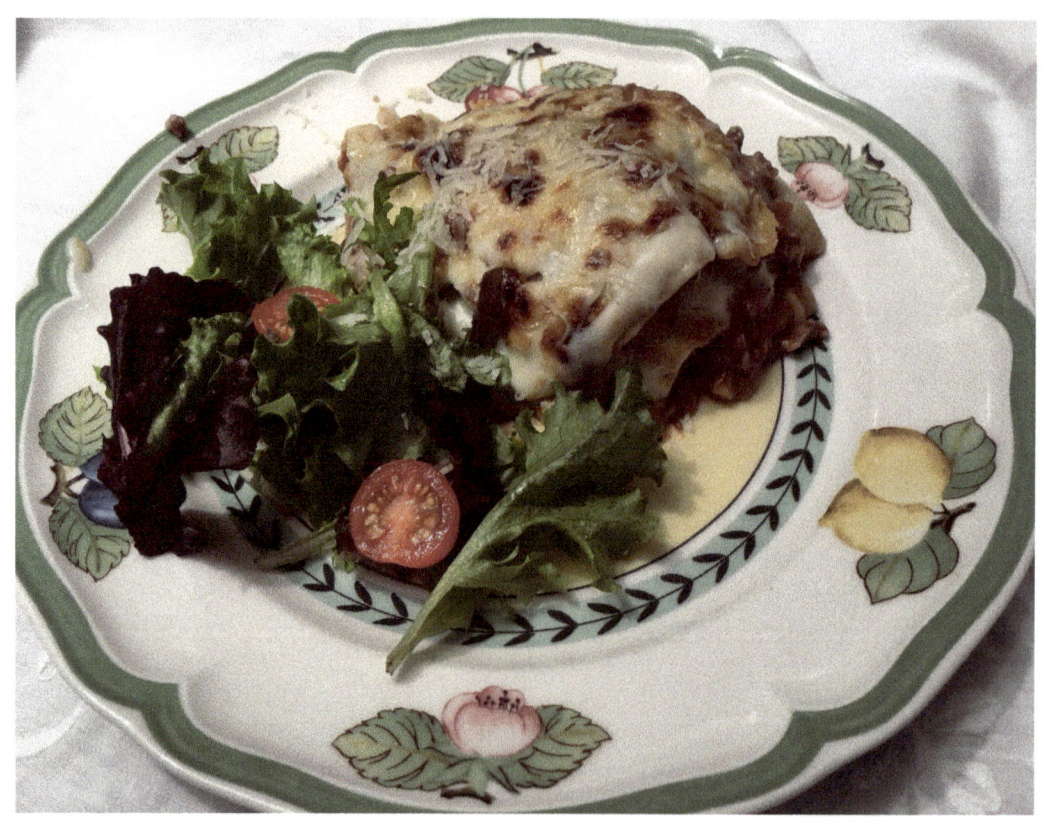

A Layered Delight

A tale of layers, rich and slow,
Where sauce and cheese in rhythm flow.
The pasta sways, the herbs do sing,
A dish where time and love do cling.

The oven glows, the edges brown,
A feast where hands set plates down.
With salad crisp and bread so near,
A meal to share in love sincere.

—*Inspired by Robert Louis Stevenson*

Lasagne

Serves 8

Ingredients

- 3 Tbsp of olive oil
- 4 celery sticks, finely chopped
- 2 onion, finely chopped
- 100 g finely chopped carrots
- 3 garlic cloves, crushed
- 140 g pack of pancetta (smoked sliced bacon cut up finely)
- 500 g beef mince (10% fat)
- 500 g pack pork mince or British veal mince
- 200 ml milk
- 2 tins chopped tomatoes
- 2 bay leaves
- 1 sprig of rosemary
- 2 thyme sprigs
- 2 tsp dried oregano
- 2 beef stock cubes
- 500 ml red wine
- 200 g dried pasta sheets, 10-12 sheets
- 70 g parmesan, finely grated
- 2 tsp sugar
- 4 Tbsp flour
- 3 heaped Tbsp tomato puree
- 1 tsp nutmeg

For the Béchamel sauce

- 2 L milk
- 1 onion, thickly sliced
- 3 bay leaves
- 3 cloves
- 150 g butter
- 150 g plain flour
- 1 tsp nutmeg

Method

This dish is best prepared the night before. Make up the white sauce and mince sauce, leave in 2 separate covered containers. This allows the sauce to become cold and they are easier to assemble in the morning, leave in the fridge during the day and remove 1 hour before cooking in the evening.

1. Grease a 3.5 litre dish.

2. First infuse the milk for the béchamel sauce. Put the milk, onion, bay and cloves into a large saucepan and bring very gently just up to the boil. Turn off the heat and set aside for 1 hour to infuse.

3. For the meat sauce, put the oil, celery, onion, carrot and garlic and pancetta in another large saucepan. Cook gently together until the vegetables are soft but not coloured.

4. Tip in all the mince, the milk and the tomatoes. Using a wooden spoon stir together and break up and mash the lumps of mince against the sides of the pan.

5. When the mince is mainly broken down, stir in all the herbs, the stock cubes and wine, and bring to a simmer. Cover and cook for 40 minutes, stirring occasionally to stop the bottom catching until the meat is tender. Taste and season with salt and pepper, add the nutmeg.

6. To finish the béchamel sauce, strain the milk through a fine sieve into one or two jugs.

7. Melt the butter in the same pan then, using a wooden spoon, mix in the flour and cook for two minutes. Stir in the strained milk, a little at a time - the mix will thicken at first to a doughy paste, but keep going, adding milk gradually to avoid lumps.

8. When all the milk has been added bring to the boil then gently simmer, stirring constantly (if you have any lumps, give it a quick whisk). Gently bubble for a few minutes until thickened. Season to taste with salt, pepper and nutmeg.

9. Tip the sauces into 2 sealed containers leave in the fridge overnight.

10. Spread a third of the meat sauce over the base of a roughly 3.5 litre baking dish. Cover with a single layer of pasta sheets, snapping them to fit if needed, then top with a third of the béchamel. Sprinkle over a third of the Parmesan,

11. Then another layer of pasta. Spoon over the second third of the meat, then pasta, followed by second third of the béchamel sauce and scatter over a little Parmesan.

12. Then another layer of pasta, final third of the meat sauce, then pasta, béchamel sauce and finally the Parmesan cheese.

13. Place in the fridge to allow the lasagne to rest for 6 hours before cooking.

14. Heat oven to 180°C.

15. Sit the dish on a baking tray to catch the spills and bake for one hour until bubbling, browned and crisp on top.

Best frozen before cooking. Wrap well in cling film and freeze up to three months. Remove from the freezer, transfer to the fridge 48 hours before you want to cook to allow it to defrost, then bake as directed, checking after 1 hour in case it needs a further 10-15 minutes (if you have frozen any leftovers, defrost in the fridge, then reheat in the microwave.)

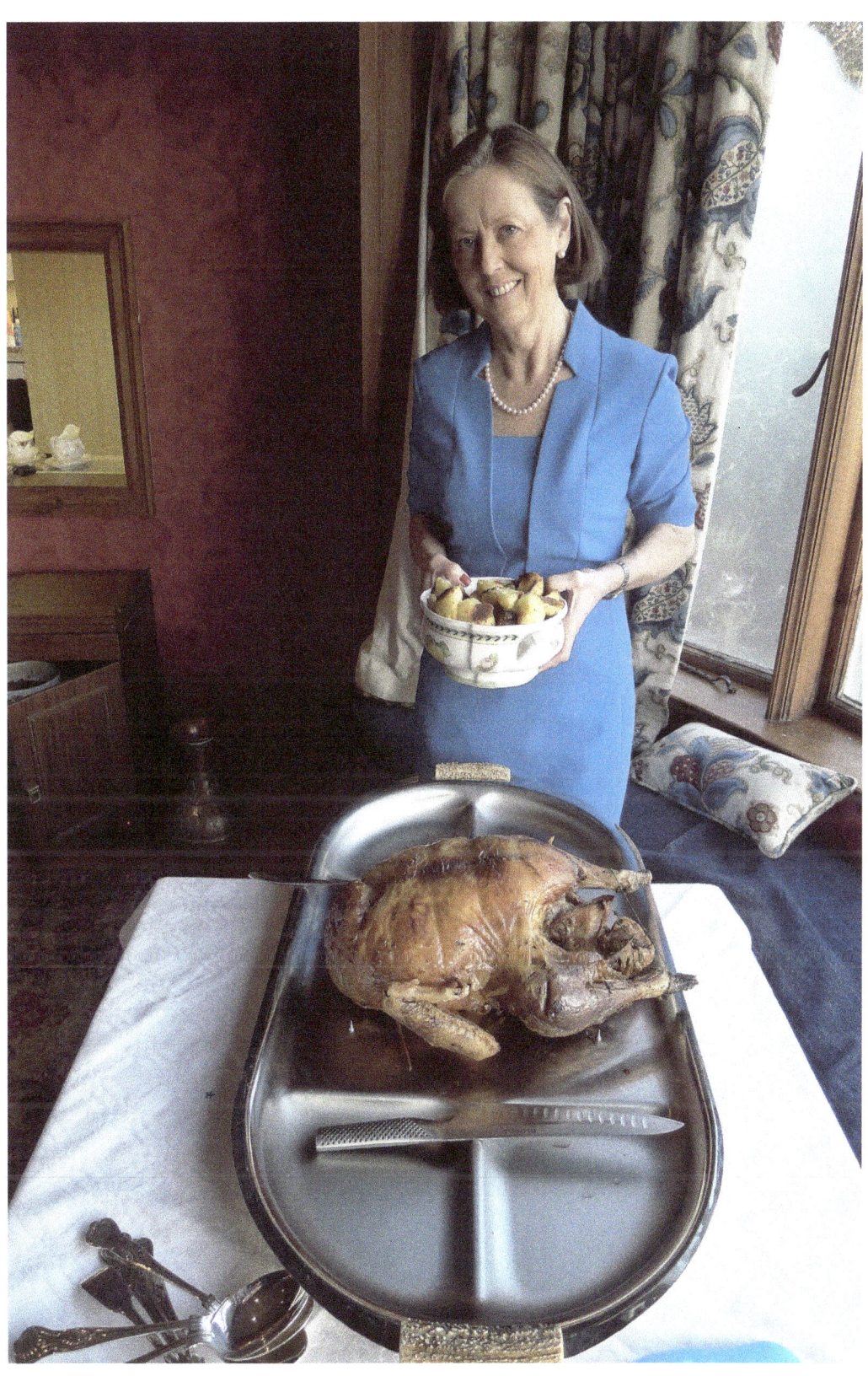

Beef

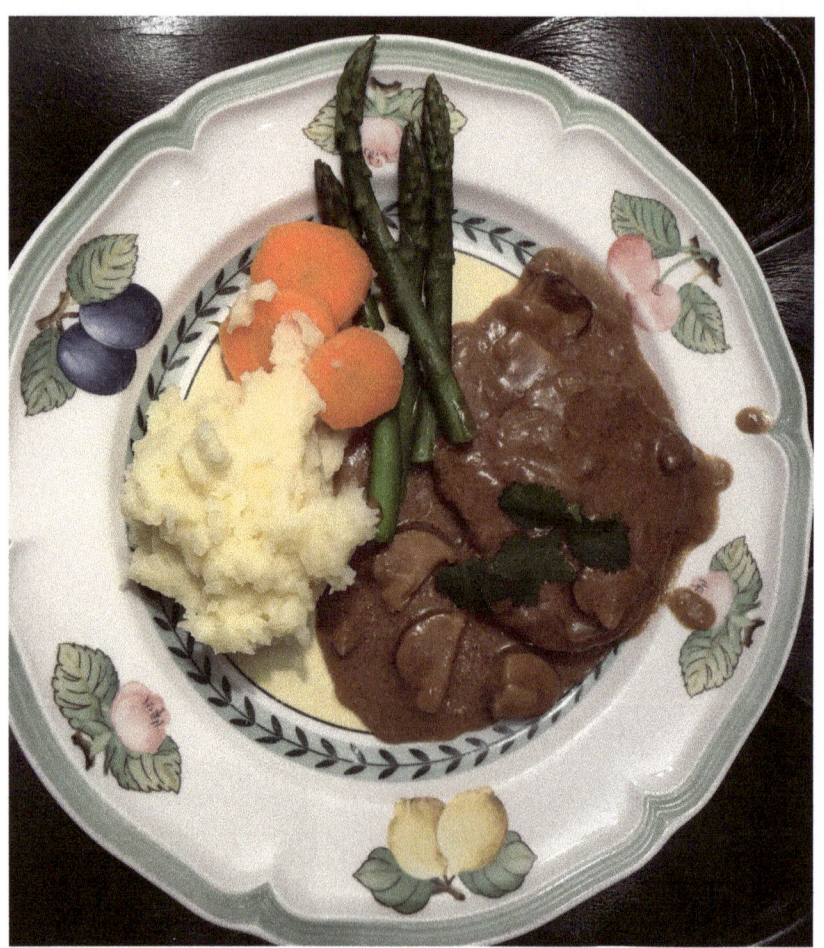

A Dish of Strength and Heart

The steaks do sizzle, rich and bold,
A tale of hearth and hands of old.
With mushrooms soft and onions bright,
A meal that hums with deep delight.

The cream pours in, the sauce runs deep,
A flavour warm, a taste to keep.
With butter's touch and thyme so fine,
A dish of comfort, strong yet kind.

—Inspired by John Buchan

Polish Nelson Steaks

Serves 4

Ingredients

4 rump steaks, about 175 g each

40 g seasoned flour

60 g butter

1 large onion, peeled and sliced

175 g mushrooms, sliced

150 ml single cream

150 ml beef stock

Salt

Freshly ground black pepper

Method

1. Coat the steaks in seasoned flour. Melt 40 g of the fat in a frying pan and fry the steaks to seal quickly on both sides. Transfer to the pan

2. Add the remaining fat to the pan and fry the onions until soft. Add the mushrooms and continue cooking for 1 minute. Add any remaining flour to the pan cook for 1 minute.

3. Add the cream and stock to the pan and bring to the boil. Add plenty of salt and pepper and pour over the steaks.

4. Cover the casserole and cook in a preheated oven, 170°C for one hour or until the steaks are tender.

5. Serve the steaks with their sauce and vegetables in a deep serving dish, garnished with chopped parsley, carrot sticks and potatoes.

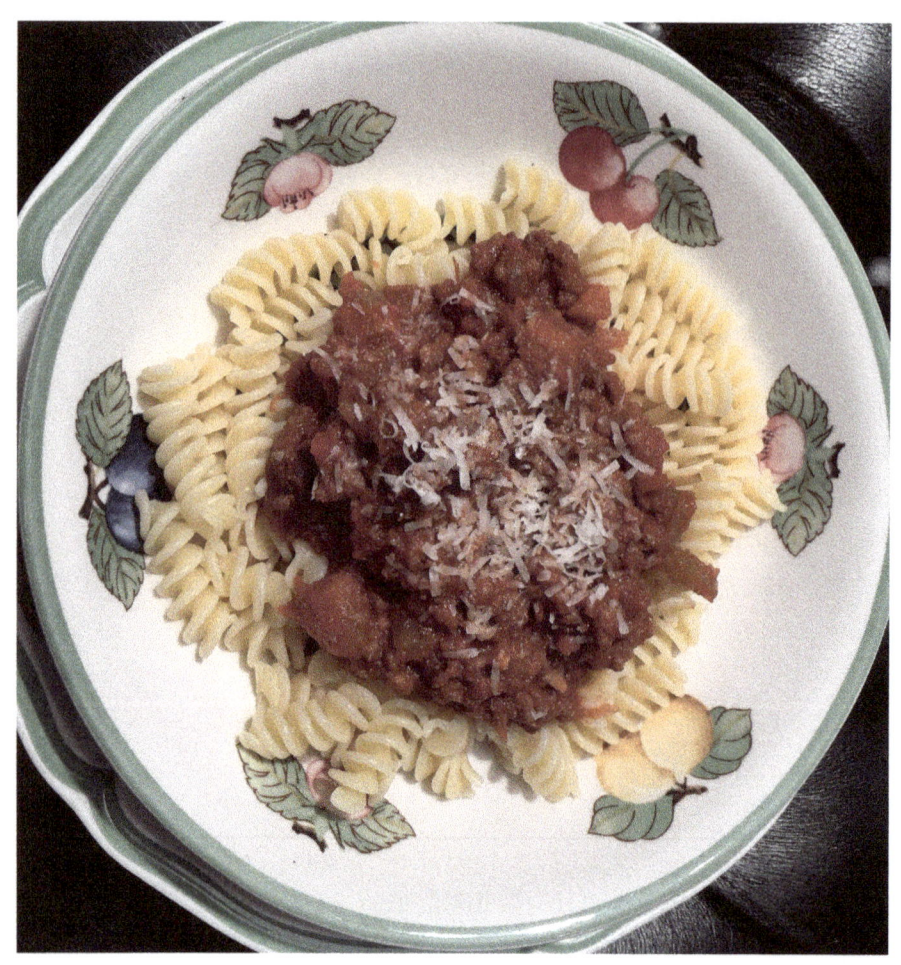

A Slow and Tender Tale

The pot is filled, the scent runs free,
A meal of depth and history.
With garlic bright and nutmeg strong,
A sauce that sings both bold and long.

The wine flows in, the milk stands near,
A dish that hums with love sincere.
With pasta firm and cheese atop,
A meal where time shall never stop.

—Inspired by Robert Louis Stevenson

Ragu Modenese

Serves 6

Ingredients

Salt and pepper

450 g minced veal

2 sticks of finely chopped celery

1 large carrot finely chopped

1 large onion finely chopped

3 cloves of garlic finely chopped

1½ tins of plum tomatoes

2 Tbsp of tomato puree

1 large glass of red wine

1 glass milk

Nutmeg

1 Tbsp oil

Method

1. In a heavy bottom pan add oil, garlic, onion, salt and mince, fry gently, until all the meat juice has evaporated .Add celery and carrot, fry until soft.
2. Add milk and grated nutmeg. Lower heat; allow the milk to fully evaporate.
3. Add wine and allow to evaporate fully.
4. Add tin tomatoes
5. Simmer for an hour, it may need more beef stock added if it becomes dry.
6. Add tomato puree for extra colour and flavour.
7. Add salt and pepper to taste.

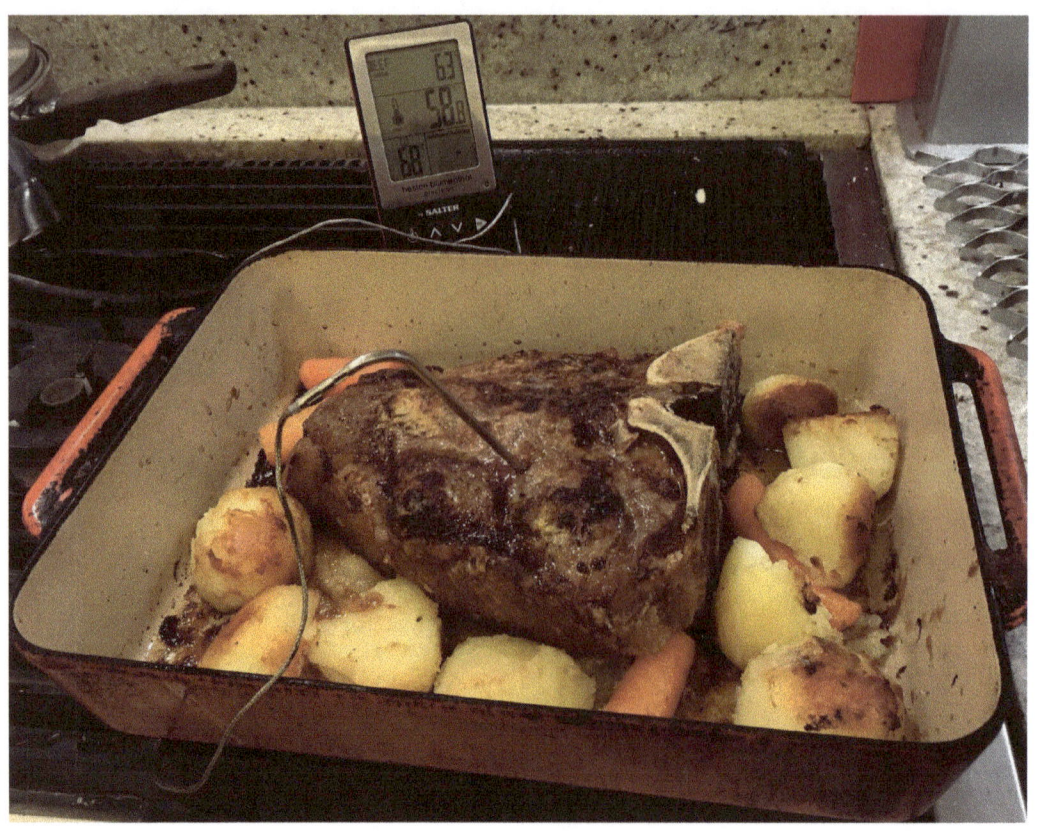

A Carver's Pride

The oven hums, the beef stands tall,
A feast to grace both great and small.
The mustard sings, the juices flow,
A meal where patience makes it so.

The carving knife in steady hand,
A dish that time shall still command.
With Yorkshire crisp and gravy deep,
A taste of strength, a past to keep.

—*Inspired by Robert Burns*

Roast Beef

Serves 4-6

300-350 g per person on the bone/rib, 225 g per person off the bone/sirloin

Ingredients

1.4 kg sirloin of beef off the bone

2 Tbsp plain flour

2 tsp of mustard, English or Dijon

1 large onion

1 tsp freshly ground pepper

2 Tbsp of vegetable oil

Method

1. Thickly slice an onion and place on the bottom of the roasting tin under the beef.
2. Spread a thin coating of mustard on the beef and then dust the surface of the meat with a mixture of flour and dry mustard, and sprinkle with freshly milled pepper (but no salt, since this encourages the juices to escape).
3. Heat the oil in a frying pan until smoking , then sear the beef all over.
4. Place in the oven at 185°C.
5. Cooking time; 15 minutes per 450 g for rare 50°C on a thermometer; plus an extra 15 minutes for medium rare, 55°C on a thermometer, 30 minutes for medium 60°C on a thermometer, 45 minutes for medium well done 65°C on a thermometer or 1 hour for well done 70°C on a thermometer.
6. Baste the meat by spooning the pan juices over it from time to time during cooking. Half way through the cooking time turn the meat over.
7. Remove from the oven and place on a carving dish. Allow 10 minutes for the meat to relax before carving. Keep the meat warm by placing tin foil over the meat.
8. As the meat relaxes, some of the juices will exude onto the carving dish; these should be added to the gravy. The meat will carry on cooking on the inside as it relaxes.

Accompaniments to roast beef - horseradish sauce, Yorkshire pudding, and roast potatoes.

Yorkshire Pudding

Serves 4-6

Ingredients

150 g plain flour
4 large eggs
175 ml of milk
25 ml of water
2 Tbsp of sunflower oil
Roasting dish 20 x 30 cm

Method

1. Preheat the oven to 210°C. Put the oil into a roasting tin.

2. Measure the flour and salt, sieve into a bowl and make a well in the centre. Add the eggs and a little milk. Whisk, until smooth, gradually adding the remaining milk. This can be done with a handheld electric whisk. Pour the mixture into a jug.

3. Transfer the roasting tin into the preheated oven for 5 minutes, until the oil is piping hot.

4. Carefully remove the heated tin from the oven and pour the batter into the tin. Quickly return it to the oven and cook for 30 minutes or until golden brown and well risen. Serve immediately.

Avoid opening the oven during cooking process as this will cause the Yorkshire Pudding to deflate.

A Rise to Glory

A batter light, a pan so bright,
A dish that swells in golden light.
The oven's breath, the oil's embrace,
A taste that time shall ne'er erase.

With beef beside and gravy near,
A meal to bring both warmth and cheer.
A bite, a pause, a sip of ale,
A dish where memories set sail.

—Inspired by Robert Burns

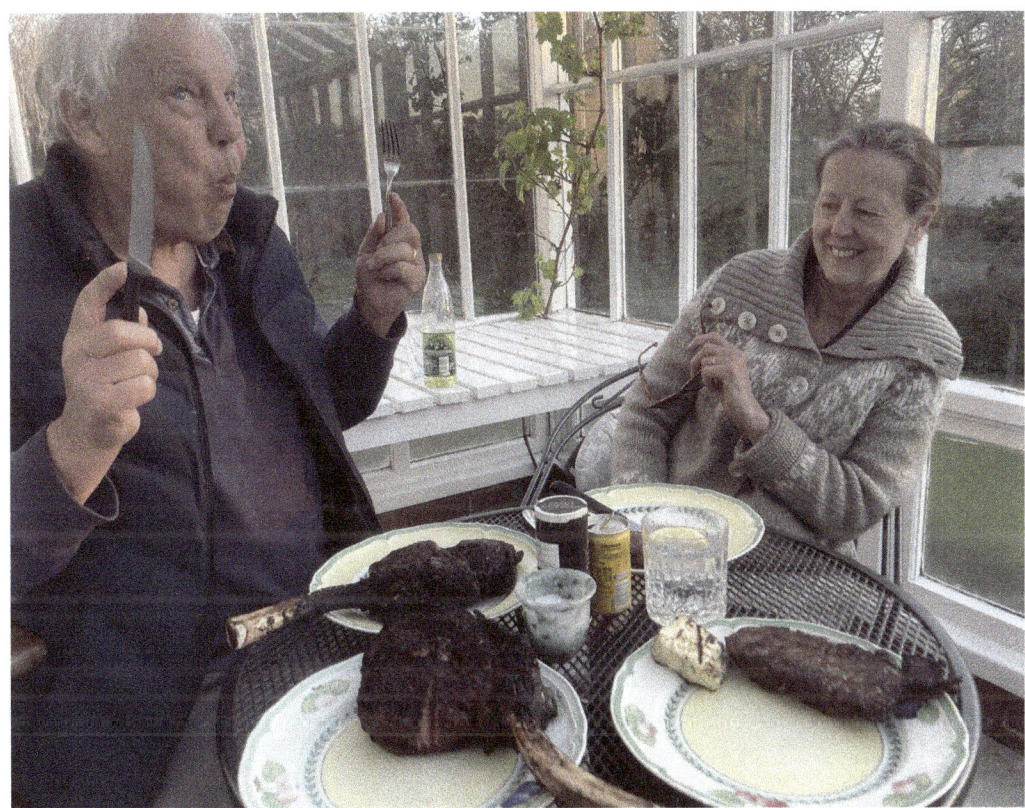

Beef

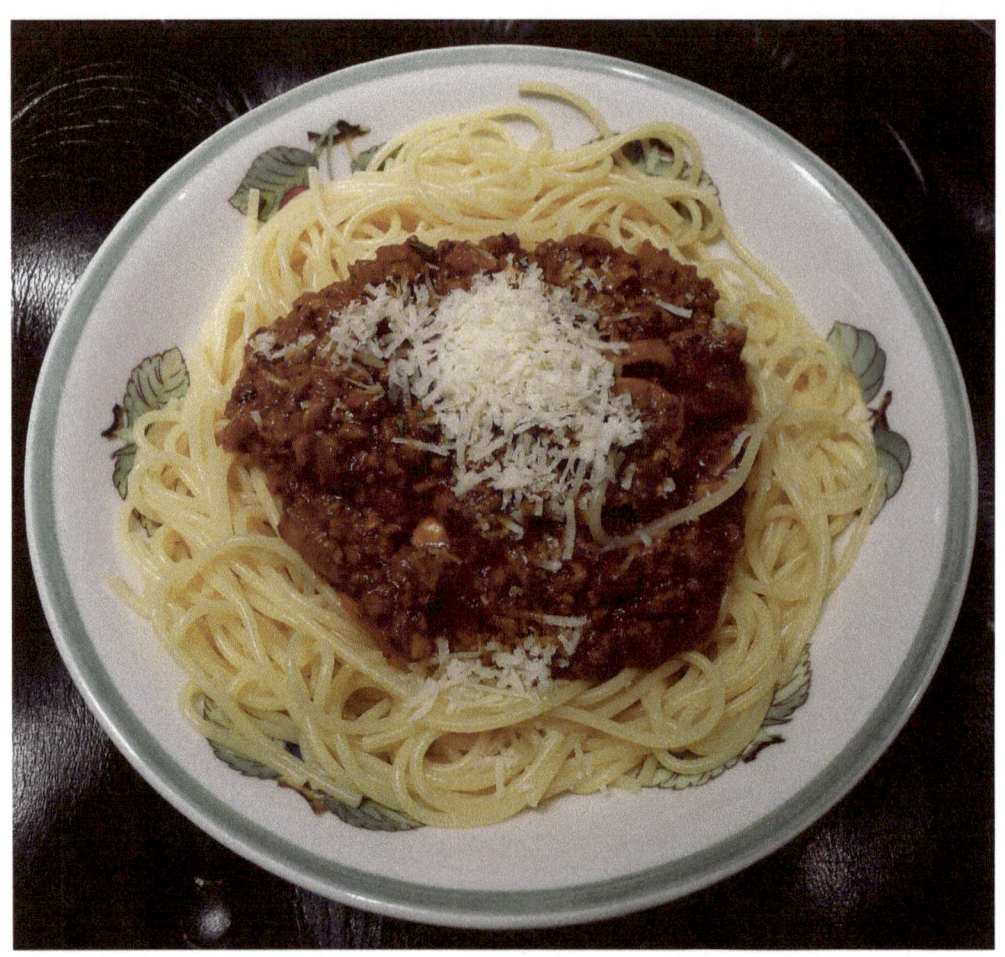

162

A Dish of Stories Told

A pot of red, a tale so bright,
Where herbs and stock and wine unite.
The pasta twirls, the sauce does cling,
A dish where joy and flavour sing.

A sprinkle fine of cheese so true,
A plate where laughter passes through.
With bread and wine and hearts held high,
A meal where time slips softly by.

—*Inspired by Robert Louis Stevenson*

Spaghetti Bolognaise

Serves 4

Ingredients

325 g spaghetti

450 g lean mince beef

1 onion, thinly sliced

2 cloves garlic

2 Tbsp olive oil

100 g mushrooms thinly sliced

2 level Tbsp flour

1 tin chopped plum tomatoes

1 level tsp salt

Freshly ground black pepper

2 tsp mixed herbs

60 g double concentrate tomato puree

¼ pt red wine

¼ pt beef stock

1 heaped Tbsp of chopped parsley

75 g parmesan cheese, grated

Method

1. Heat the oil in a large pan and gently fry the onions for about 5 minutes. Add the chopped garlic and minced beef, stirring until the meat is thoroughly browned.

2. Add the mushrooms and fry for a few minutes. Mix in the flour cook for a few minutes. Add the tomatoes and their juices, seasoning, mixed herbs and tomato puree.

3. Pour over the red wine and beef stock, bring to the boil. Lower the heat and place a lid on the pan and cook gently for 45minutes-1 hour. Until tender. Then add the parsley. Taste, adjust seasoning.

4. Cook the spaghetti, drain, serve in bowls, sprinkled the grated Parmesan cheese on top of the meat.

5. Serve with garlic bread and a green salad.

Beef

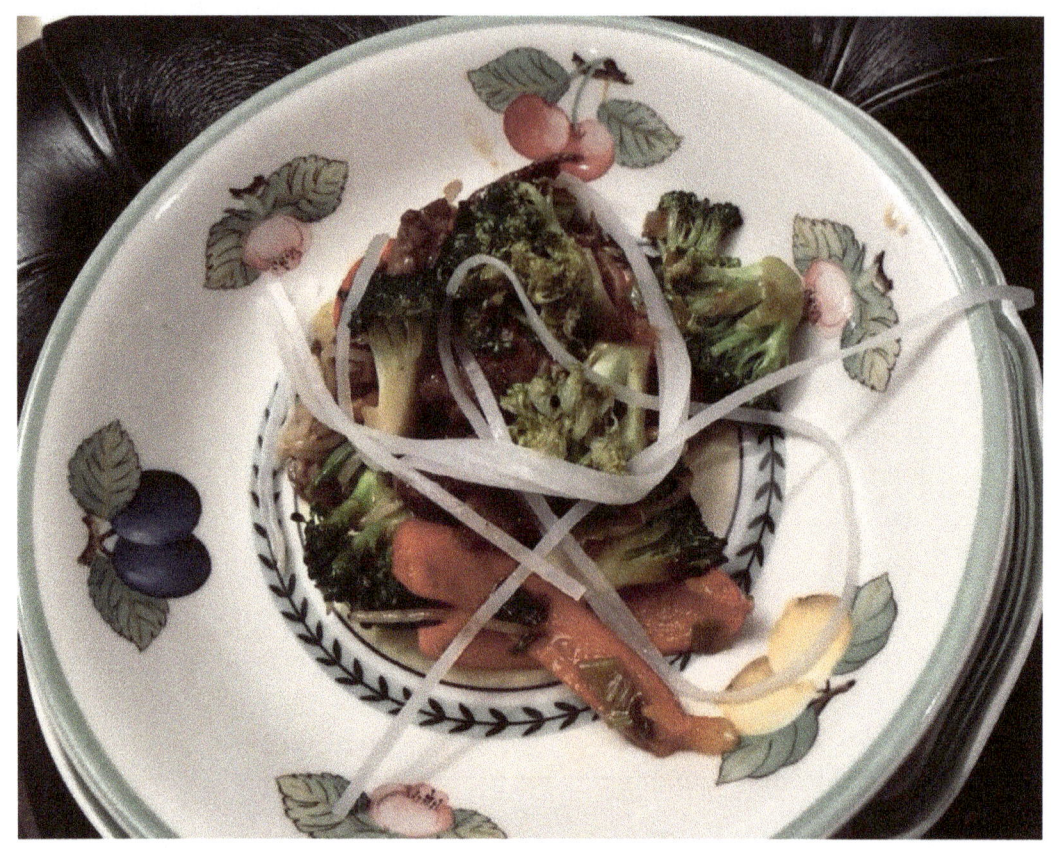

A Dance of Heat and Spice

A flick of flame, a stir so fast,
A dish where heat and flavour last.
With ginger's spark and soy so deep,
A taste where fire and motion keep.

The peppers crisp, the noodles twine,
A meal both bold and light, divine.
With chopsticks raised and laughter bright,
A dish that sings through every bite.

—Inspired by Contemporary Scottish Poets

Stir-fry Beef

Serves 4

Ingredients

- 450 g sirloin or fillet of beef cut into thin strips
- 1½ Tbsp cornflour
- Freshly ground pepper
- 3 Tbsp dark soy sauce
- 2 Tbsp of sesame oil
- 1 Tbsp olive oil
- 1 red pepper cut into thin strips
- 2.5 cm root ginger grated
- 2 cloves of garlic crushed
- 100 g bean sprouts
- 4-5 Tbsp of sherry
- 2 Tbsp water
- 1 broccoli head, broken down into small florets
- 1 tsp Chinese 5 spices; salt
- 1 bunch of spring onions sliced diagonally
- 1 packet of fresh egg noodles

Method

1. Put the beef in a bowl to marinate for 30 minutes with the cornflour, salt, freshly ground pepper, soy sauce and the Chinese 5 spices.
2. Meanwhile, split the broccoli into florets, slice the onions and the red pepper, crush the garlic and grate the ginger.
3. Put the sesame oil into a wok, fry the sliced spring onions for a few minutes then add the garlic, and ginger for 1 minute. Add the red pepper. Fry for 2 minutes.
4. Pour in the water and sherry; you may need more, if you like a lot of sauce. Add the broccoli florets; (at this stage you may want to add any other vegetables,) After 4 minutes add the bean sprouts and noodles. Simmer with a lid on for 1 minute, don't overcook the vegetables as you need the vegetables with a crunch.
5. Meanwhile, fry the marinated steak in another frying pan, with some oil olive, if you want it rare only cook for a short time, cook longer for medium etc.
6. Stir in the noodles, cook for 3 minutes. Add the steak to the vegetables, and serve in bowls, and hand round with soy sauce.

Beef

Flint Family Cookbook

Lamb

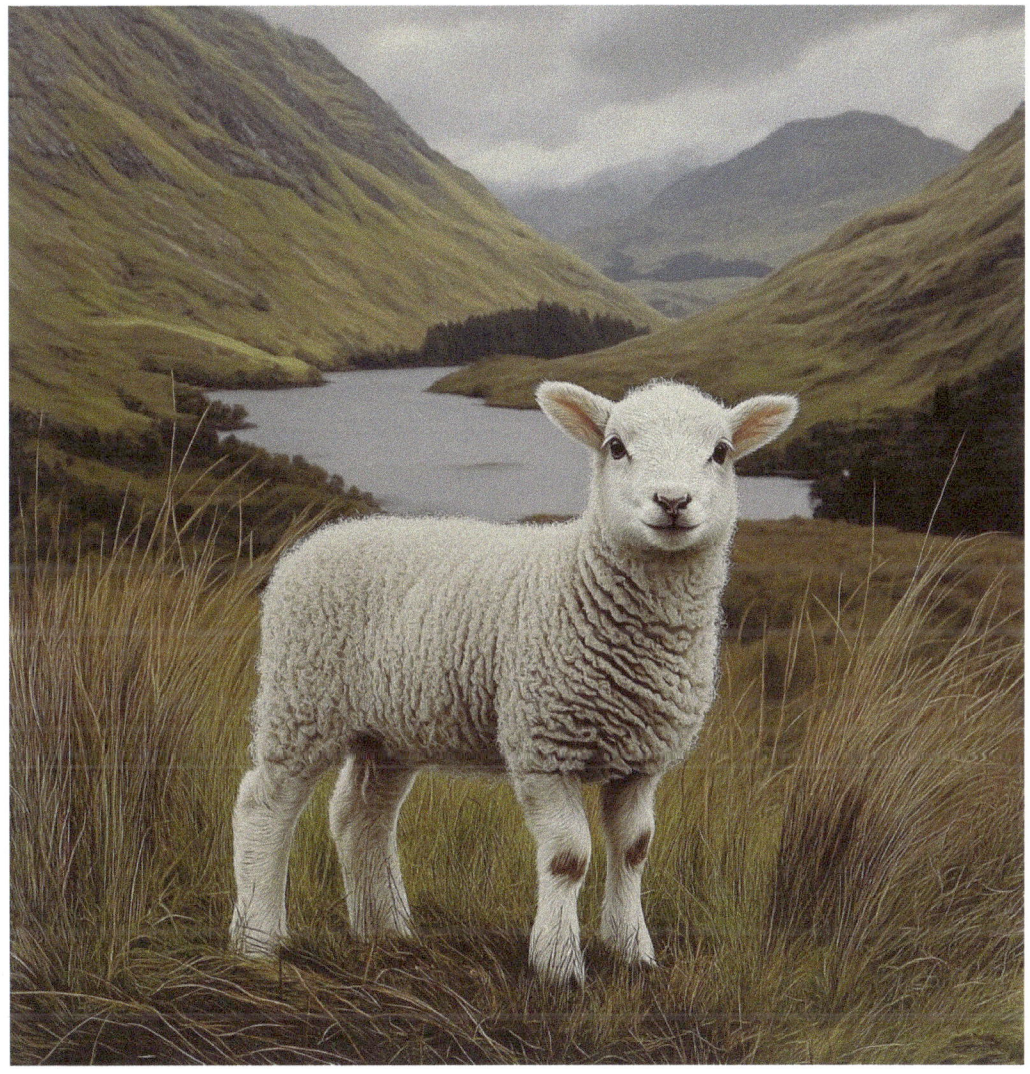

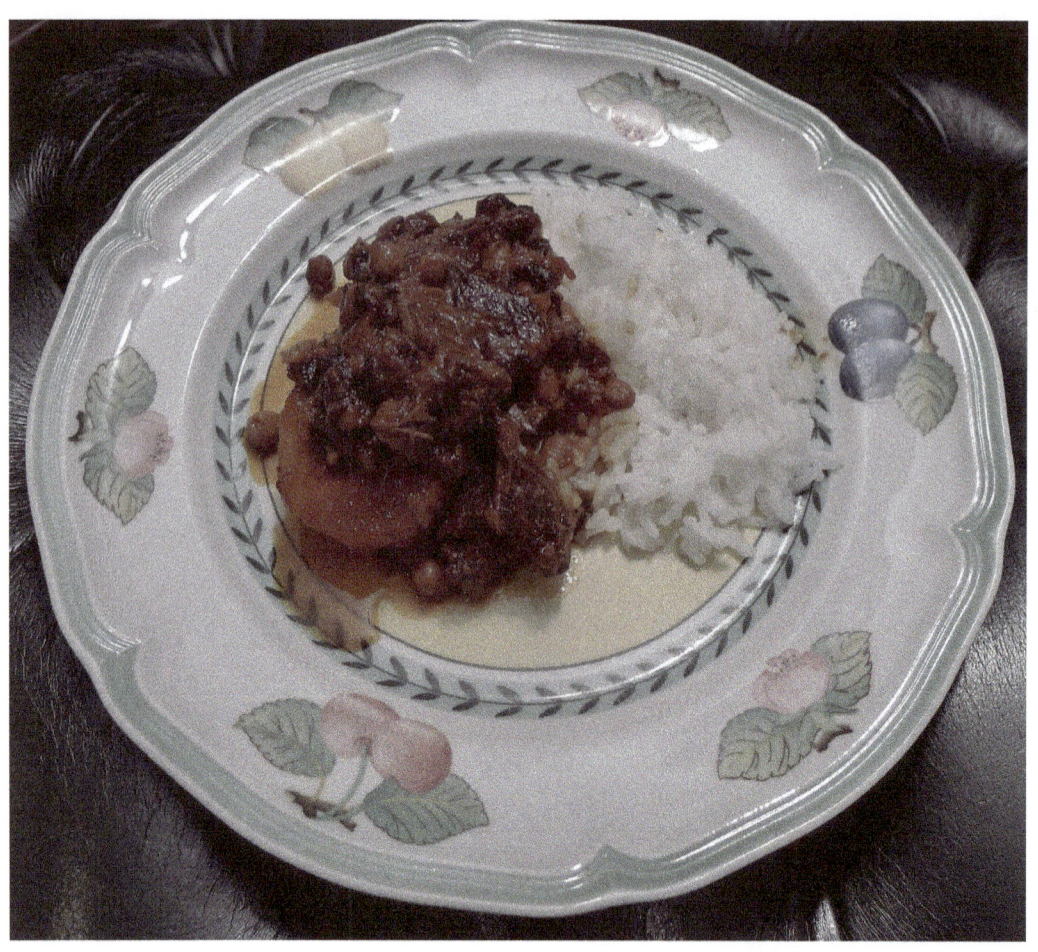

A Song of Spice and Time

A whisper bold, a saffron sigh,
The cinnamon hums, the almonds fly.
With apricots bright and honey's glow,
A tale of lands where warm winds blow.

The lamb drinks deep of spice and sun,
A dish where time and patience run.
With couscous light and herbs so free,
A feast of ancient mystery.

—Inspired by Sir Walter Scott

Lamb Tagine

Preparation time 50 minutes, cooking time approx. 2 hours. Serves 6

Ingredients

1 Tbsp ground ginger
1-2 tsp coarsely ground black pepper
2 tsp ground cinnamon
1 tbsp turmeric
1½ Tbsp paprika
½ tsp chilli powder
1.1 kg (2 ½ lb) cubed boneless lamb
450 g onions
3 plump garlic cloves
½ tsp salt
5 Tbsp olive oil
175 g (6 oz) ready-to-eat dried apricots
50 g (2 oz) sultanas
85 g (3 oz) toasted flaked almonds
1 tbsp honey
300 ml tomato juice
400 g can chopped tomatoes
300 ml (½pt) hot lamb stock
Fresh coriander to garnish
Couscous to serve

Method

1. Preheat the oven to 170°C/Gas 3. If using a fan oven, cook from the cold at 150°C. Put the spices into a small bowl and mix them well. Put the lamb cubes in a large mixing bowl and tip in the spices.

2. Coat the lamb cubes evenly in the spice mixture. Your hands are the best tools for this job, but if you prefer not to get them messy, use two large spoons instead. Peel and grate the onions using a grater and chopping board. Peel and chop the garlic cloves, then crush them with a knife to a paste with the salt.

3. Put the casserole dish on high heat and add a tablespoon of oil. When the oil is hot, add a quarter of the lamb and cook until the cubes are brown on the underside. Turn the cubes over and cook until all the sides are browned. Remove them with a slotted spoon and set aside. Brown the rest of the lamb in batches, adding another tablespoon of oil with each batch. Browning the meat will take about 15 minutes in total.

4. When all the meat is browned and set aside, reduce the heat and add the remaining tablespoon of oil. Wait a few seconds until hot, then add the onions and garlic. Stir well until the ingredients are well coated in the pan juices, then cook them until they are soft but not browned, stirring often. This will take about 10 minutes.

5. Return the lamb to the casserole and stir in the remaining ingredients. Bring to the boil, cover and place the casserole dish in the oven. Cook for 2 hours or until the lamb is tender, stirring halfway through. About 10 minutes before the end, prepare the couscous and chop the coriander, reserving a sprig. Serve the lamb tagine sprinkled with chopped coriander and the couscous topped with a sprig of coriander.

Lamb

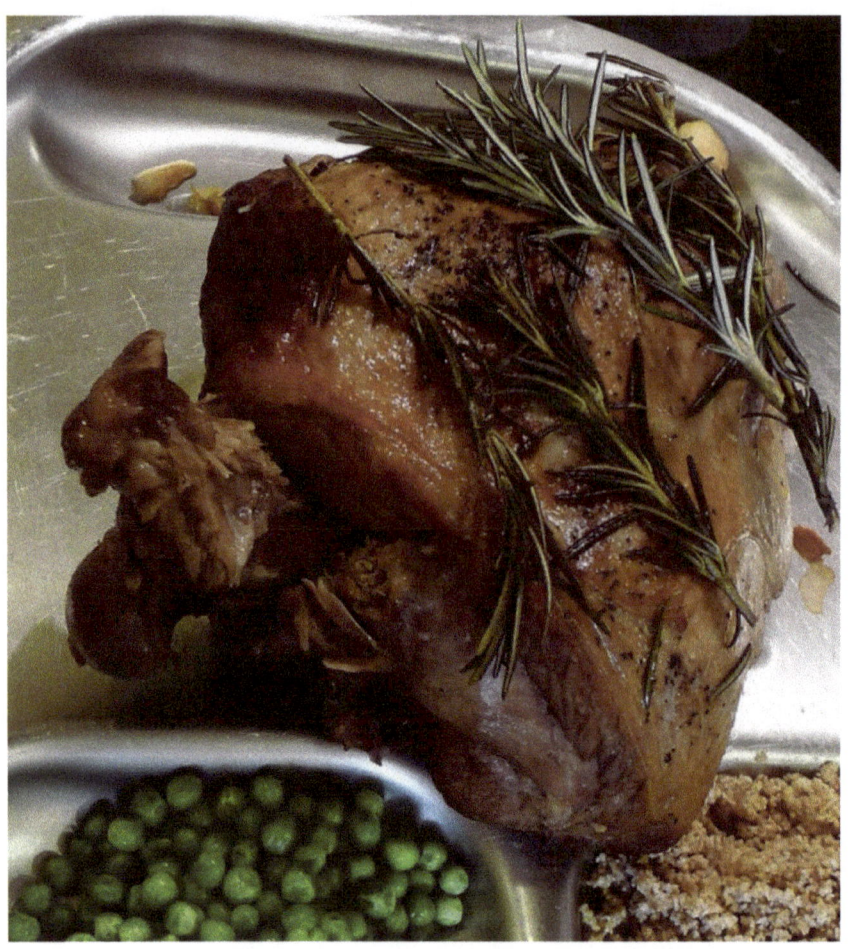

A Roast of Patience and Grace

The oven hums, the hours pass slow,
As rosemary scents the lamb below.
A tender fall, a bone drawn free,
A dish of time, of legacy.

The wine runs deep, the garlic sways,
A feast to last through autumn's days.
With sauce so rich and herbs so bright,
A meal to bring the heart delight.

—*Inspired by Robert Burns*

Slow-Cooked Leg or Shoulder of Lamb

Cooking time 4 hours. Serves 6–8
With rosemary

Ingredients

- 2 Tbsp of olive oil
- Salt and freshly ground pepper
- 2.5 kg leg of lamb on the bone
- 2 medium onions, thinly sliced (or 5 shallots)
- 1 big carrot, roughly chopped
- 3 celery sticks
- 150 g chopped tomatoes (optional)
- 500 ml dry white wine
- 2 heads of garlic, halved
- 2 bay leaves
- 15 single sprigs of rosemary
- A pinch of chilli flakes
- A few squeezes of lemon juice
- A handful of flat-leaf parsley, finely chopped
- 2 sheets of greaseproof paper and tin foil

Method

1. Preheat oven to 170°C. Heat the oil in a large frying pan. When the oil is hot, add the lamb and seal. Brown the lamb all over.

2. Place the lamb on top of the roughly chopped vegetables, bay leaves, rosemary sprigs, parsley, garlic, and chilli flakes. Add the wine and season well with salt and pepper.

3. Wet greaseproof paper under a tap, wring/crumple dry, and smooth out a little. Place the damp paper over the lamb and cover it tightly with a layer of tin foil, tucking it around the outside edge of the tin so the meat is hermetically sealed.

4. Put in the oven and cook for 4 hours. When it is done, you should be able to pull the bones from the meat. Carefully lift the joint from the tin onto a chopping board or serving dish, cover, and keep warm.

5. Remove most of the fat from the cooking juices and strain the rest of the sauce through a sieve into a saucepan, pressing down to get all the flavour from the vegetables and herbs: you can force some of them through the sieve to thicken the sauce a bit if you want. If the juices are too thin, put the pan on the hob and bubble away for a few minutes, but don't expect it to be like thickened gravy.

6. Add a few squeezes of lemon juice to taste–you want to brighten the sauce's flavour, not make it overly lemony. Check the seasoning and reheat if necessary. Hand round in a gravy bowl alongside the meat.

7. Serve with petit pois, roast or mashed potato, chopped carrots and skirlie or with mint sauce and red currant jelly.

Flint Family Cookbook

Vegetables

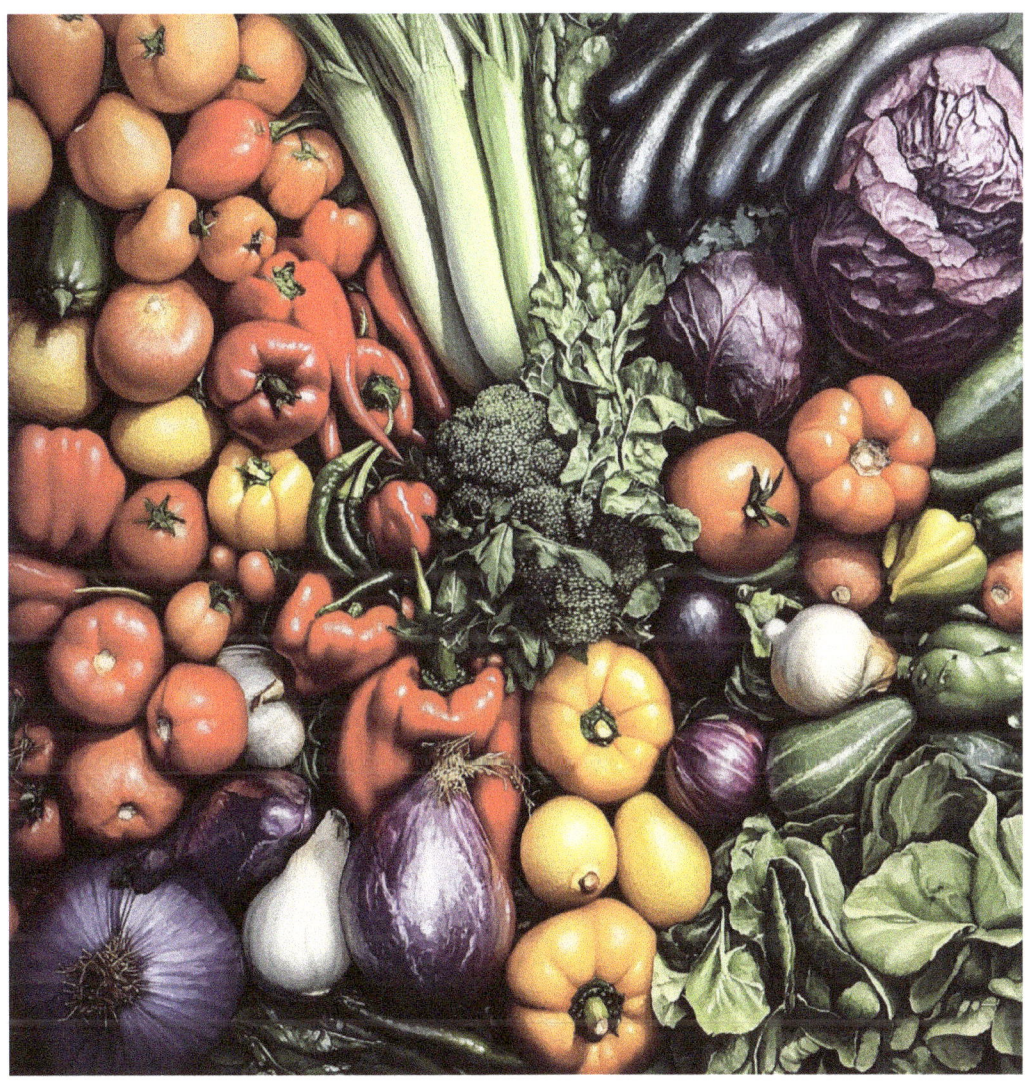

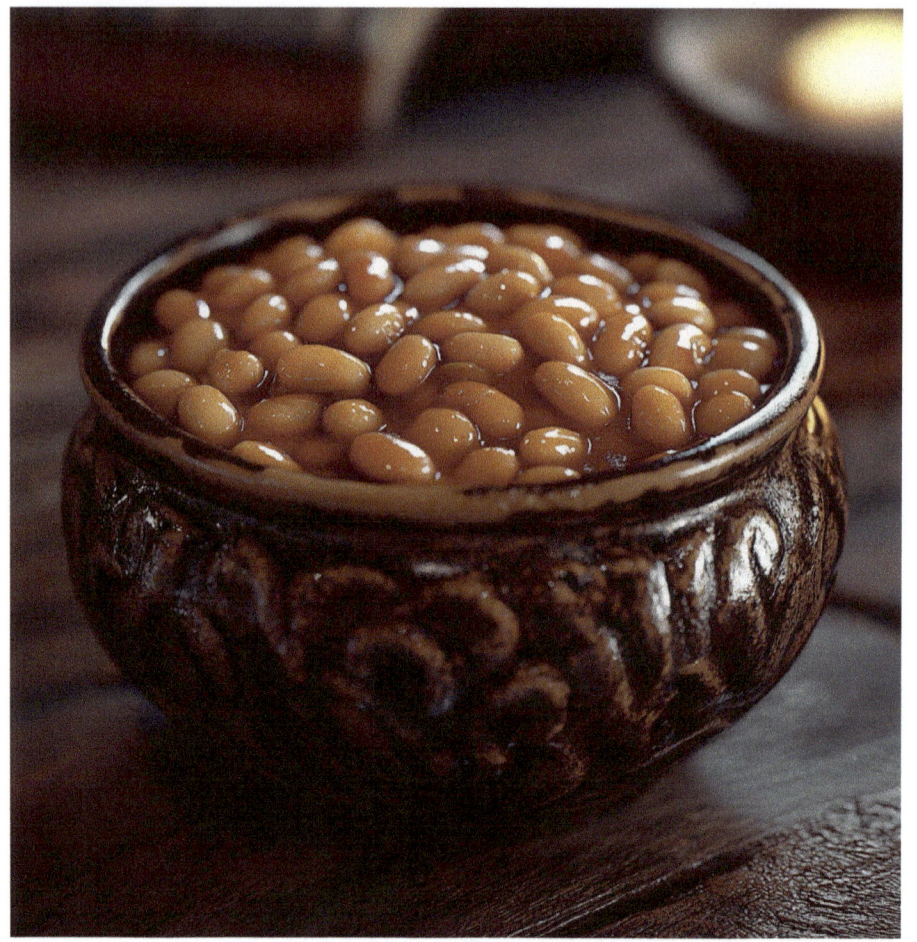

A Slow and Steady Warmth

*A pot so deep, a flame so low,
Where beans and treacle softly flow.
A taste that lingers, sweet yet bold,
A comfort served from days of old.*

*With shallots kissed by butter's grace,
A dish that holds both time and place.
A spoonful warm, a humble cheer,
A bite to bring the heart sincere.*

—*Inspired by Robert Burns*

Boston Baked Beans

My quick version of Boston baked beans

Serves 2-3

Ingredients

1 large tin of baked beans
2 shallots, finely chopped
2 tsp of treacle
10 g butter, melted

Method

1. Melt the butter in a small saucepan. Add the chopped shallots, and cook until transparent, about 10 minutes.

2. Add the beans and cook over medium heat for 5 minutes, until heated through. Finally, add the treacle, cook for 3 minutes, and serve

Vegetables

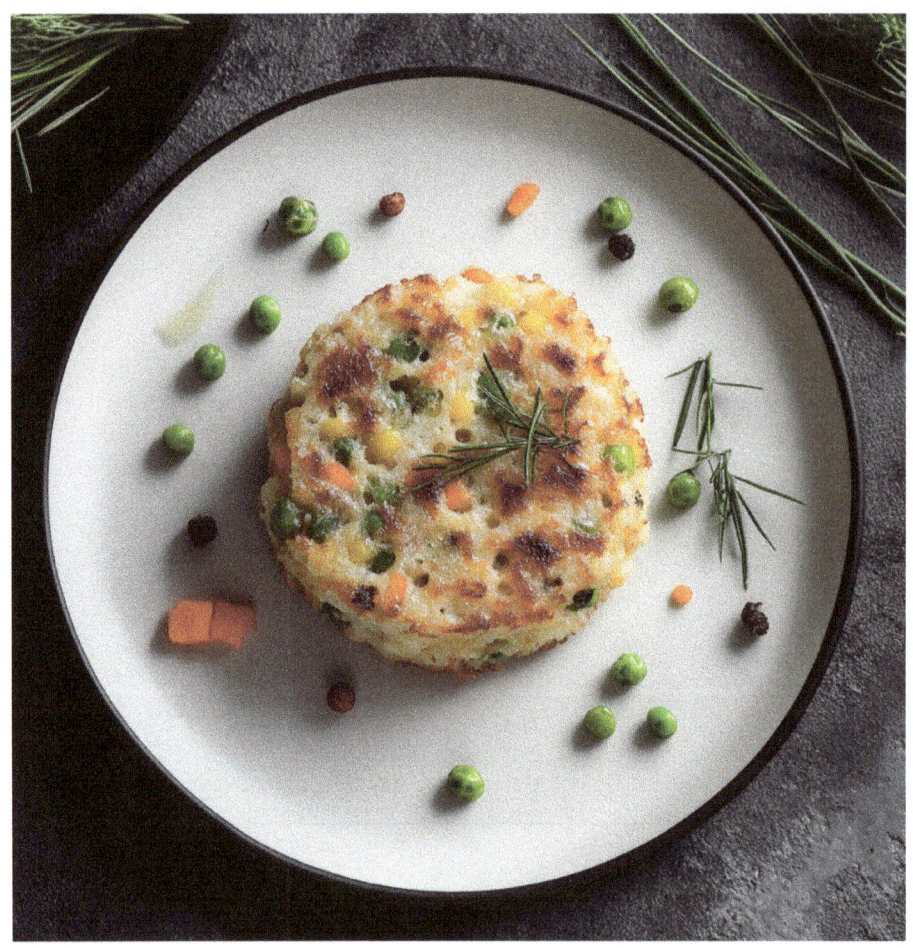

176

A Crisp Delight

A golden crust, a heart so light,
A bite of cheer, a crisp delight.
The cabbage hums, the garlic sings,
A dish where winter comfort clings.

A sizzle bright, a nutmeg's grace,
A meal that knows no time nor place.
So lift your fork, embrace the cheer,
A taste of home, both warm and near.

—*Inspired by John Buchan*

Bubble and Squeak Cakes

Serves 4

Ingredients

500 g potatoes

2 egg yolks

75 g butter

225 g Savoy cabbage, finely shredded

2 garlic cloves, thinly sliced

A generous grating of fresh nutmeg

Salt and pepper

2 Tbsp sunflower oil

Method

1. Boil the potatoes in salted water until soft. Drain and mash. Add the egg yolks and 25 g butter. Season the potatoes with salt and pepper.

2. Heat the rest of the butter in a large frying pan. Fry the cabbage and garlic with the nutmeg over medium heat for 5 minutes until the cabbage is tender. Mix into the mashed potato.

3. Shape the potato mixture into 4 round cakes. Heat the oil in a large frying pan and fry the cakes for 5 minutes until browned on both sides. Carefully lift the cakes from the pan and serve.

Vegetables

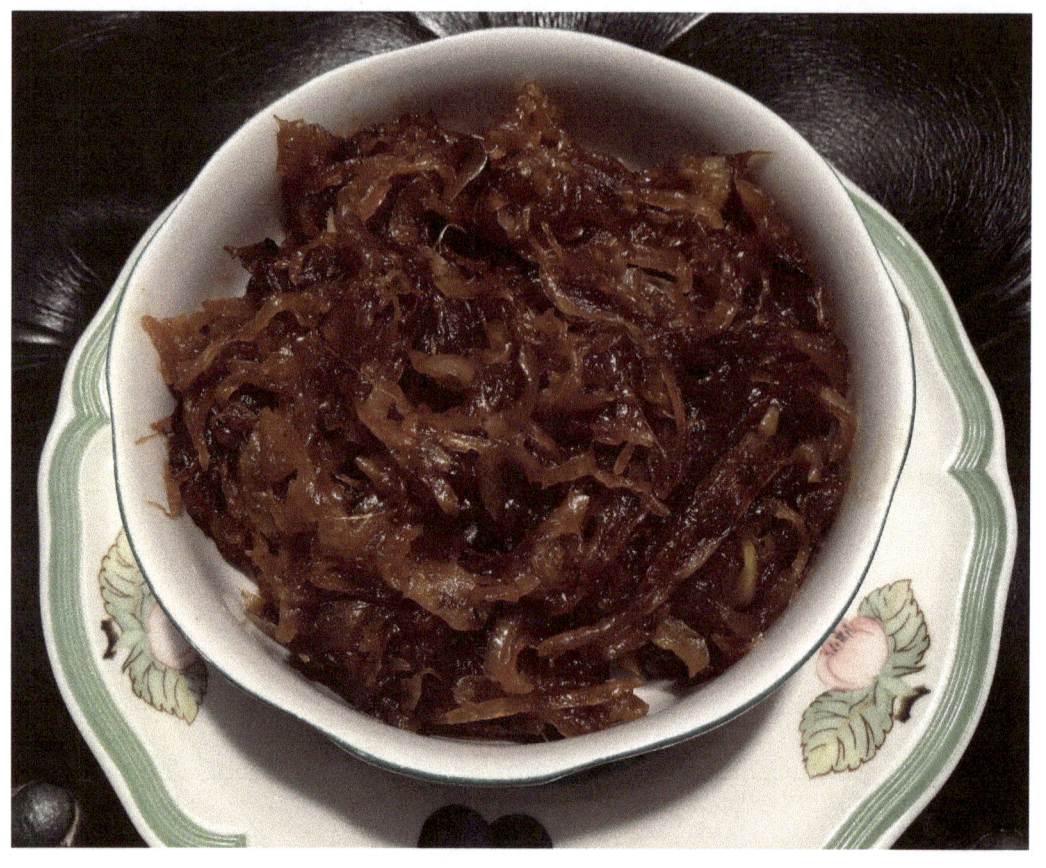

A Slow and Golden Tale

*A whisper low, a gentle stir,
As onions melt to gold and blur.
With butter's warmth and sugar's kiss,
A pot of patience, pure and bliss.*

*A spoonful deep, a taste so fine,
A hint of sherry, aged like wine.
A spread of warmth, a touch so sweet,
A tale of time in layers steeped.*

—*Inspired by Contemporary Scottish Poets*

Confit D'Oignons

Serves 8

Ingredients

40 g butter

900 g onions, peeled and finely sliced

100 g Demerara sugar

3 Tbsp sherry vinegar

1½ Tbsp Crème de Cassis

2 tsp of salt

Method

1. Melt the butter in a medium-sized saucepan. When it starts to turn light brown, add the onions. Stir together and cook gently for 5 minutes, stirring with a wooden spoon now and again.

2. Add the remaining ingredients, including the salt, stir together, then simmer uncovered for 1½-2 hours. The time required will depend on the size of your pan, the heat, and even the onions; some are more watery than others. Stir occasionally to prevent the mixture from sticking and scorching. The finished "marmalade" should look dark golden and sticky.

3. Use the onion confit as required while hot or transfer to a bowl and cover when cold. Due to the high sugar content, this will keep for 2 weeks in the refrigerator. Make a larger quantity if you want to have some on hand in the future to add interest to meat, fish or cheese dishes.

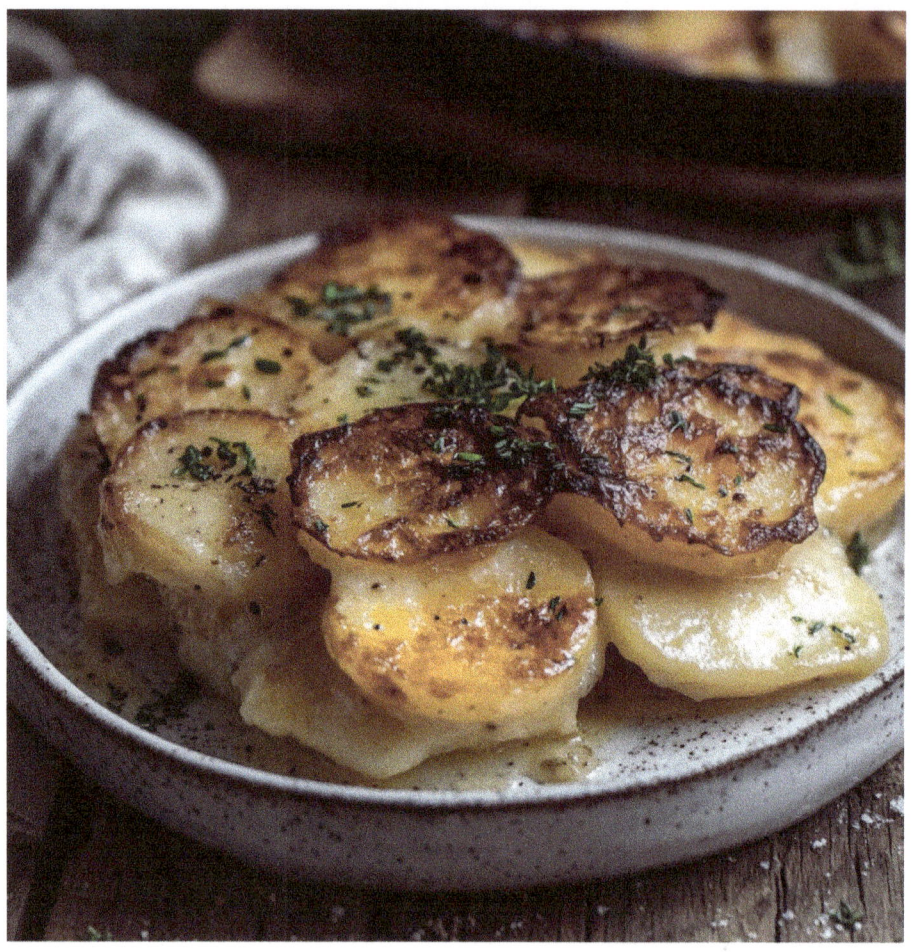

A Creamy Embrace

A golden top, a heart so deep,
Where cream and spice together steep.
The oven hums, the layers meld,
A dish where time and love are held.

With parmesan and warmth so light,
A plate to grace the coldest night.
A bite, a sigh, a moment free,
A meal of quiet luxury.

—Inspired by Robert Louis Stevenson

Gratin Dauphinoise

Serves 5

Ingredients

675 g potatoes, peeled weight (large baking potatoes save time)

175 ml milk

2 tsp of salt

65 ml double cream

15 g fresh parmesan cheese, grated

Method

1. Preheat oven to 180°C.

2. Thinly slice the potatoes in a food processor fitted with the slicing blade. Alternatively, use a mandolin or a very sharp knife.

3. Place the potato slices in a wide pan. Add the milk and salt. Mix thoroughly with a large spoon. Cover with a lid, place over medium heat, and bring to a boil. Check now and again. Once boiling, add the cream. Stir it thoroughly but carefully, as you do not want to break up the potato slices.

4. Continue cooking for 3-5 minutes, or until the starch in the potatoes combines with the milk and cream to produce a thick, creamy mixture.

5. Transfer the potato slices and their creamy sauce to an ovenproof gratin dish. Sprinkle the grated parmesan cheese over the top.

6. Bake in a preheated oven for 40-60 minutes, by which time the potatoes will be tender and the top golden brown. At this stage, they can be served straightaway as an accompaniment to a main course, or they will happily wait for a while, covered with tin foil in a low oven.

7. NB Alternatively, let them become cold and set. Cover and refrigerate overnight. Stamp out rounds using a pastry cutter or cut into small squares or triangles. Place on a lightly buttered baking tray and reheat at 180°C for 10-15 minutes until piping hot. This gives a neater result than serving in spoonfuls.

Do not use a nonstick pan when cooking the potatoes with the milk. They will scorch when cooked, and a certain proportion will stick to the pan. (Your pan will be difficult to clean, but it helps if you soak it for a while.)

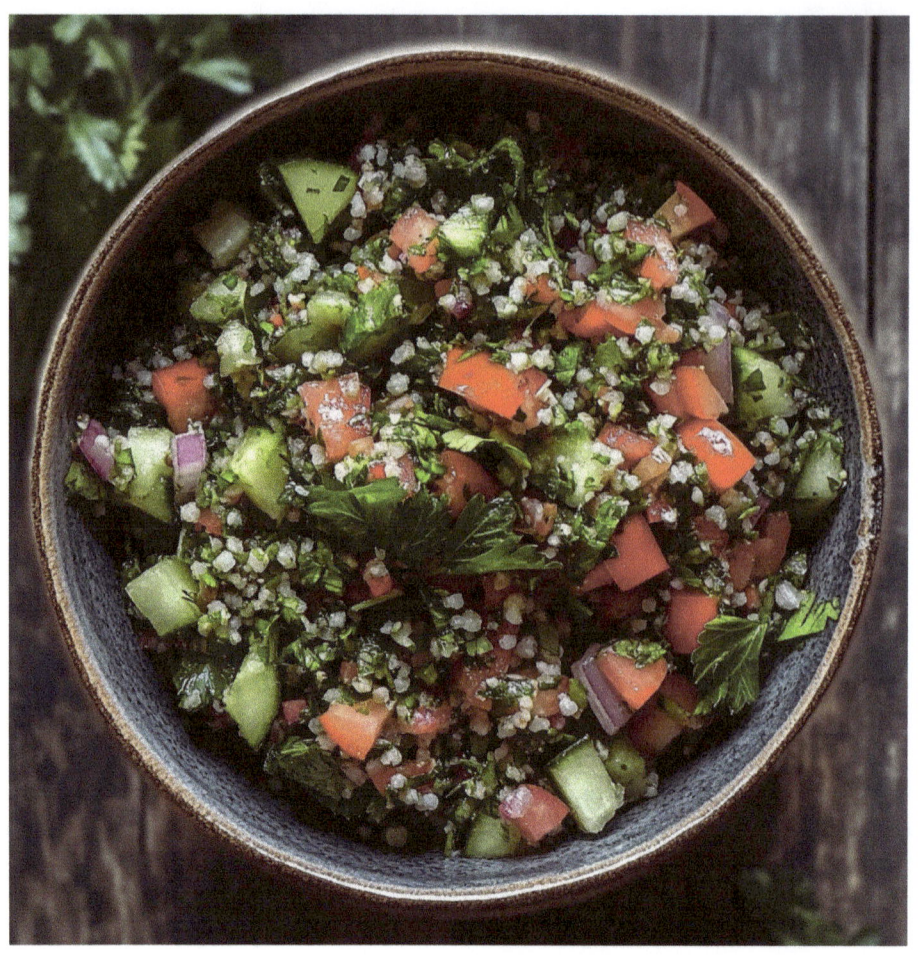

A Garden's Whisper

The parsley sways, the mint sighs bright,
A dish of green in morning light.
The wheat so soft, the lemon bold,
A tale of lands both bright and old.

With olive's kiss and hands so free,
A plate where herbs and grains agree.
A taste of sun, a song so light,
A meal to make the spirit bright.

—*Inspired by Contemporary Scottish Poets*

Herby Tabbouleh

Serves 4-6

Ingredients

125 g bulgur wheat, soaked in cold water overnight

1 red onion finely chopped

2 tomatoes, skinned, seeds removed, finely diced

2 large bunches flat leaf parsley, roughly chopped

1 bunch mint, roughly chopped

1 bunch coriander, roughly chopped

1 lemon juice only

1 Tbsp extra virgin olive oil

1 Tbsp runny honey

Method

1. Drain the bulgur wheat and place into a large bowl. Add the other ingredients and stir until well combined.
2. Season, to taste, with salt and freshly ground pepper.

This can be served with a tagine recipe or as a salad.

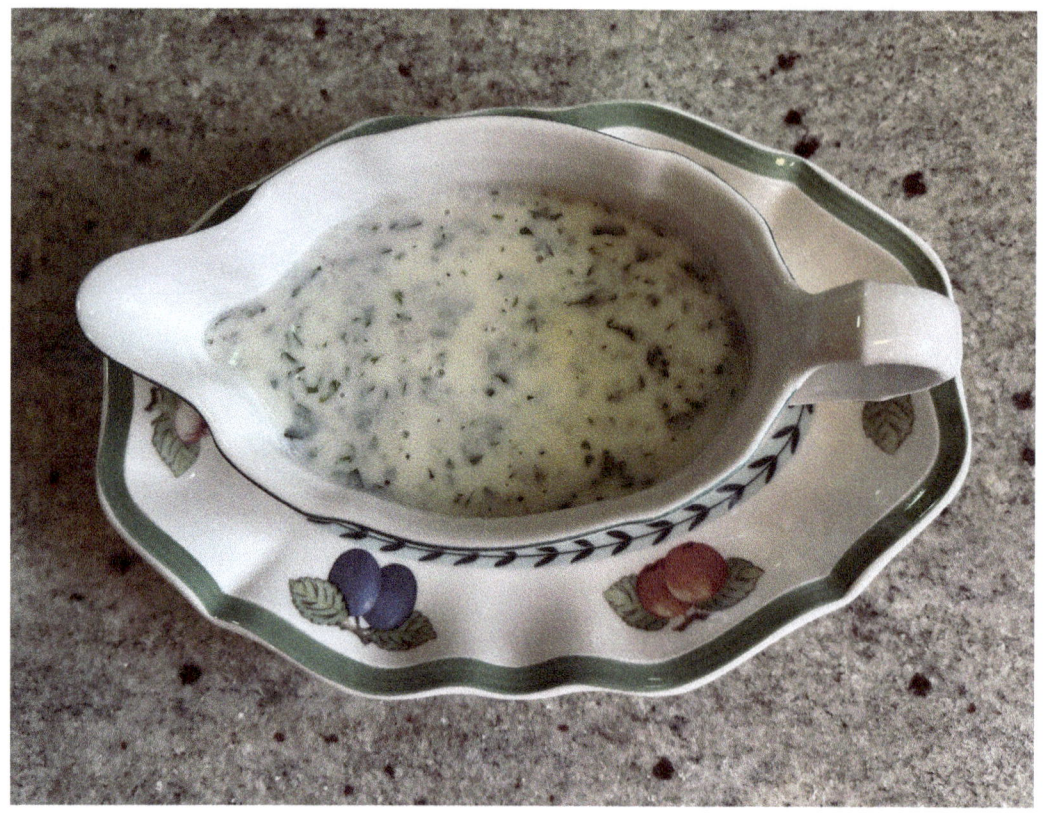

184

A Sauce of Soft Embrace

A gentle pour, a tender flow,
A sauce of green, so light, so low.
With milk and herbs, a velvet stream,
A taste that hums like quiet dreams.

A ladle full, a plate made bright,
A whisper soft, a touch so light.
With fish or bread, it sings its tune,
A dish to warm both heart and spoon.

—Inspired by John Buchan

Parsley Sauce

(Shown with salmon and haddock fishcakes)

Serves 4-6

Ingredients

425 ml milk
1 bay leaf
1 sliced onion, 5 cm thick
Pinch of mace
A few chopped parsley stalks
10 whole black peppercorns
25 g plain flour
40 g butter
4 heaped Tbsp of parsley
1 Tbsp single cream
1 tsp lemon juice
Salt and freshly ground black pepper

Method

1. Place the milk and the following 5 ingredients in a saucepan, bring everything slowly to a simmering point, then pour the mixture into a bowl and leave it aside to get completely cold.

2. When ready to make the sauce, strain the milk into a jug, discarding the flavourings. Melt the butter in a saucepan, add the flour, mix together until there are no lumps. Gradually add the milk, whisking all the time over a low heat. Turn the heat up to a medium heat until thickened.

3. Then, turn the heat to its lowest possible setting and let the sauce cook for 5 minutes, stirring occasionally.

4. When ready to serve the sauce, add the parsley, cream and lemon juice. Taste and add the seasoning. Then, serve in a warm jug to pour over the fish.

When chopping herbs always use a sharp knife.

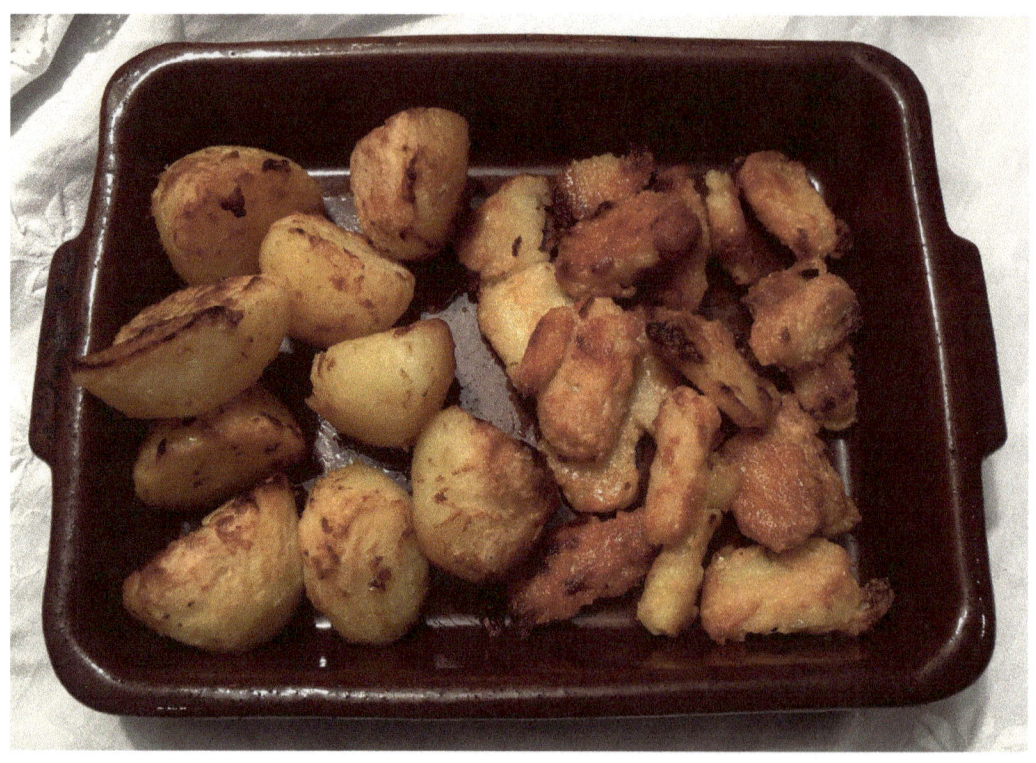

A Golden Crust, A Tender Bite

A coat of gold, a heart so sweet,
A dish where crisp and comfort meet.
The cheese melts slow, the edges brown,
A feast to bring the winter down.

The butter hums, the oven sings,
A warmth that every cold day brings.
With hands held high, the plates are filled,
A meal to soothe, a heart rebuilt.

—*Inspired by Robert Burns*

Parsnips Baked in Parmesan Cheese

Serves 8

It can be prepared well in advance, up to 24 hours, or it can be prepared and frozen, and it will cook perfectly if allowed to defrost first.

Ingredients

1.25 g parsnips or sweet potatoes

175 g plain flour

50 g parmesan cheese

Salt and freshly milled black pepper

1 Tbsp ground nut oil & a knob of butter

Method

1. Preheat the oven to 200°C.

2. Combine the flour, parmesan cheese, salt, and pepper in a mixing bowl. Peel the parsnips and cut them into half, then cut each half into four lengthways. Cut out some of the woody centres.

3. Now, pop the parsnips in a saucepan and pour in boiling salted water. Put on a lid, bring them to a boil, turn down the heat, and simmer for 3 minutes.

4. Meanwhile, have a large kitchen tray ready. As soon as you are ready, drain them in a colander. While they are still steaming, drop a few at a time (with some kitchen tongs) into the flour and parmesan mixture, shaking the bowl and moving them around to get a good, even coating.

5. As they are coated, transfer them to the tray. Ensure you do them all swiftly, as the flour mixture will only coat them while they are still steamy!

6. They are ready to cook, store in the refrigerator, or freeze when they're all coated. Any leftover flour and parmesan can be sifted and kept in the fridge or frozen for another time.

7. To bake them, place a large solid roasting tin in the oven to preheat, and in it, put enough groundnut oil to cover the base and a knob of butter for flavour. Then, when the oil is hot, remove the tin from the oven and quickly place the parsnips side by side in the tin.

8. Tilt the tin and baste all the parsnips with hot fat. Place the tin back in the oven and bake for 20 minutes. Then, turn the parsnips over, drain off any surplus fat, and continue to bake for 15-20 minutes or until they are crisp and golden.

If your roast potatoes are on the high shelf, these can be below on the lower shelf.

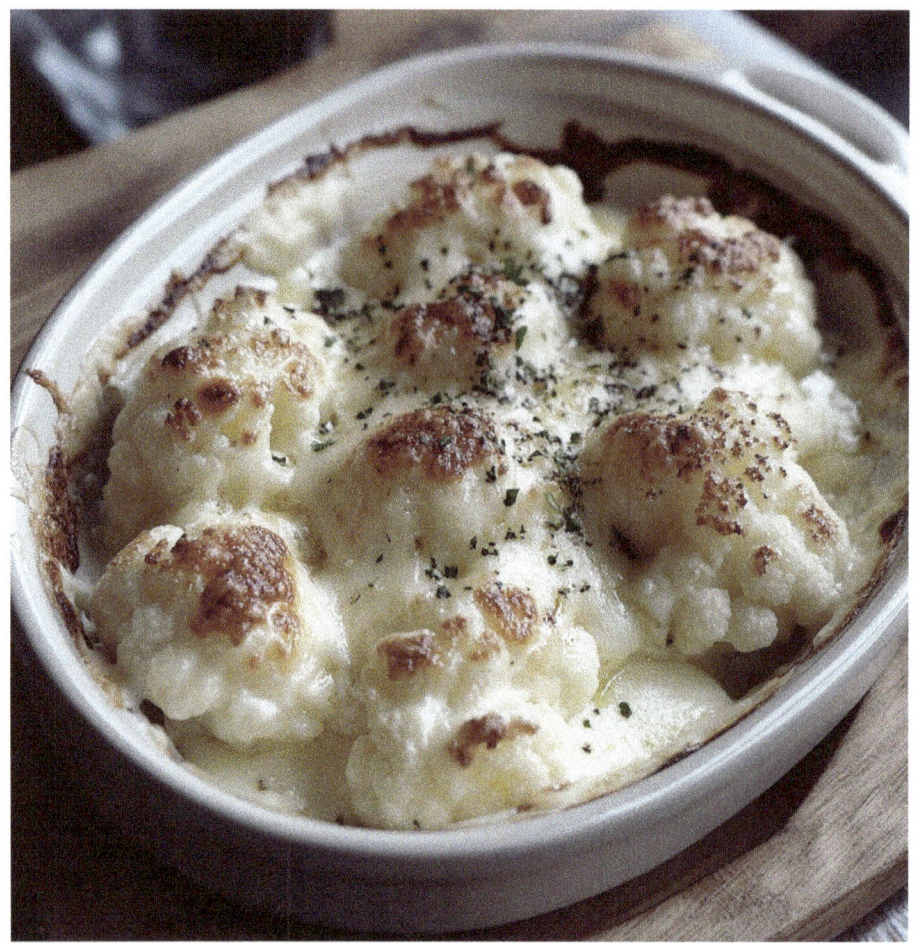

A Creamy, Golden Dream

A dish so bright, a sauce so bold,
A taste of warmth, a tale retold.
With Gruyère deep and mustard mild,
A comfort shared by kin and child.

The nutmeg hums, the crust glows bright,
A meal to grace the winter night.
So take a fork, embrace the cheer,
A dish that brings the heart sincere.

—*Inspired by Robert Louis Stevenson*

Perfect Cauliflower Cheese

Serves 4

Ingredients

1 head cauliflower, trimmed and broken into florets (broccoli can be used instead)

For the béchamel sauce

25 g butter

25 g plain flour

400 ml full-fat milk

Pinch English mustard powder

200 g gruyere cheese, grated

55 ml double cream

Salt and pepper

Pinch of nutmeg

For the topping

50 g parmesan cheese

Method

1. Preheat the oven to 180°C.

2. For the cauliflower, cook the florets in a large pan of boiling water for about 10 minutes or until tender. Drain and set aside.

3. Meanwhile, for the béchamel sauce, melt the butter in a clean saucepan and beat it in the flour until smooth. Slowly whisk in the milk until smooth, and then stir in the mustard powder, grated cheese and double cream. Keep stirring until the cheese has melted and the mixture is thick and creamy. Season to taste with salt and freshly ground pepper.

4. Place the cauliflower florets into an ovenproof casserole dish and pour over the cheesy sauce. Sprinkle over a pinch of freshly ground nutmeg.

5. Sprinkle over the parmesan cheese. Bake for 15 minutes or until the topping is golden brown and bubbling.

Vegetables

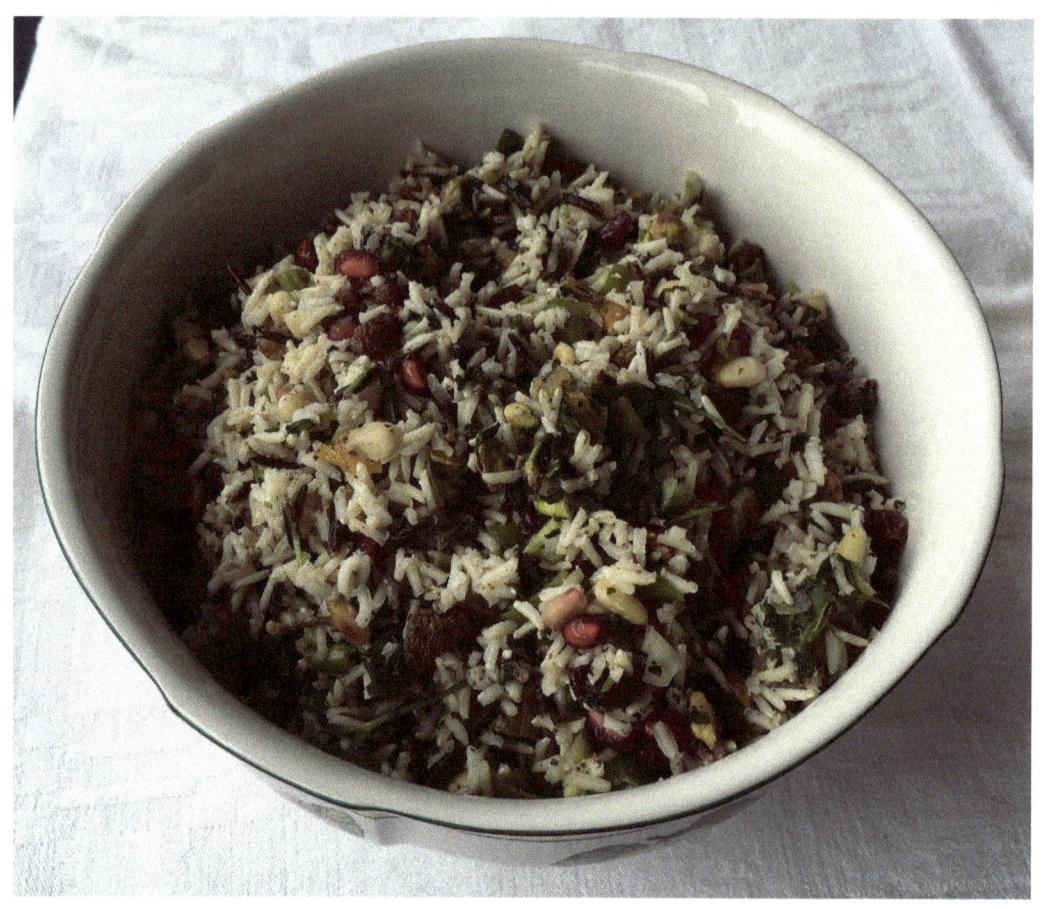

A Dance of Jewel and Grain

The rice stands light, the fruits shine bold,
A dish where East and West unfold.
With lemon bright and herbs so free,
A meal of sun and history.

The nuts do crunch, the spices twine,
A plate where taste and colour shine.
A bowl to share, a tale untold,
A feast where warmth and love take hold.

—*Inspired by Sir Walter Scott*

Persian Rice Salad

Serves 10

Ingredients

150 g basmati or other long-grain rice

75 g wild rice or red Camargue rice

2 Tbsp pine nuts

2 Tbsp pistachios or pecans

2 Tbsp flaked almonds

75 g sultanas

75 g dried apricots or dates, finely chopped

Seeds of 2 pomegranates, pith removed

4 spring onions, finely sliced

3 Tbsp flat-leafed parsley, chopped

2 Tbsp fresh coriander, chopped

2 tsp sumac powder (optional)

Zest of 2 lemons

Juice of 1 lemon

Sea salt and freshly ground black pepper

Method

1. Cook the different kinds of rice in separate pans of boiling salted water according to the instructions, and take care not to overcook. Drain the rice and refresh it under cold running water until cold.

2. Heat a deep frying pan or skillet. Add the pine nuts and toast, shaking them occasionally to prevent burning.

3. Mix the different kinds of rice and add the toasted pine nuts and all the other salad ingredients, seasoning to taste with salt and pepper.

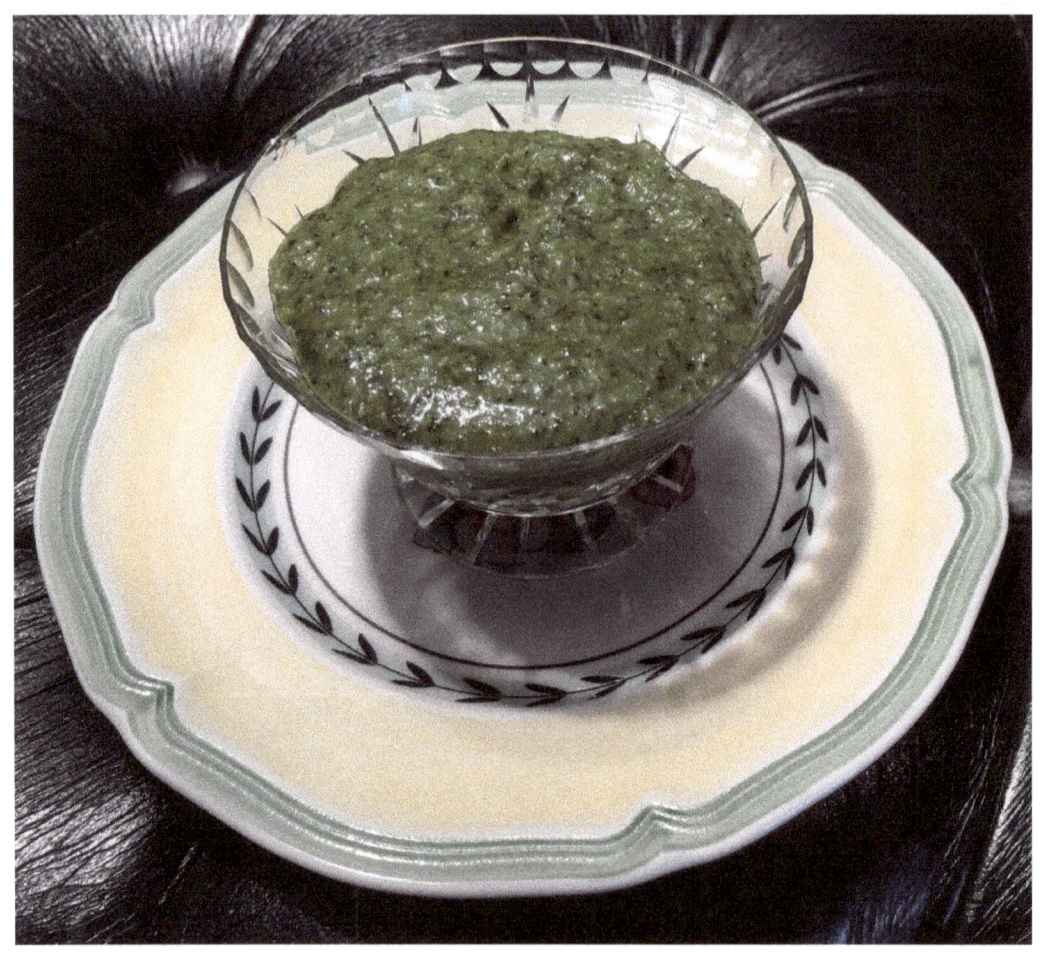

A Blend of Green and Gold

A crush of leaves, a swirl of bright,
A mix of boldness, rich yet light.
With garlic's hum and nuts so free,
A taste of summer's memory.
The oil runs deep, the cheese stands tall,
A spoonful brightens, softens all.
A touch of time, a simple grace,
A spread to warm the coldest place.

—*Inspired by Contemporary Scottish Poets*

Pesto

Ingredients

170 g basil leaves

100 g pine nuts

200ml extra virgin olive oil

5 g parsley

200 g parmesan cheese

5 extra large cloves

½ tsp salt

Method

1. Place the pine nuts into a food processor with 100ml olive oil. Blend until you have a smooth paste. Add the garlic and whiz until smooth.

2. Add the parmesan cheese with a little more olive oil if necessary. Blending well.

3. Add the basil leaves a handful at a time and blend well, adding the remaining olive oil.

4. Add the parsley and salt.

This should give you 5 portions.

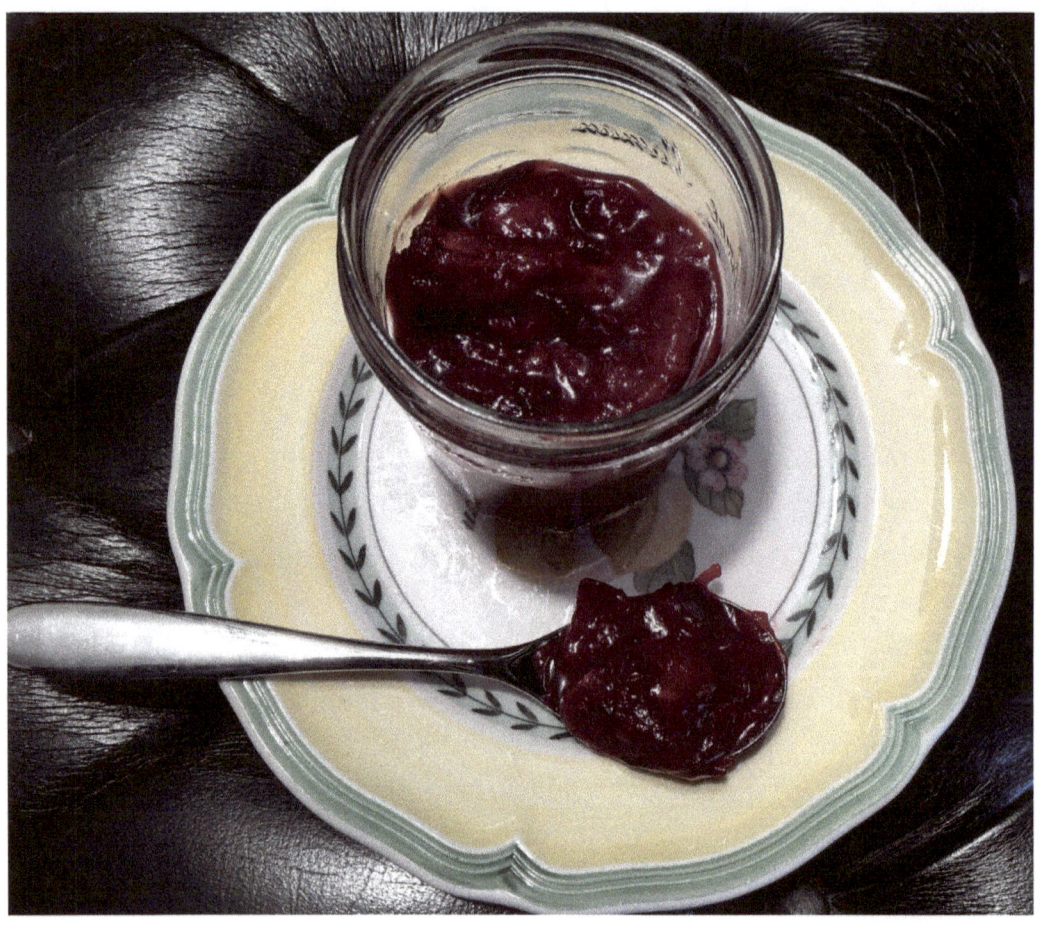

A Sweet and Tangy Dance

The plums fall ripe, the spices call,
A chutney rich, a feast for all.
With vinegar's bite and sugar's kiss,
A taste that lingers, bold yet bliss.
The cinnamon hums, the shallots blend,
A sauce where sweet and sharp suspend.
With meats or cheese, a touch so bright,
A jar of joy, both day and night.

—Inspired by Robert Louis Stevenson

Plum Chutney

Makes about 350 g, or 1 medium jar

Ingredients

500 g dark red plums

2 shallots chopped

1 Tbsp olive oil

100 ml white wine vinegar

3 Tbsp water

1 cinnamon stick

100 g Demerara sugar

Method

1. Cut the plums in half down the crease; twist the halves in opposite directions and pull them apart. Prise out the stones and discard them. Roughly chop the flesh.

2. Place the chopped shallots in a heavy-based saucepan with the oil and heat until sizzling. Sauté gently for 5 minutes until softened.

3. Add the plums, vinegar, water, cinnamon and sugar. Stir until the sugar is dissolved, then simmer for about 25 minutes, stirring occasionally, until softened and slightly thickened.

4. Meanwhile, preheat the oven to 130°C. Place a clean jam jar in the oven to warm. When the plum chutney is ready, spoon it into the jar. Seal it with a lid and leave to cool completely.

Vegetables

Flint Family Cookbook

Desert

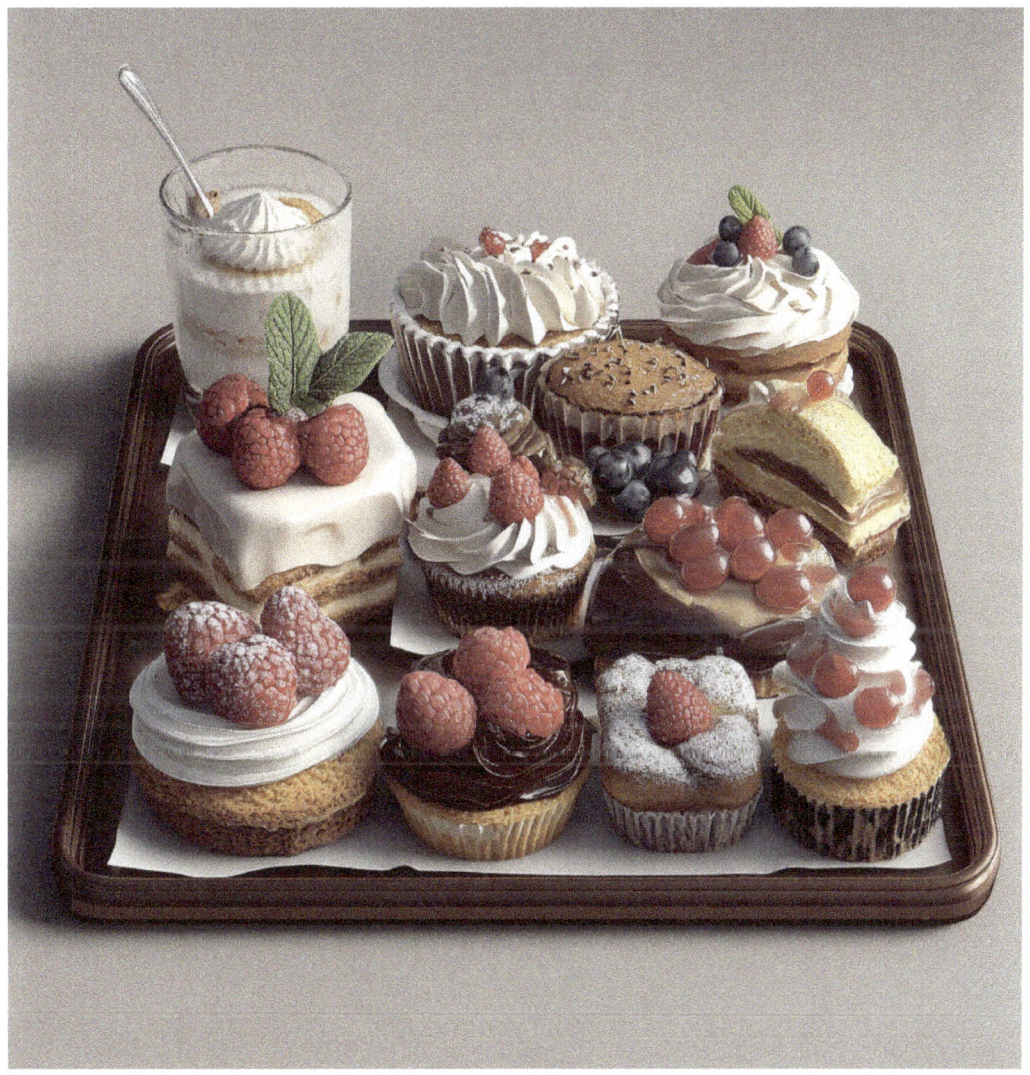

Desert

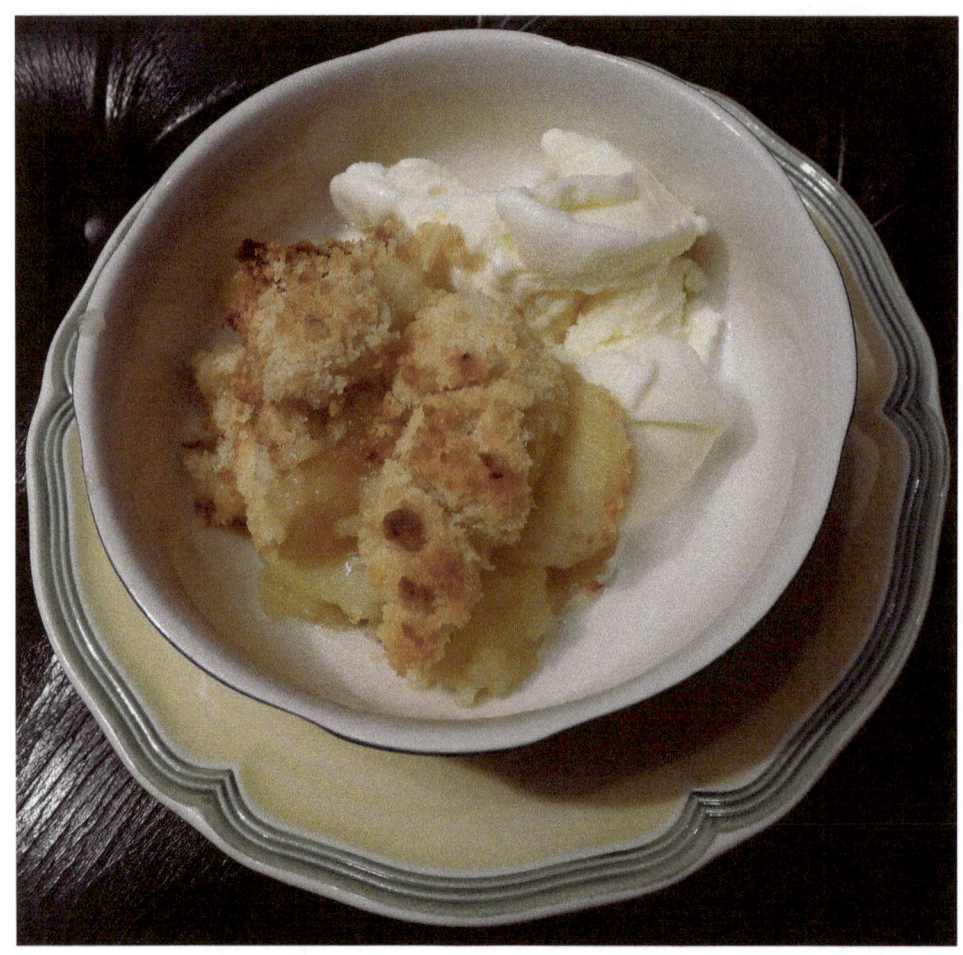

A Crumble's Warm Embrace

The apples stew, their scent runs deep,
Beneath a golden, sugared sweep.
The butter hums, the spice takes flight,
A dish to warm the coldest night.

A spoonful rich, a comfort pure,
A taste that makes all hearts secure.
With custard poured or cream so wide,
A simple joy, well satisfied.

—*Inspired by Robert Burns*

Apple Crumble

Serves 6

Ingredients

100 g butter

200 g plain flour

200 g caster sugar

750 g prepared fruit (sliced cooking apples peaches, rhubarb, plums or gooseberries)

Method

1. Add the butter and flour to one large bowl. Rub the butter into the flour until the mixture resembles fine breadcrumbs, and then stir in 100 g of sugar.
2. Mix the remaining sugar with the prepared fruit and put into a large pie dish.
3. Spoon the crumble mixture over the fruit and lightly press it down.
4. Bake at 180°C for about 45 minutes, until the fruit is soft.
5. Serve with custard or double cream.

Variations

1. Add sultanas to the apples.
2. Add 7 g ground ginger, mixed spice or cinnamon to the flour before rubbing in the fat.
3. Serve with custard or fresh cream.

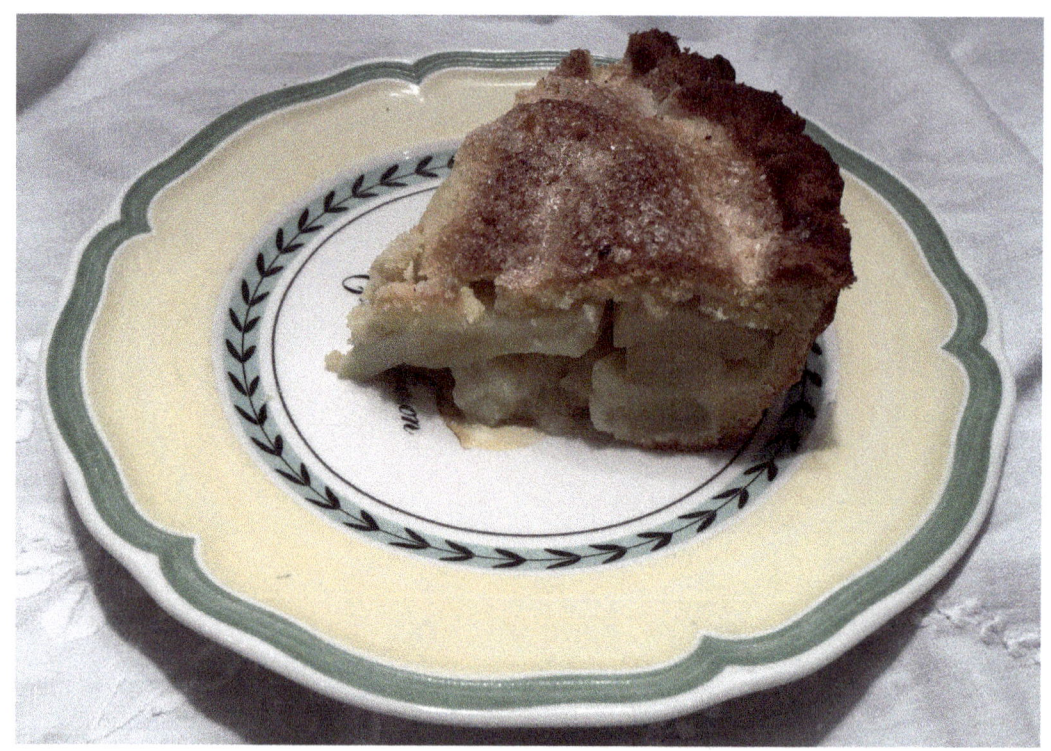

A Slice of Home

The crust stands tall, so crisp, so light,
A golden dome, a sweet delight.
The apples melt, the sugar sways,
A feast of love from bygone days.

With lemon bright and butter deep,
A dish that memory shall keep.
A slice, a sigh, a taste so true,
A pie that holds the past in view.

—Inspired by John Buchan

Apple Pie

Serves 8

Ingredients

For the pastry

300 g plain flour
Good pinch of salt
¾ tsp baking powder
3 Tbsp caster sugar
200 g unsalted butter, chilled and diced
Finely grated zest of 1 small lemon
1 medium free-range egg yolk
4 Tbsp milk

For the filling

50 g unsalted butter softened
3 Tbsp caster sugar
Plus, extra for sprinkling
Finely grated zest of 1 small lemon
1 Tbsp lemon juice
850 g dessert apple (about 8 medium)
If using Brambly apples, more sugar will be required, about 100 g
Makes 1 large apple pie
You will need a 1 x 26 cm pie plate or a deep oven-proof plate

Method

1. Put the flour, salt, baking powder and caster sugar into the bowl of a food processor and pulse a few times to mix the ingredients. Add the pieces of butter and run the machine until the mixture looks like fine breadcrumbs. Add the lemon zest and pulse a couple of times.

2. Mix the egg yolk with the milk. With the machine running, add the yolk mix through the feed tube. Stop the machine as soon as the dough comes together in a ball. If there are dry crumbs and the dough feels dry and hard, add more milk, a tsp at a time. (Alternatively, make the pastry by hand)

3. Turn out the dough, flatten it into a disc about 3 cm thick and wrap it in cling film. Chill for about 20 minutes until firm.

4. Meanwhile, make the filling. Put the soft butter, sugar, lemon zest, and juice in a bowl and beat with a wooden spoon until soft and creamy—don't worry if it looks a bit curdled. Set aside until needed.

5. Peel, core, and slice the apples into a mixing bowl. If you are using different varieties, make sure they are well mixed.

6. Heat the oven to 190°C and put a baking sheet in the oven to heat up.

7. Lightly dust the worktop and your rolling pin with flour. Cut off one-third of the pastry for the lid and roll out the rest to a circle about 1 cm larger than the pie dish.

Desert

8. Wrap the pastry loosely around the rolling pin and lift it over the pie dish. Unroll to drape over the dish, then flour your fingers and gently press the pastry onto the base and rim. Leave any excess pastry hanging over the rim for now.

9. Carefully arrange the apple slices in neat layers on the pastry, mounding them up and adding dabs of the butter mixture, evenly spaced, between each layer. If using cooking apples, add the extra sugar at this stage. Finish with a layer of apples, and leave the pastry rim clear of filling. Brush with cold water.

10. Roll out the rest of the pastry into a large circle to cover the mound of apples. Roll it around the pin and drape it over the pie. Gently but firmly press the pastry onto the dampened rim to seal the two layers together.

11. Use a sharp knife to trim off any pastry hanging over the rim of the plate.

12. With the back of a small knife, knock up the edge by making small horizontal cuts into the pastry rim so it looks like the pages of a book, Then scallop the pastry edge, place two fingers on the edge and gently draw a knife between them, continue doing this all the way round.

13. Cut a small slit or steam hole in the centre of the pastry lid. If you like, gather up the pastry trimmings, re-roll and cut out leaves; stick them onto the pie lid with a dab of water. Lightly brush the pastry with water and sprinkle with sugar.

14. Set the pie on the heated baking tray in the oven and bake for about 20 minutes until the pastry starts to colour. Turn down the oven to 180°C and bake for 20-25 minutes until the pastry is golden.

15. Leave to cool for 15 minutes, then serve with custard or ice cream. If there are any leftovers, gently warm them before serving so that the buttery filling starts to melt again.

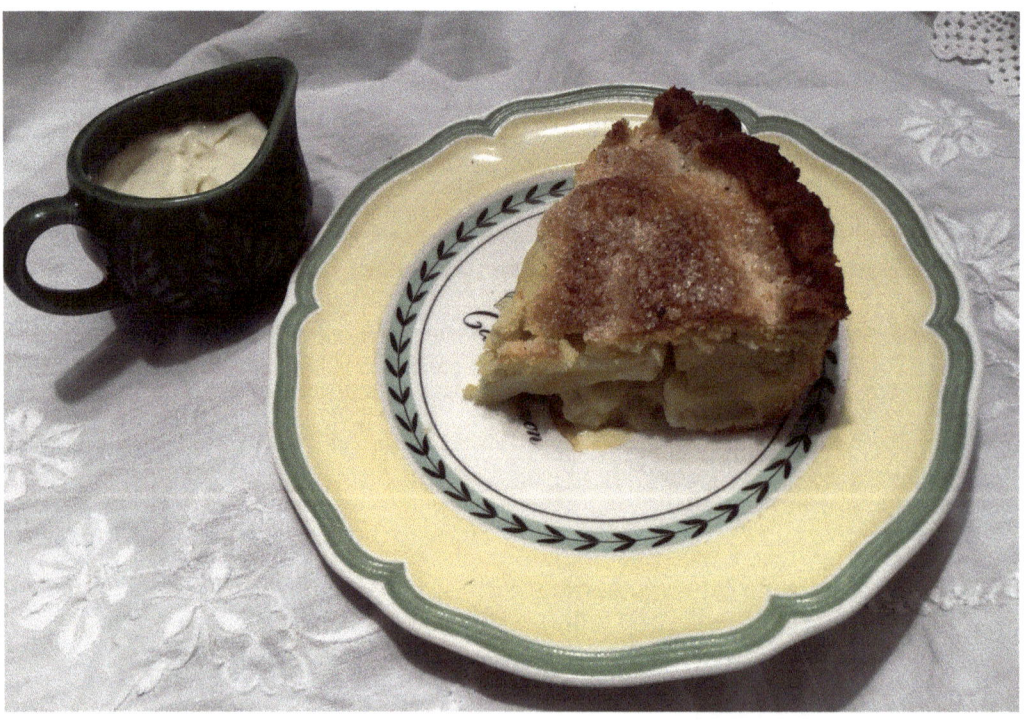

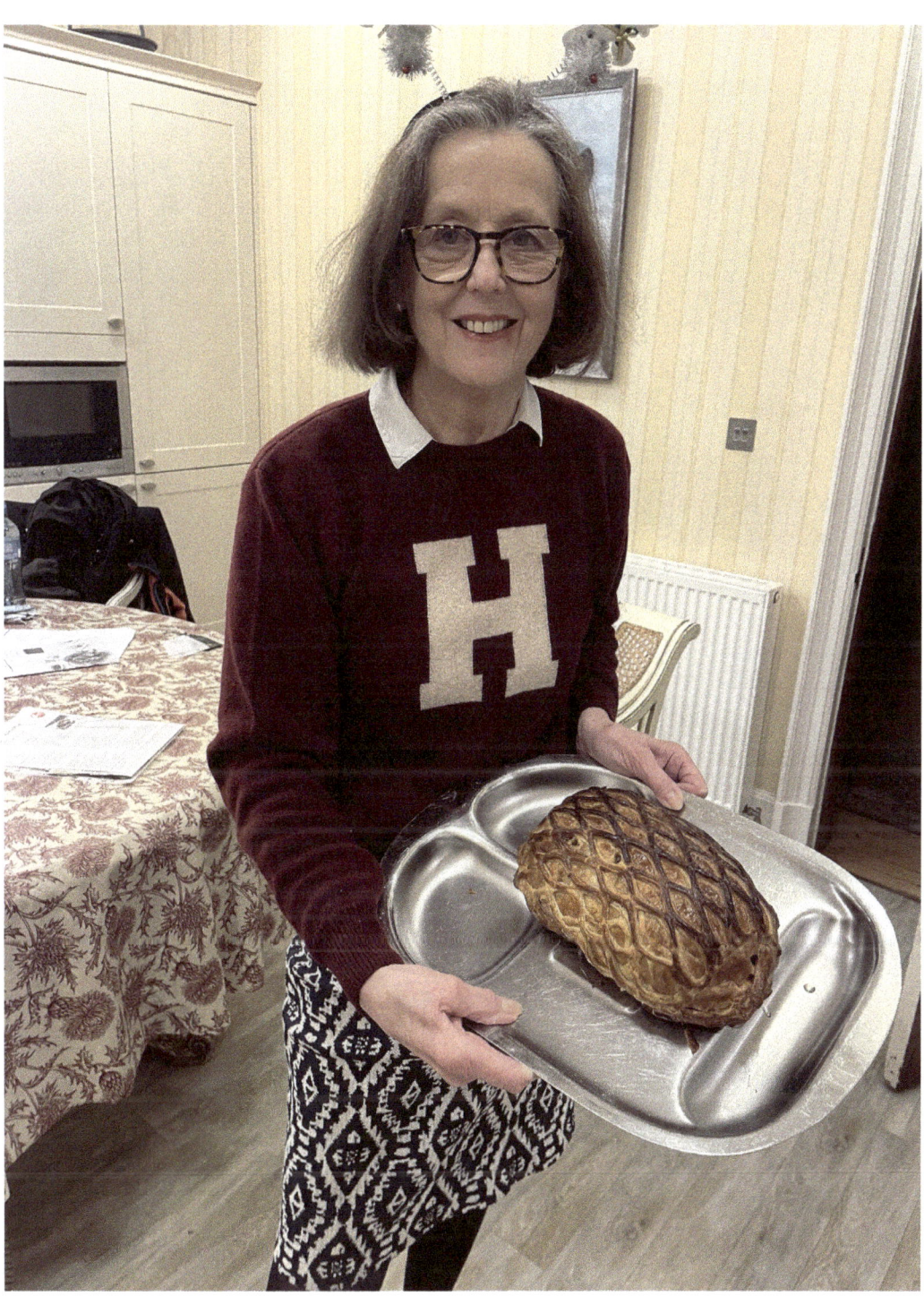

Desert

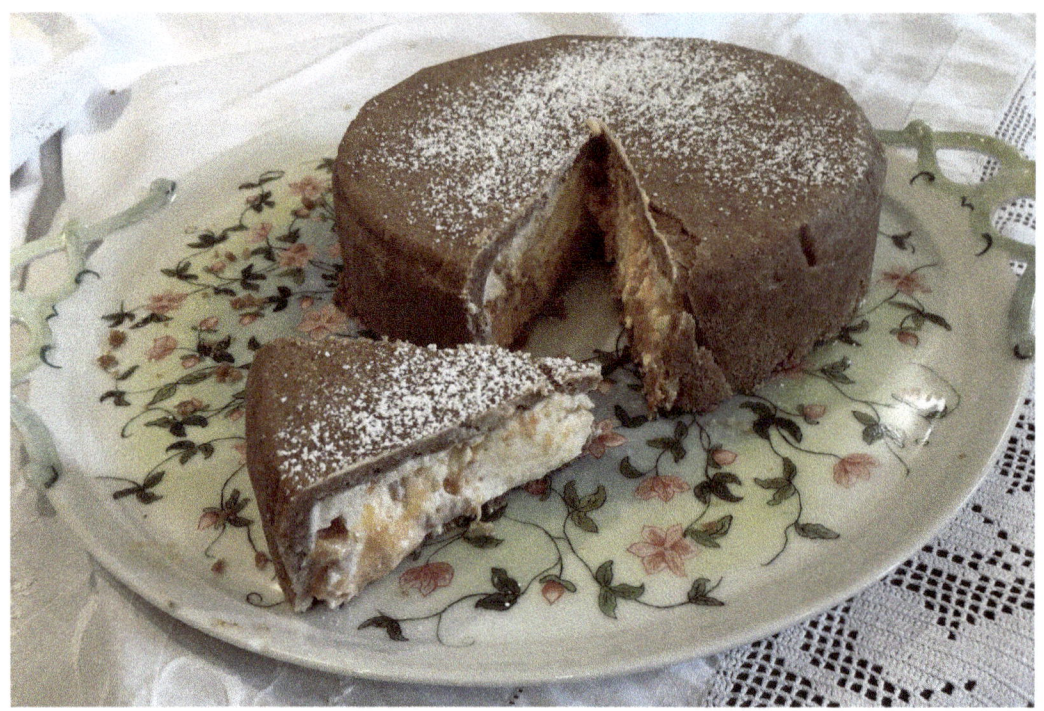

A Bite of Summer's Glow

The biscuit hums, the cream stands bright,
A golden fruit in softened light.
With apricots both tart and sweet,
A dish where sun and sweetness meet.

A swirl, a spoon, a flavour bold,
A taste of summer's warmth retold.
A slice to lift, to shine, to cheer,
A treat to bring the heart sincere.

—*Inspired by Contemporary Scottish Poets*

Apricot Cheesecake

Serves 10-12

Ingredients

450 g fresh apricots

75 g granulated sugar

350 g digestive biscuits

175 g butter

5 ml (1 level tsp) ground mixed spice

50 g caster sugar

5 sheets gelatine

225 g cream cheese

225 ml double cream, lightly whipped

Grated rind of 1 lemon

397 g (14 fluid oz) can condensed milk

Icing sugar

Method

1. Grease and line the base of a 21.5 cm spring-release tin. Halve and stone the apricots and poach gently in sugar syrup and 200 ml water. Do not overcook the apricots, as they will become too soft. Drain and cool, then cut into small cubes.

2. Finely crush the biscuits. Melt the fat and stir in the biscuit crumbs, spice, and sugar. Use three-quarters of the crumbs to line the base and sides of the prepared tin. Set in the refrigerator for 30 minutes.

3. Add the grated lemon rind and place it to one side. Prepare the gelatine according to the instructions.

4. Blend together the rind, cheese, condensed milk, sugar, double cream, and cooled gelatine until smooth. Gently fold in the chopped apricots. Pour everything into the crumb case, sprinkle the remaining crumbs over the top, and refrigerate overnight.

5. Turn out upside down and dredge heavily with sifted icing sugar.

Desert

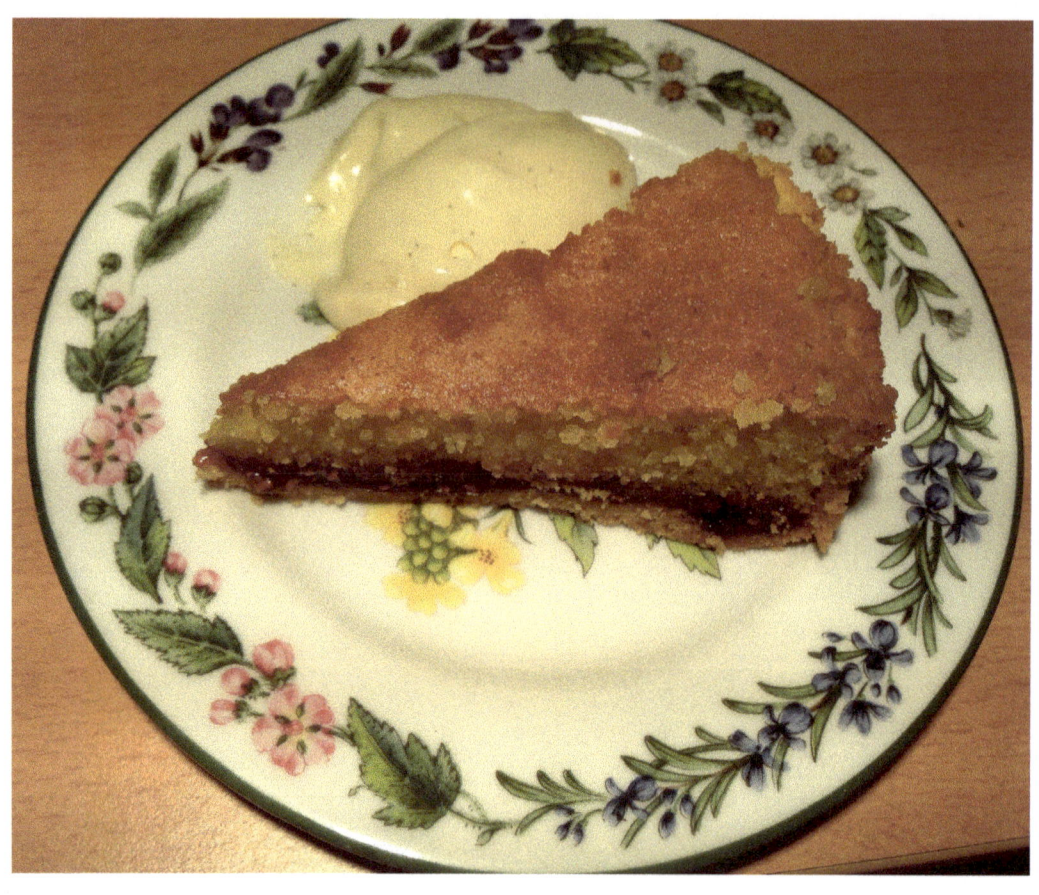

A Tale in Almond Gold

A pastry crisp, a jam so bright,
A touch of almonds, soft yet light.
The oven hums, the sugar sways,
A treat to mark the finest days.

With custard rich or cream so fair,
A dish to savour, sweet and rare.
A taste of home, a joy so free,
A slice of love in history.

—Inspired by Robert Louis Stevenson

Bakewell Tart

Old fashion method

Serves 6-8

Method

Sweet short-crust pastry (see pastry recipe)

3-4 Tbsp raspberry jam

75 g butter

75 g caster sugar

150 g cake crumbs

75 g ground almonds

3 medium eggs

Juice ½ a lemon

Method

1. Line the base of a pie dish with the sweet pastry; spread the bottom of the dish with jam. Keep the pastry trimmings, roll them into a long pencil shape, twist them, and put them to one side.
2. Cream the butter and sugar well; add the yolks a little at a time. Then add the almonds, cake crumbs, and lemon juice and mix together.
3. Stiffly beat the egg whites and gently fold them into the cake mixture. Spread over the jam and bake in an oven at 170°C for about 40 minutes. Remove from the oven, place the pastry twists on top of the tart, and cook for 15-20 minutes.
4. Serve with ice cream, cream or custard.

Desert

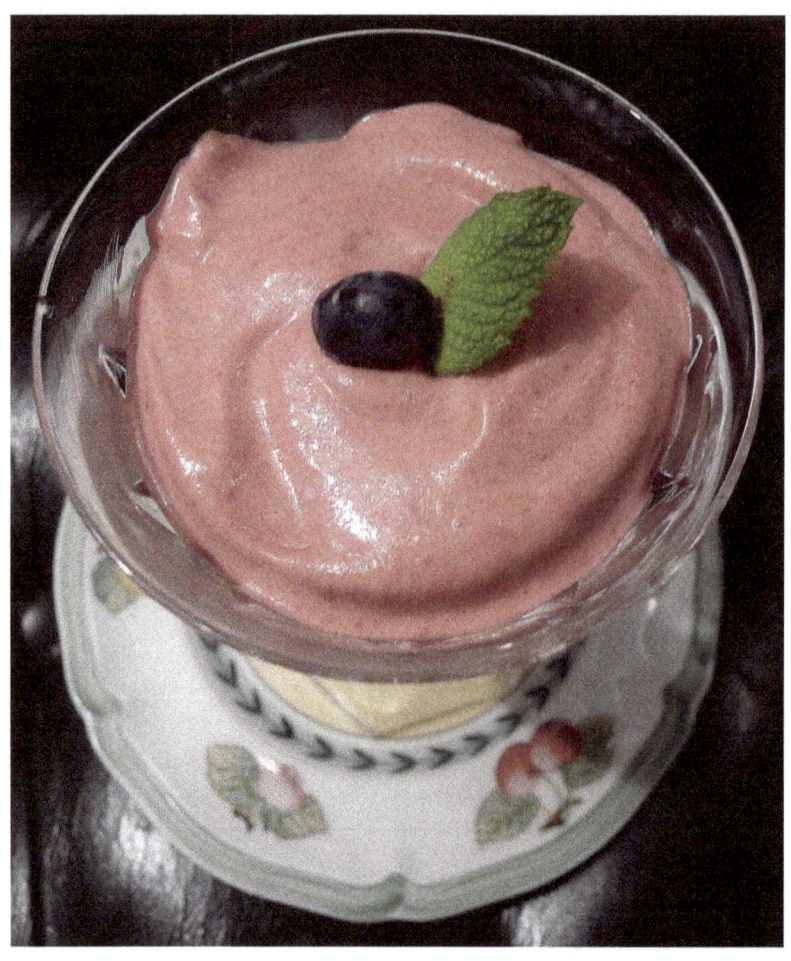

A Cloud of Purple Light

A berry's kiss, a sugar's cheer,
A taste of summer's fleeting year.
With cream so light and tart so sweet,
A dish where fruit and velvet meet.

A swirl, a sigh, a mousse so fair,
A touch of colour, light as air.
A spoonful rich, a dream untold,
A taste of brightness, soft yet bold.

—Inspired by Contemporary Scottish Poets

Blackcurrant Mousse

Serves 6

Ingredients

600 g blackcurrant, cleaned

75 g caster sugar

2-3 Tbsp of caster sugar, to sweeten

1 Tbsp of lemon juice

300 ml double cream

1 egg white

3 egg yolks

Method

1. Rinse the blackcurrants in a colander to remove dust or dirt. Put the blackcurrants in a pan and sprinkle over the 75 g of caster sugar.

2. Stir in the lemon juice and heat gently for two minutes or until the blackberries soften and release their juices. Remove and reserve 12 blackcurrants for decorations and continue cooking the rest.

3. Simmer the blackcurrants gently for 15 minutes, stirring regularly until soft and squidgy. Remove from the heat and press the berries and juice through a sieve over a bowl, using the bottom of a ladle to help you extract as much of the puree as possible. Leave the puree to cool and discard the seeds. You should end up with 300-325 ml of puree. Leave to cool completely.

4. Put the cream in a large bowl and whip with an electric whisk until soft peaks form. When the whisk is removed from the bowl, the fruit's acidity will thicken the cream further. Fold into the blackcurrant puree.

5. Place the egg yolks and sugar into a mixing bowl and beat on full speed for 5 minutes until thick and light yellow in colour. Fold into the puree.

6. Finally, whip the egg white until the soft peak stage, and add to the puree.

7. Divide between 6 bowls or one large bowl.

8. Place in the fridge overnight.

9. Decorate with a blob of cream, mint leaf and blackcurrant.

Desert

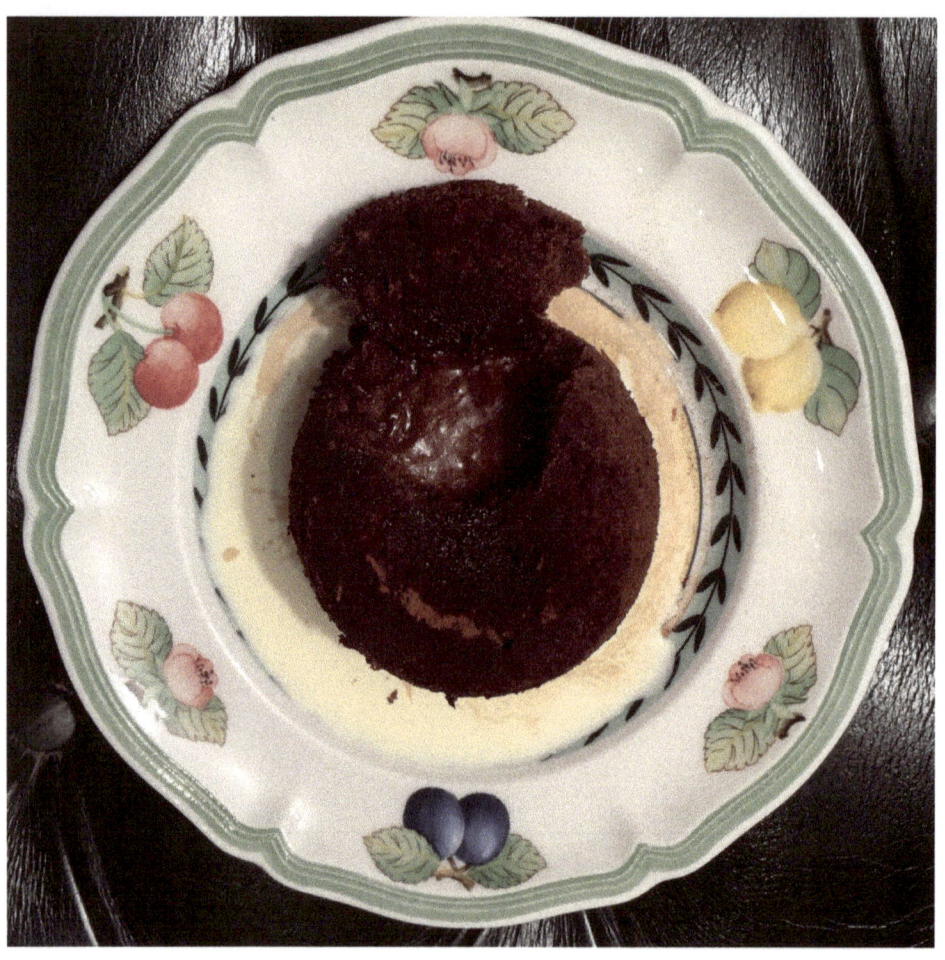

210

A Heart of Hidden Fire

A bite so crisp, a heart so bright,
Where cocoa melts in molten light.
The spoon dips deep, the richness flows,
A warmth that only chocolate knows.

A dish of depth, of silk, of cheer,
A taste to bring delight so clear.
A moment hushed, a pause so free,
A dream of chocolate ecstasy.

—Inspired by Robert Louis Stevenson

Chocolate Fondant

Serves 2

Ingredients

50 g unsalted butter, plus extra, softened, for greasing

1 Tbsp cocoa powder, sieved, for dusting

50 g dark chocolate (70% cocoa solids) chopped into small chunks

1 egg, plus 1 egg yolk

25 g caster sugar

1 heaped Tbsp plain flour

Method

1. Preheat the oven to 200°C.

2. Grease 2 x 150 ml dariole moulds. Add the cocoa powder to one and then transfer it to the other, turning it as you go until the mould is evenly coated. Repeat with the other mould, discarding the excess cocoa.

3. Melt the chocolate and the butter together in a bowl set over a pan of barely simmering water (or in a microwave, in short bursts) with a pinch of salt. Stir to combine and set aside to cool briefly.

4. Using electric beaters, whisk together the egg, egg yolk, and sugar until tripled in volume. It should hold a trail for 2-3 seconds.

5. Sift over the flour and gently fold in. Add a little of the egg mixture to the melted chocolate, then, in two batches, carefully fold in the remainder.

6. Divide the mixture between the moulds, cleaning the edges with kitchen paper if needed.

7. Bake in the oven for 10 minutes, until well risen and a crust has formed on the top. They should still have a slight wobble. Turn out onto plates and serve at once, dusted with cocoa powder.

Make ahead. The prepared fondants can be kept in the fridge, covered tightly with cling film, up to 24 hours in advance. Bake from chilled, as per the recipe.

Desert

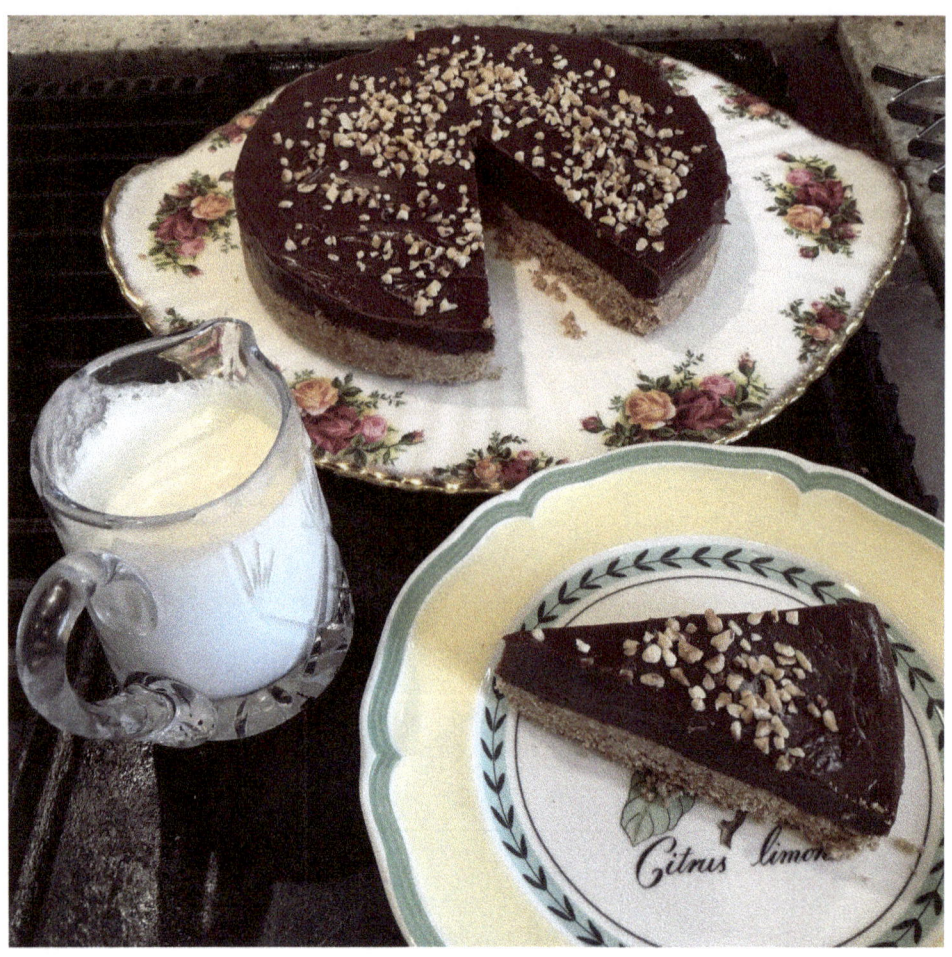

A Nutty, Silken Dream

A base so firm, a top so light,
A swirl of chocolate, rich yet bright.
The hazelnuts do softly crunch,
A taste that lingers past the lunch.

A feast of silk, a treat so wide,
A slice of joy, a bite with pride.
With hands held high and plates set near,
A dish to bring the heart sincere.

—Inspired by John Buchan

Chocolate Hazelnut Cheesecake

Serves 8-12

Ingredients

250 g digestive biscuits

75 g soft unsalted butter

400 g jar Nutella or equivalent chocolate nut spread at room temperature

100 g chopped toasted hazelnuts

500 g cream cheese at room temperature

60 g icing sugar, sifted

22 cm springform cake tin

Method

1. Break the biscuits into the bowl of a food processor. Add the butter and 1 Tbsp (15 ml) of the Nutella and blitz until the mixture starts to clump. Add 25 g of the toasted hazelnuts and pulse until you have a damp, sandy mixture.

2. Tip this into your springform tin and press it into the base, either using your hands or the back of a spoon. Place in the fridge to chill while you prepare the filling.

3. Beat together the cream cheese and icing sugar until smooth and soft. Then, patiently scrape the rest of the Nutella out of its jar into the cream cheese mixture and continue beating until combined.

4. Take the springform tin out of the fridge. Carefully scrape and smooth the Nutella mixture over the biscuit base, scattering the remaining hazelnuts on top to cover. Place the tin in the fridge for at least 4 hours or overnight.

5. For best results, serve straight from the fridge. Just before you eat, up-spring the cake from the tin, still on its base. To cut it, dip a sharp knife in cold water, wiping and dipping again between each cut.

You could slide it off the base if you are feeling confident.

Desert

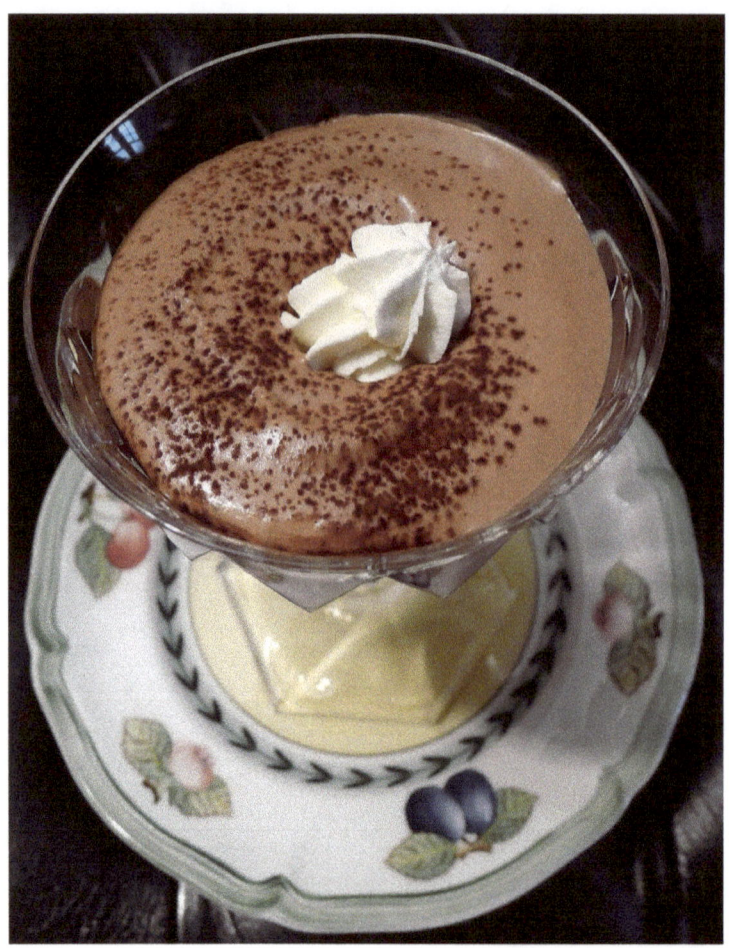

Chocolate Rum Mousse

A Whispered Indulgence
A velvet bite, a touch so bold,
A sip of warmth, a tale retold.
The chocolate sways, the rum hums near,
A dish to bring both joy and cheer.

A spoonful rich, a dream so bright,
A taste that lingers through the night.
A feast of silk, of depth, of grace,
A mousse where time and flavour trace.

—Inspired by Contemporary Scottish Poets

Chocolate Rum Mousse

Serve 6

Ingredients

100 g plain chocolate

150 g milk chocolate

3 egg yolks

1 egg white whisked to soft peak stage

1 tsp vanilla essence

2 level tsp espresso coffee (dissolved in 1 Tbsp hot water)

300 ml double cream

2 Tbsp dark rum

Method

1. Slowly melt the 2 chocolates in the top of a double saucepan over low heat.
2. Remove from the heat and allow to cool.
3. Beat the egg yolks lightly. To this add the rum, coffee and vanilla essence. Then gently mix into the melted chocolate.
4. Whip the cream until reasonably thick, and fold into the chocolate mixture.
5. Beat egg white until stiff and fold into the mixture.
6. Pour mixture into a serving dish. Chill for at least 2 hours or, better still, overnight.
7. To serve, sprinkle with cocoa powder and a swirl of whipped cream.

This is a medium set. For a lighter chocolate mousse, add 2 egg whites.

Desert

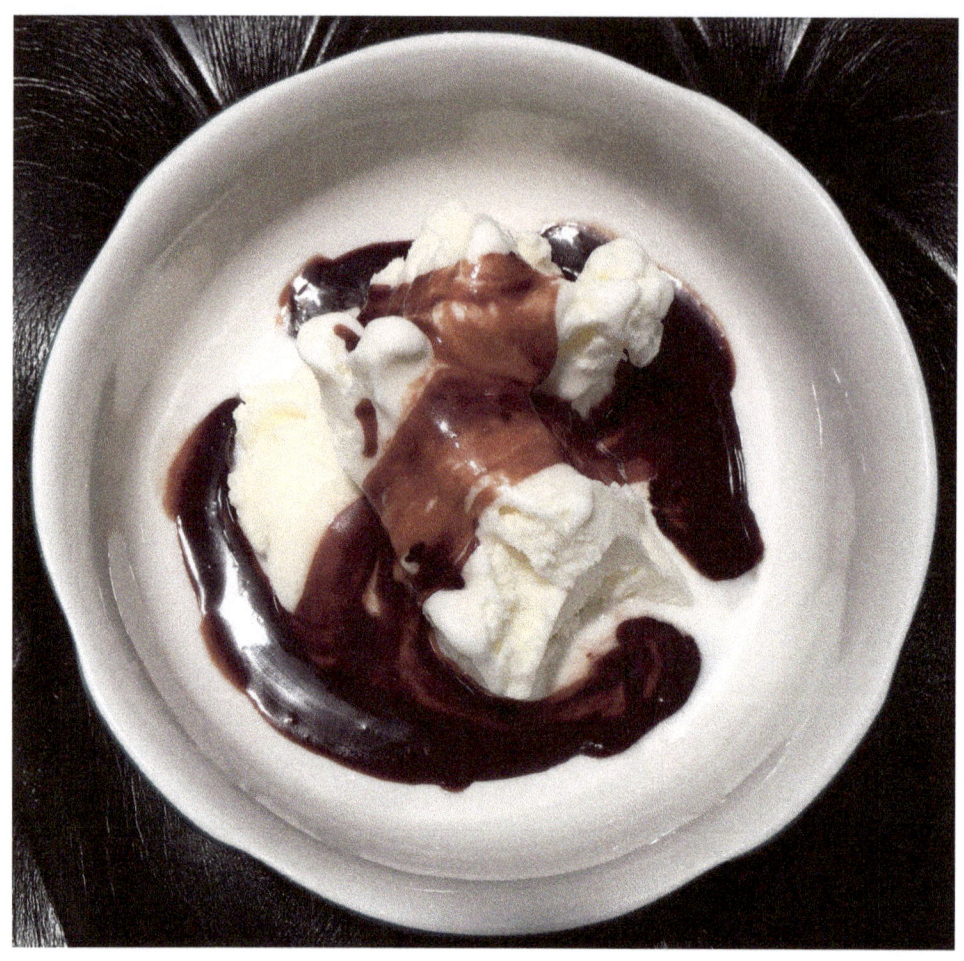

A Stream of Sweet Delight

A golden swirl, a velvet pour,
A sauce of bliss and nothing more.
The butter hums, the cocoa sighs,
A treat that makes the spirit rise.

With syrup rich and cream so light,
A drizzle warm, a pure delight.
Upon the ice, it melts away,
A taste to sweeten any day.

—Inspired by Robert Louis Stevenson

Chocolate Sauce

Serves 2-3

Ingredients

40 g butter
2 Tbsp syrup
2 Tbsp cocoa powder
2 Tbsp cream
Ice Cream

Method

1. Melt the butter over a low heat. Add the cocoa powder and syrup. When blended, add the cream and pour it over the ice cream.

Dad's favourite recipe!

Desert

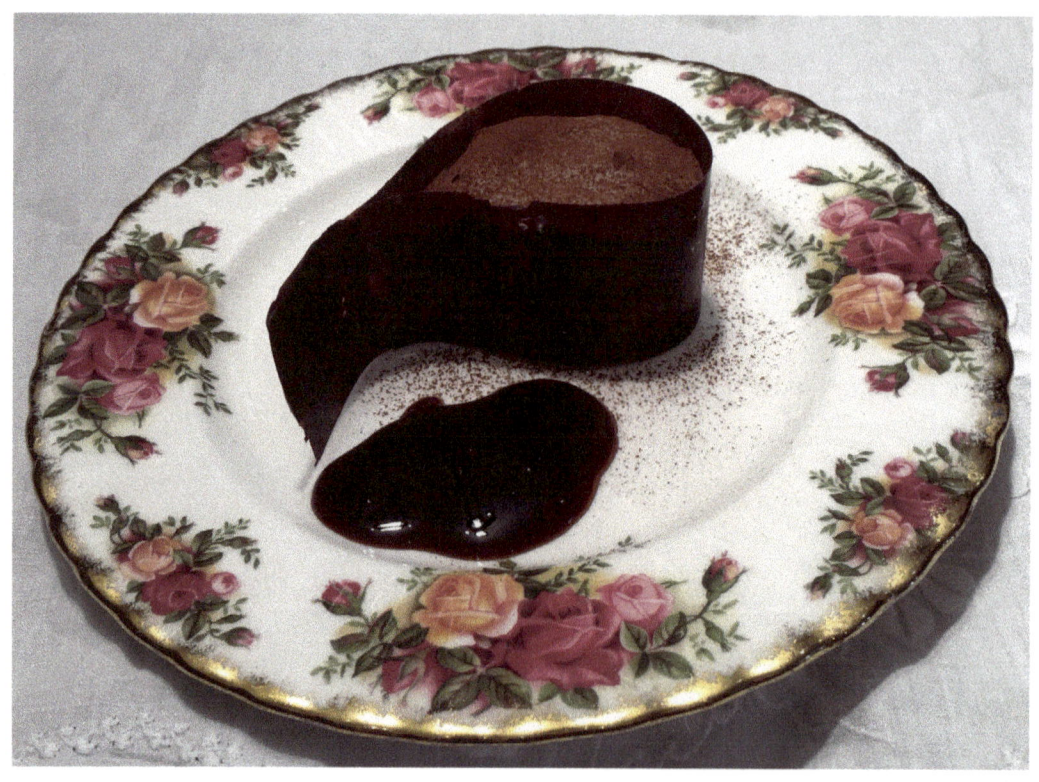

A Teardrop Rich with Cocoa Dreams

A whisper dark, a satin gleam,
A mousse so light, a cocoa dream.
A careful hand, a tempered grace,
A chocolate tear in perfect place.

With wine so deep and sauce so fine,
A taste that lingers, bold like time.
A spoon, a sigh, a bite so bright,
A gift of chocolate, pure delight.

—*Inspired by John Buchan*

Chocolate Tears

Serves 8-10

Ingredients

For the chocolate collar

175 g Menier plain chocolate

Mousse

175 g Bourneville plain chocolate

275 ml double cream chilled

2 eggs, size 2, separated

1 Tbsp of caster sugar

1 Tbsp of cocoa powder

Sauce

300 ml Banyuls or Maderia wine

50 ml unsweetened prune juice

2 level tsp of arrowroot

Method

1. Line a tray with a sheet of silicone paper

2. Break the Menier chocolate into a bowl and melt over a pan of gently simmering water.

3. Stir now and again, and when it is completely smooth remove it from the pan.

4. Do not overheat or the chocolate will become dull and dry.

5. Lay a strip of celluloid, 4 x 26 cm on a flat surface and spread one-eighth of the chocolate thinly over the entire surface using a palette knife.

6. Without damaging the surface, carefully lift it onto its side and curve it into a teardrop shape so that the two ends meet, chocolate sides touching for about an inch of their length. Slide the ends together so that they match perfectly.

7. Holding the two edges together, lift the teardrop and transfer it onto the silicone paper-lined tray. Ease it into a tear shape. Repeat with the others and refrigerate.

8. Break the chocolate into a bowl for the mousse and add 2 tablespoons of the double cream. Set the bowl over a pan of simmering water and let it melt. When smooth, remove the bowl from the heat and let it cool for a minute or two.

9. Separate the egg whites and yolks, placing the whites into a spotlessly clean bowl. Mix the yolks thoroughly into the chocolate, and then allow to cool.

10. Using an electric hand-held mixer or balloon whisk, beat the egg whites until stiff. Gently but thoroughly fold the whipped egg whites into the chocolate mixture.

Desert

11. Pour the remaining cream into the empty bowl and beat until stiff. Gently but thoroughly fold it into the chocolate mixture.

12. Remove the teardrop from the refrigerator. Fit a piping bag with a large plain nozzle. Fill the piping bag with the chocolate mousse, close it, and pipe it into the chocolate shells. Do not grasp the piping bag around the mousse, as the heat of your hand will soften it.

13. Smooth the top of the mousse with a palette knife, so it is level with the chocolate shell—Refrigerate, preferably overnight.

14. To make the sauce, place the Banyuls in a pan, bring it to a boil, and let it ignite by lighting it with a match or shaking it over a gas flame. Let it burn itself out, and then reduce its volume by half.

15. Add the prune juice and simmer until 210 ml remain.

16. Place the arrowroot in a small container, add 2 or 3 teaspoons of cold water, and mix together until smooth. Pour a little hot liquid onto it, stir, and pour into the pan. Stirring constantly, bring back to the boil and simmer for a few minutes. Pour into a bowl and allow to cool. Cover when cold.

17. To serve, dust the tops of the teardrops with sieved cocoa powder. Gently remove each one from the Bakewell paper, then, starting at one corner of the plastic strip, carefully peel it away.

18. Transfer the chocolate to a serving plate. Hold the chocolate with another piece of clean plastic to avoid spoiling it with fingerprints.

19. Spoon a little sauce beside the inner curve. Serve immediately.

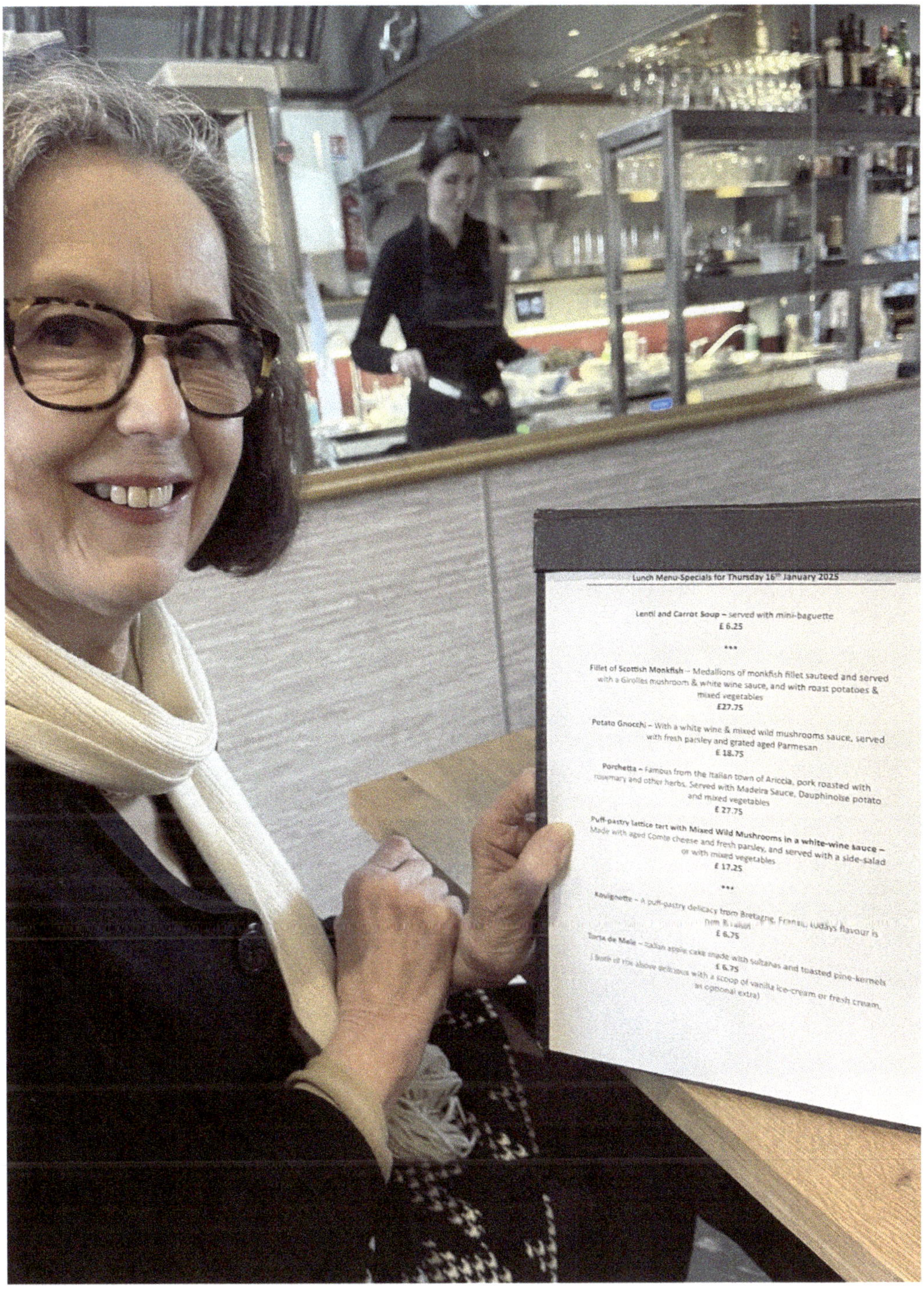

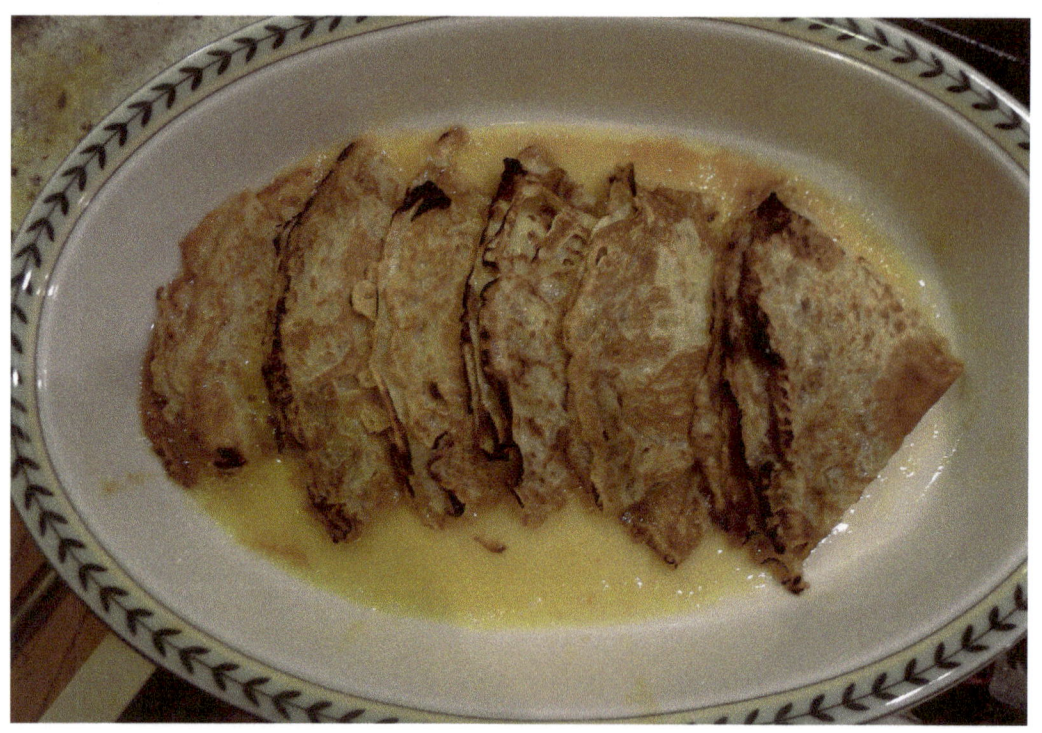

A Dance of Fire and Citrus

The orange glows, the butter sings,
A crepe that waltzes as it clings.
The liqueur flares, the sugar sways,
A dish to mark the finest days.

A flame, a cheer, a fork held high,
A taste that makes the spirits fly.
A moment bright, a citrus tune,
A plate of joy beneath the moon.

—Inspired by Robert Burns

Crepes Suzette

Serves 8

Ingredients

For the crepes

165 g plain flour

1 Tbsp caster sugar

Finely grated zest of 1 medium orange

3 large eggs beaten

300 ml whole milk

100 ml water

1½ Tbsp of butter & 1½ Tbsp of vegetable oil for frying

Filling

125 g butter, cut into small cubes

125 g icing sugar sieved

Grated rind of 1 orange

4 Tbsp brandy/or orange liqueur

For the sauce

Juice of 2 medium oranges (5 fluid oz), plus grated rind of one orange and strips of orange for garnish

Juice and finely grated zest of 1 lemon

2 Tbsp caster sugar

2 Tbsp Cointreau or Grand Marnier

1 Tbsp of Brandy to ignite the crepes

Method

1. First, make the crepes. Stir the sieved flour, sugar, and orange zest in a mixing bowl. Make a well in the centre, add the eggs, and mix with a spoon, gradually adding the milk. When all the milk has been incorporated, beat the mixture for 2 minutes until smooth.

2. Now melt the butter in a small saucepan, add this to the mixture and pour into a jug.

3. Heat a small amount of vegetable oil in a heavy-based frying pan or deep pancake pan until hot. Pour a little batter, tilting the pan to coat the base as thinly as possible. When the batter turns slightly darker and feels firm, flip it over with a large palette knife to cook the other side. Transfer the crepe to a warm plate, cover with cling film or a large saucepan lid, and continue with the remaining batter to make 16 crepes.

4. After each pancake, coat the pan with a thin lining of oil.

To make the filling

1. Put the butter and icing sugar in a food processor and cream together. Then, slowly, tsp by tsp, add the brandy or orange liqueur.

Desert

2. Spread out the pancakes and divide the buttercream evenly between them. Spread it out to make a thin covering over each pancake, and fold each in half, then in half again, to form a triangle.

3. Butter a large oven-proof dish and arrange the triangles to overlap in it. (If you are going to freeze, cover it with foil or cling film. Defrost overnight in the fridge.

4. When ready, put the dish in a low oven at 130°C for 20 minutes or until the buttery filling has melted. Meanwhile, make the sauce.

5. To make the sauce

6. Mix the orange and lemon juice, lemon zest, and 2 tablespoons of liqueur in a pan with the sugar. Heat gently over low heat until the sugar has dissolved, and then bring to a boil.

7. Pour the sauce over the pancakes. Take 1 Tbsp of brandy in a ladle, heat on the gas burner set alight, and pour over the crepes. Serve immediately; blow out the flames if the pancakes are becoming too scorched.

8. Serve with cream or ice cream.

The crepes can be made (to the end of step 6) several hours ahead of serving.

Flint Family Cookbook

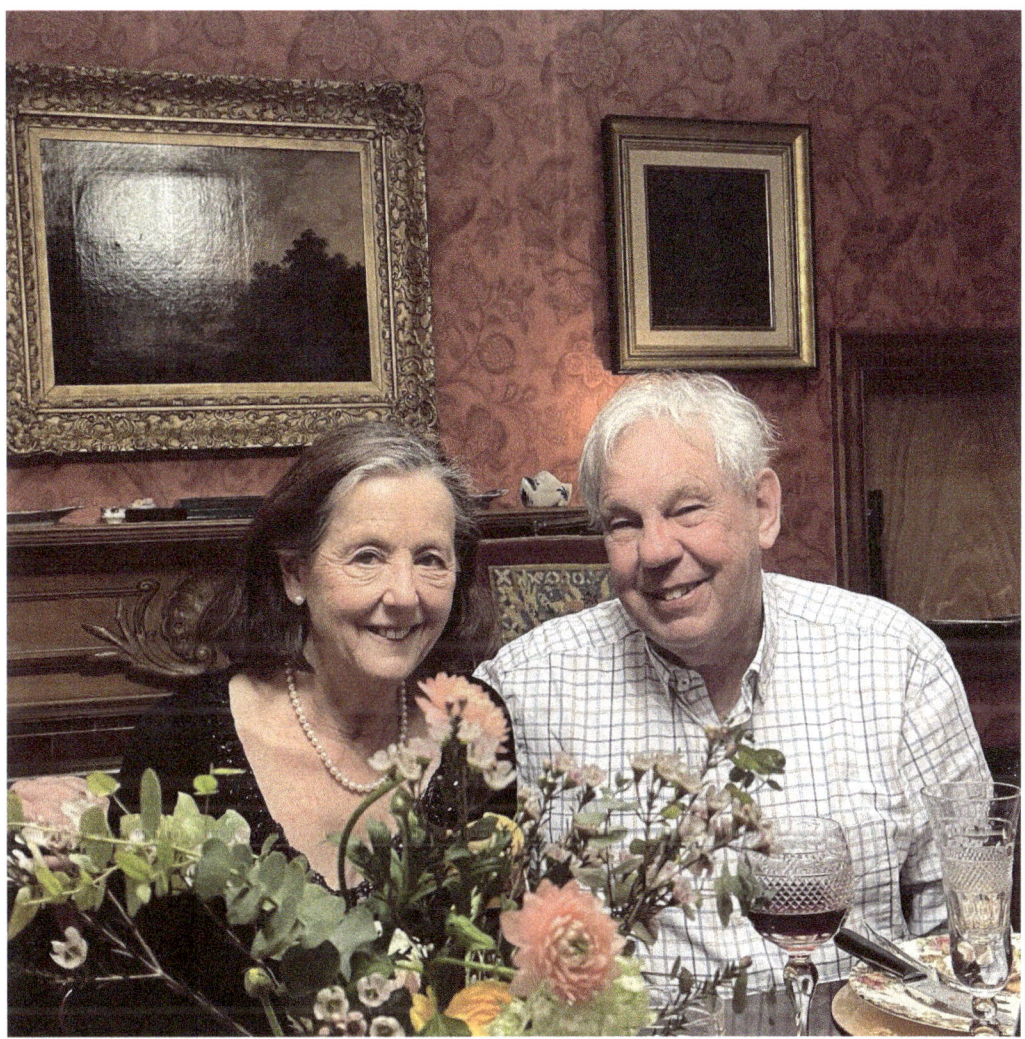

Desert

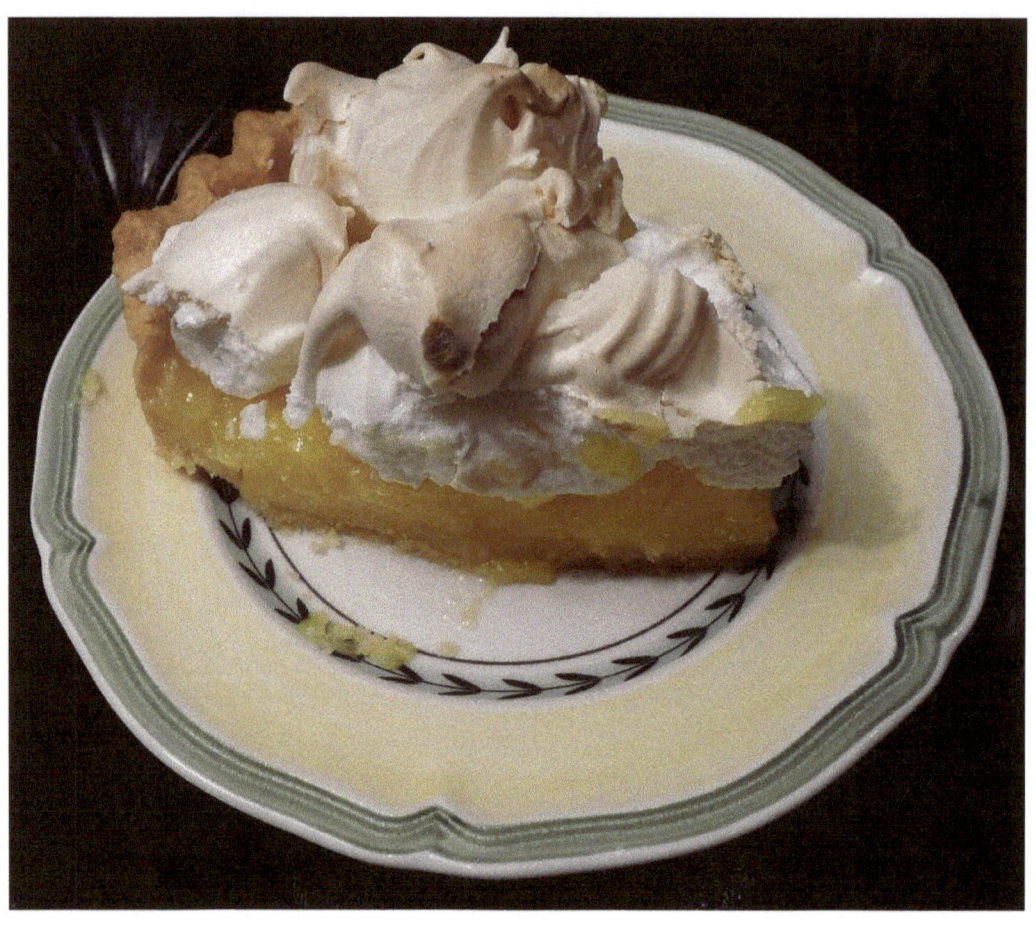

226

A Sky of Soft and Gold

A golden crust, a lemon bright,
A peak of white like clouds in flight.
The tartness hums, the sugar sways,
A dish of sun and golden days.

A bite, a cheer, a dream so wide,
A pie where sweetness melts inside.
A taste of light, a sigh so free,
A treat where joy and tart agree.

—*Inspired by John Buchan*

Lemon Meringue Pie

Serves 8

Ingredients

Sweet pastry
200 g plain flour
125 g cold butter
1 egg
2 tsp caster sugar

Lemon Filling
50 g cornflour
276 ml (10 fluid oz) cold water
200 g caster sugar
4-5 large lemons / 276 ml (10 fluid oz), zest and juice
4 free-range egg yolks
40 g butter

For the meringue topping
5 free-range egg whites
285 g caster sugar

Method

1. Preheat the oven to 200°C.
2. Make the pastry by placing the plain flour in a food processor, adding the cold butter, and whizzing until it resembles fine breadcrumbs. Add the egg with the caster sugar to the flour mix. Whizz until it begins to come together. Tip out of the food processor and lightly bring together. Shape into a round disc and wrap in baking paper for 30 minutes to relax.
3. On a lightly floured work surface, roll out the pastry to the thickness of a pound coin. Grease a 20cm-diameter shallow loose base-bottom tin. Line the tin with the pastry. Prick the bottom with a fork, line it with greaseproof paper, and fill it with baking beans. Chill for 30 minutes.
4. Place the pastry in the centre of the oven and bake for 15 minutes. Remove the paper and beans and continue to bake for 5-10 minutes or until the pastry has become dry but not coloured. Remove from the oven and allow the pastry to cool completely.
5. Reduce the oven temperature to 150°C. Mix the cornflour into a smooth paste with enough cold water to make a thin paste, then set aside. Pour the remaining water, lemon juice, zest and sugar into a large pan and gently heat, stirring until the sugar dissolves.
6. Add the cornflour paste, increase the heat, boil, and cook for about 1 minute, stirring continuously, until smooth and thick. Lower the heat and cook for three minutes until thick and glossy.
7. Add the butter and stir until melted. Stir in the egg yolks and mix vigorously. Pour the filling into the cooked pastry case and level the surface.

Desert

8. In a large bowl, whisk the egg whites until stiff peaks form. Then, gradually whisk in the sugar, a Tbsp at a time, until thick and glossy. Spoon the meringue over the filling, leaving only the rim of the pastry case uncovered.

9. Bake for 25-35 minutes until the meringue is golden and crisp. Do not overcook; you can always use a blow torch to finish browning the meringue. Leave to cool before removing it from the tin. Serve cold.

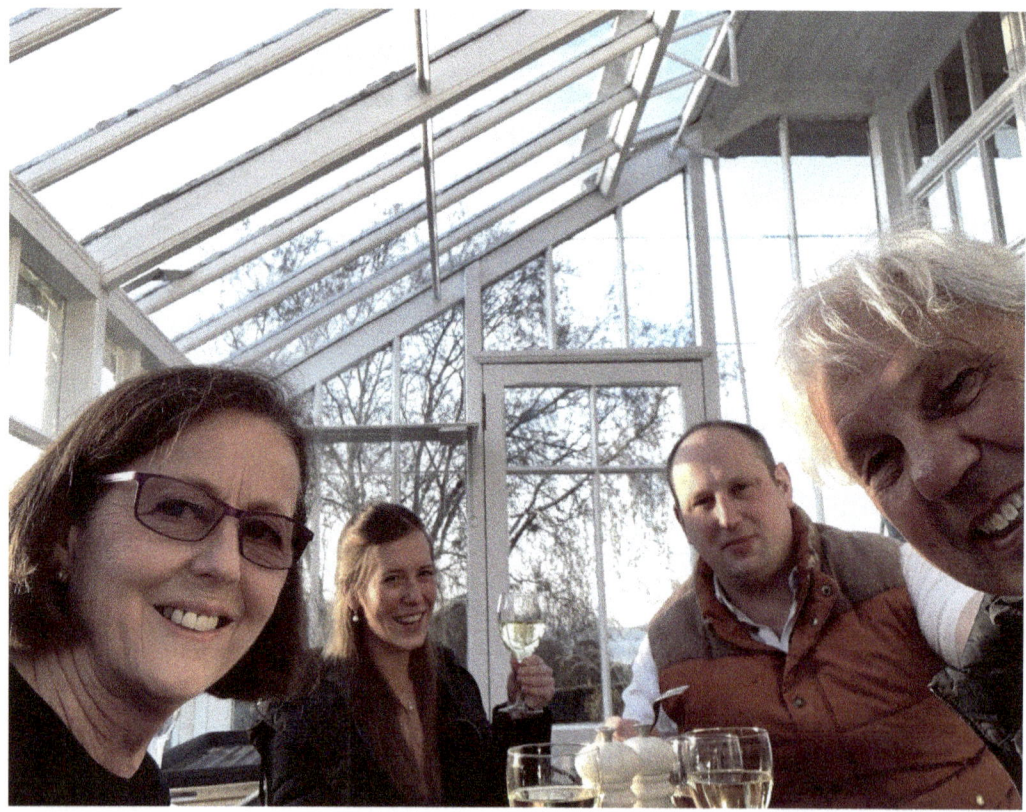

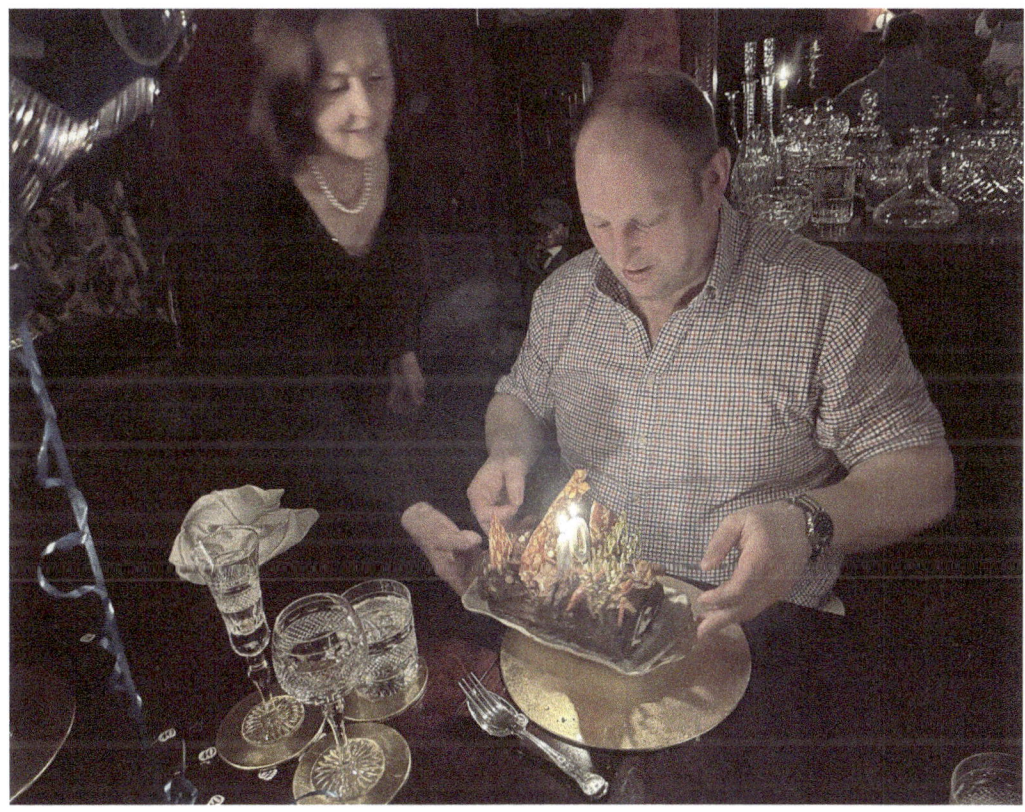

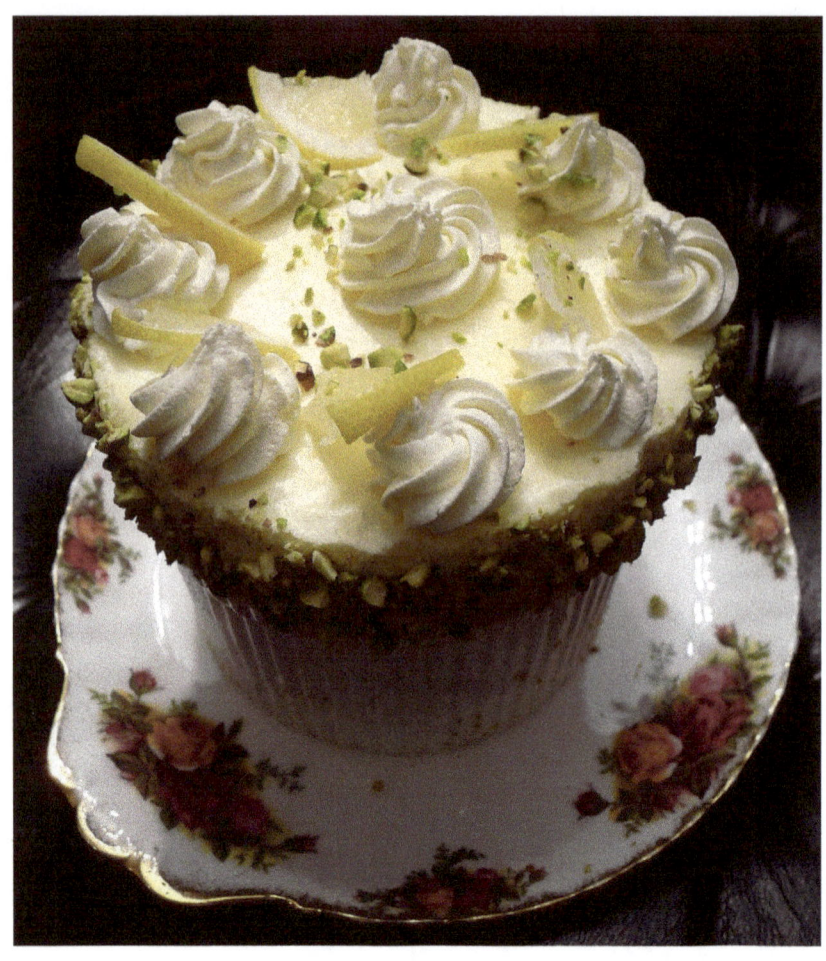

A Cloud of Citrus Light

A whisper soft, a golden glow,
A soufflé light as drifting snow.
With lemon bright and sugar sweet,
A dream upon the tongue to meet.

A spoon, a sigh, a breath so free,
A taste of sky and memory.
With pistachio's touch and cream so wide,
A dish where simple joys reside.

—Inspired by Robert Louis Stevenson

Lemon Soufflé

Serves 6-8

This needs to be made 24 hours in advance.

Ingredients

3 lemons
4 sheets of platinum leaf gelatine
4 eggs, medium, separated
125 g caster sugar
450 ml double cream

Decoration
50 g pistachio nuts finely chopped
2 thinly sliced pieces of lemon, each cut into 4
50 g pistachio nuts
150 ml double cream lightly whipped

Method

1. First, prepare the soufflé dish. Cut a strip of double greaseproof paper long enough to fit around the outside of a 900 ml (1½pt) soufflé dish and deep enough to stand about 7.5 cm(3") above the top.
2. Tie tightly with string so that the paper is held firmly around the dish and will not allow the mixture to run out.
3. Finely grate the rinds of the lemons and place them in a large bowl.
4. Squeeze the juice from the lemons and strain into a small basin.
5. Add the egg yolks and sugar to the lemon rind, beating with an electric whisk for about 8 minutes until the mixture is thick, mousse-like, and lightens in colour.
6. Soften the leaf gelatine in water as per the instructions on the packet.
7. Remove the softened gelatine from the water and gently squeeze. Add to the lemon juice and gently warm. Let it cool and then gently add to the mousse mixture.
8. Lightly whip 450 ml of double cream until it holds its shape. Gently fold into the mousse mixture with a large wooden spoon.
9. Whisk the egg whites until they flop over in soft peaks. Stir one large spoonful at a time into the mousse mixture this will lighten the texture.
10. Pour the mixture slowly into the dish. Gently shake the soufflé dish to level the surface.
11. Refrigerate overnight.
12. Using a palette knife, carefully ease the paper away from the sides of the soufflé. Hold the knife blade against the greaseproof paper to stop the soufflé from tearing, then gently ease away the paper.

Desert

13. Whip the remaining cream until it holds its shape. Spoon into a piping bag fitted with a 1 cm star nozzle.

14. To decorate, chop the pistachio nuts and gently press them around the soufflé edges. Pipe 8 stars on top and place a piece of lemon rind next to each star.

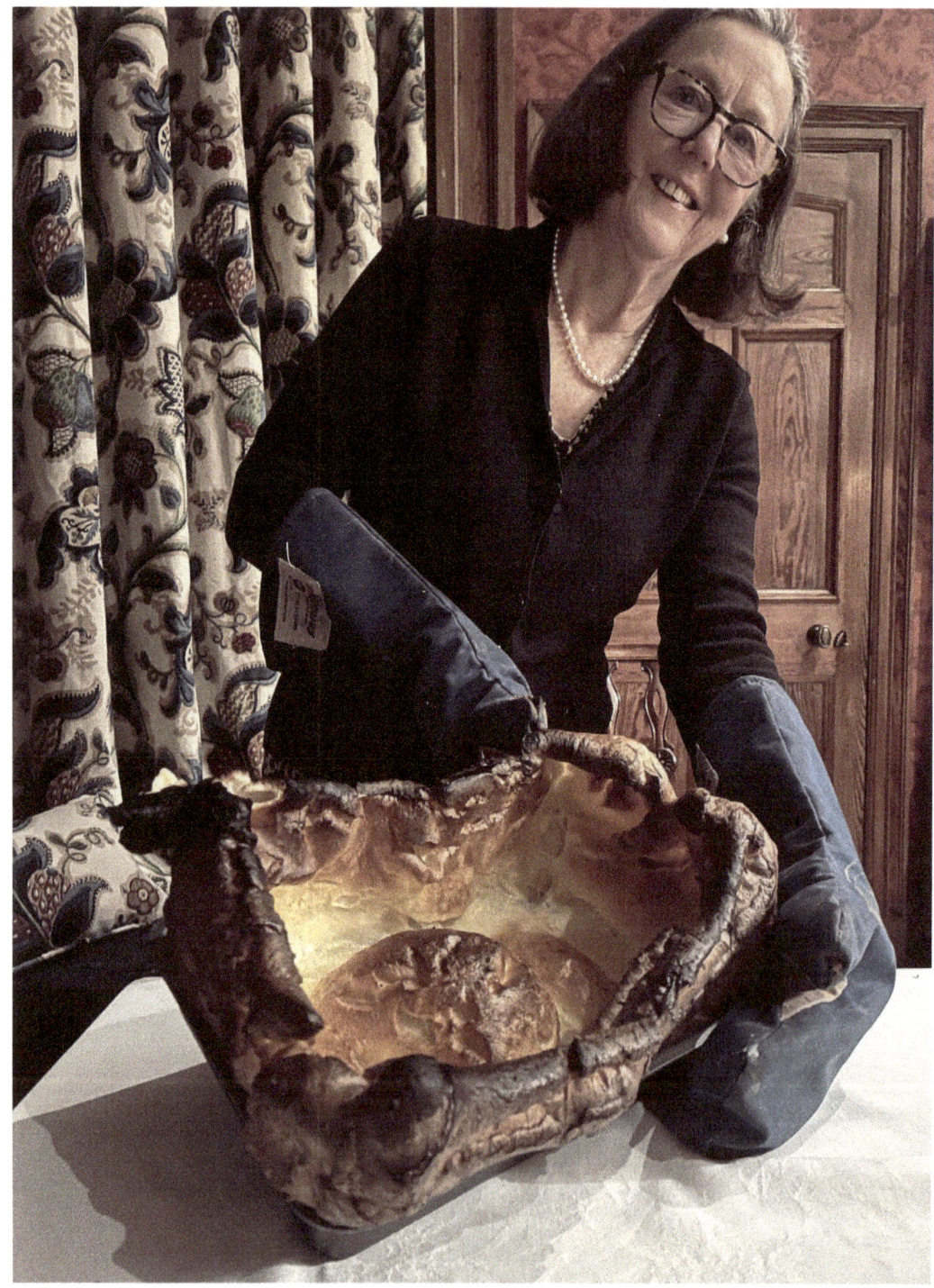

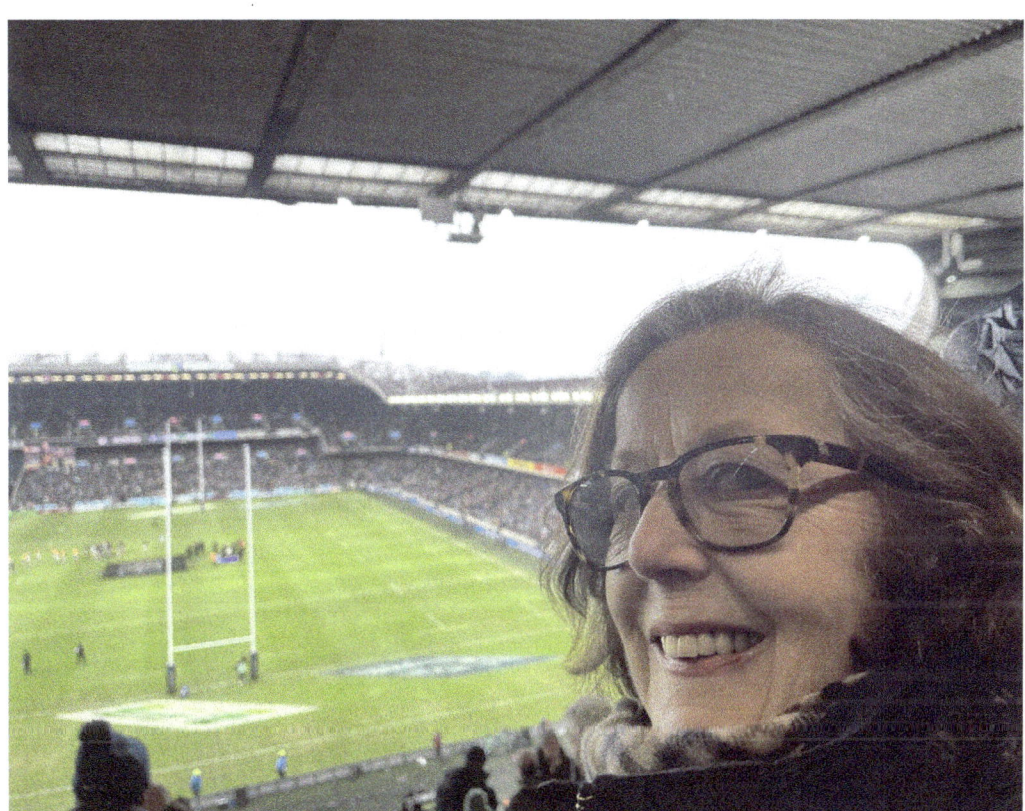

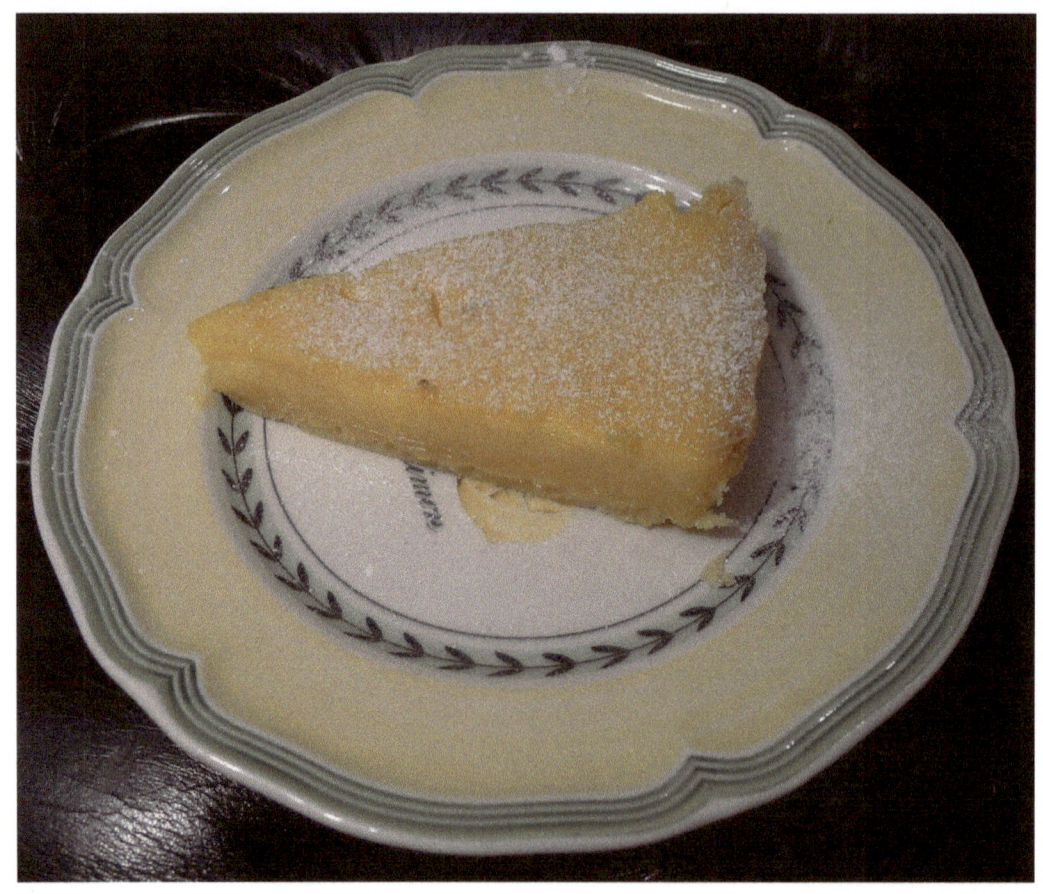

A Slice of Sun

The crust stands crisp, the lemon sings,
A golden wave where sharpness clings.
With sugar's kiss and citrus bright,
A bite of pure and sweet delight.

The oven hums, the filling sways,
A tart to mark the finest days.
With dust of sugar, light and free,
A taste of sun for you and me.

—*Inspired by John Buchan*

Lemon Tart

Serves 6-8

Ingredients

Sweet Pastry

200 g (7 oz) plain flour

125 g (4½ oz) cold butter, cut into chunks

1 Tbps golden caster sugar

1 egg, beaten

Filling

6 free-range eggs

250 g (9 oz) golden caster sugar

3-5 waxed lemons, finely grated zest of 3 and juice of all strained (170 g, 6 fluid oz)

150 ml carton double cream

Icing sugar for serving

Method

1. Preheat the oven to 190°C / Gas 5 /Fan oven to 170°C and put the mixture on a baking sheet.

2. To make the pastry, place the flour, sugar, and butter in a food processor and pulse until the mixture resembles fine bread crumbs. With the motor running, gradually add the beaten egg and blend until the mixture forms a ball. Do not over-blend, or the pastry will be tough.

3. Tip onto a floured board, knead briefly, then roll out to a 5mm thickness, regularly turning the pastry and flouring the surface. Use it to line the prepared tin. Trim the edges neatly, prick the base lightly with a fork, and chill for 30 minutes.

4. Meanwhile, use a wooden spoon to beat the eggs one at a time in a large bowl. Add the sugar until well blended, and then stir in the lemon and zest juice. Leave to stand.

5. Cover the pastry with greaseproof paper and baking beans. After 10 minutes, remove the beans and greaseproof paper and return the pastry to the oven for another 10-12 minutes until the base is cooked. Remove the pastry and reduce the heat to 120°C.

6. Meanwhile, strain the filling, skim off the surface froth, and gently stir in the cream. Slowly pour into the case. If you have a sliding oven shelf, this can be done with the tart still on it. Bake until barely set, with a slight wobble in the centre, 30-35 minutes. Cool for at least 45 minutes.

7. Serve the same day with a light dusting of sifted icing sugar.

Desert

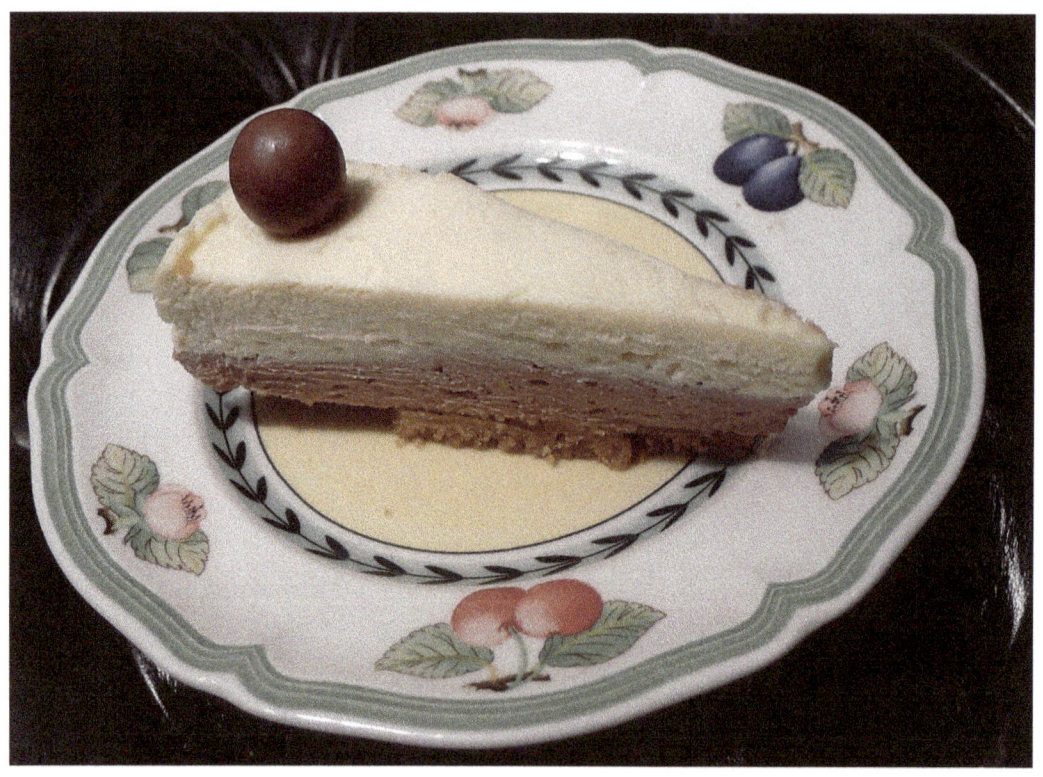

236

A Swirl of Sweet and Bold

A layer smooth, a bite so deep,
A cake where chocolate secrets keep.
The malt hums low, the cream stands tall,
A taste that sweetly conquers all.

The base holds firm, the top so light,
A dish of joy in shade and bright.
With chocolate bold and biscuits neat,
A treat where rich and soft compete.

—*Inspired by Robert Burns*

Malt Chocolate Cheesecake

Serve 10

Ingredients

200 g malted milk biscuits, crushed to crumbs

100 g salted butter, melted

5 Tbsp caster sugar

2 300 g tubs full-fat soft cheese Philadelphia

300 ml double cream

300 g white chocolate, melted

200 g bar milk chocolate, melted

2 Tbsp malt or Horlicks powder

37 g white chocolate Maltesers

Method

1. Line the base and sides of a deep, 20-22 cm loose-bottom round tin with baking parchment.

2. Mix the biscuits, melt the butter and 2 tablespoons of the sugar, and press into the base. Chill while you make the base.

3. Divide the cream cheese and cream evenly between 2 bowls. Add the white chocolate to one and milk chocolate, malt and 3 tablespoons sugar to the other. Beat each with an electric whisk until smooth and blended.

4. Spread the milk chocolate mixture evenly in the tin. Wipe around the edge to give a smooth edge. Spoon over the white chocolate mix over the top and gently smooth.

5. Decorate with the Maltesers and chill for at least 5 hours until firm (make the day before).

Desert

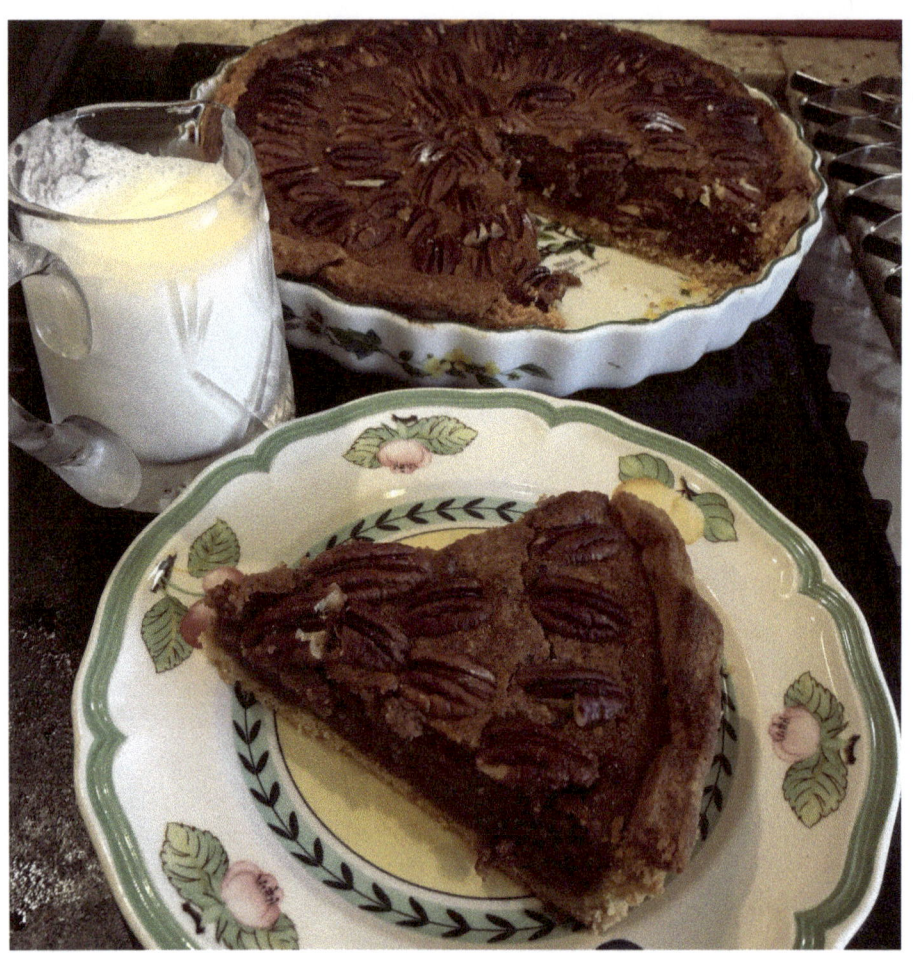

A Taste of Fire and Gold

The crust so warm, the pecans bright,
A pie of autumn's deep delight.
The maple sways, the bourbon sings,
A feast where sweetness gently clings.

A slice so rich, a taste so wide,
A bite to bring the heart with pride.
With cream so soft and nuts so deep,
A pie where love and flavour keep.

—Inspired by John Buchan

Maple Pecan Pie

Serves 10-12

Ingredients

250 g plain flour

225 g unsalted butter, cubed and chilled

100 g light muscovado sugar

125 g dates, stoned and roughly chopped

Grated zest and juice of ½ a lemon

100 ml maple syrup, plus 6 Tbsp extra

1 tsp vanilla extract

4 medium eggs

300 g pecan nut halves

284 ml carton double cream

2 Tbsp bourbon whiskey

Method

1. Put the flour and a large pinch of salt into a processor. Add 125 g of cubed butter and whiz to a fine crumb. Add 2 tablespoons water and whiz until the mixture just comes together. Turn the dough onto a lightly floured surface, shape it into a disc, and roll it out to fit a 27 x 3.5 cm (10" x 1½") loose-bottom flan case.

2. Preheat the oven to 180°C.

3. Prick the pastry all over, cover with greaseproof paper and fill with baking beans. Bake for 25 minutes, then uncover and bake for 5 minutes or until the base looks dry and light golden.

4. Meanwhile, whiz the rest of the butter in a processor. Add sugar dates and whiz to cream together. Add lemon zest, juice, syrup, vanilla extract, eggs, and 200 g nuts. Whiz until the nuts are finely chopped—the mixture will look curdled.

5. Pour into a pastry case and top with the rest of the nuts.

6. Bake for 40-45 minutes or until almost set in the middle. Cover the nuts with greaseproof paper for the last 10 minutes if the nuts turn very dark. Cool slightly before removing them from the tin. Brush them with 4 tablespoons of maple syrup.

7. Lightly whip the double cream with the whiskey and the remaining 2 tablespoons maple syrup. Serve with the pie.

Desert

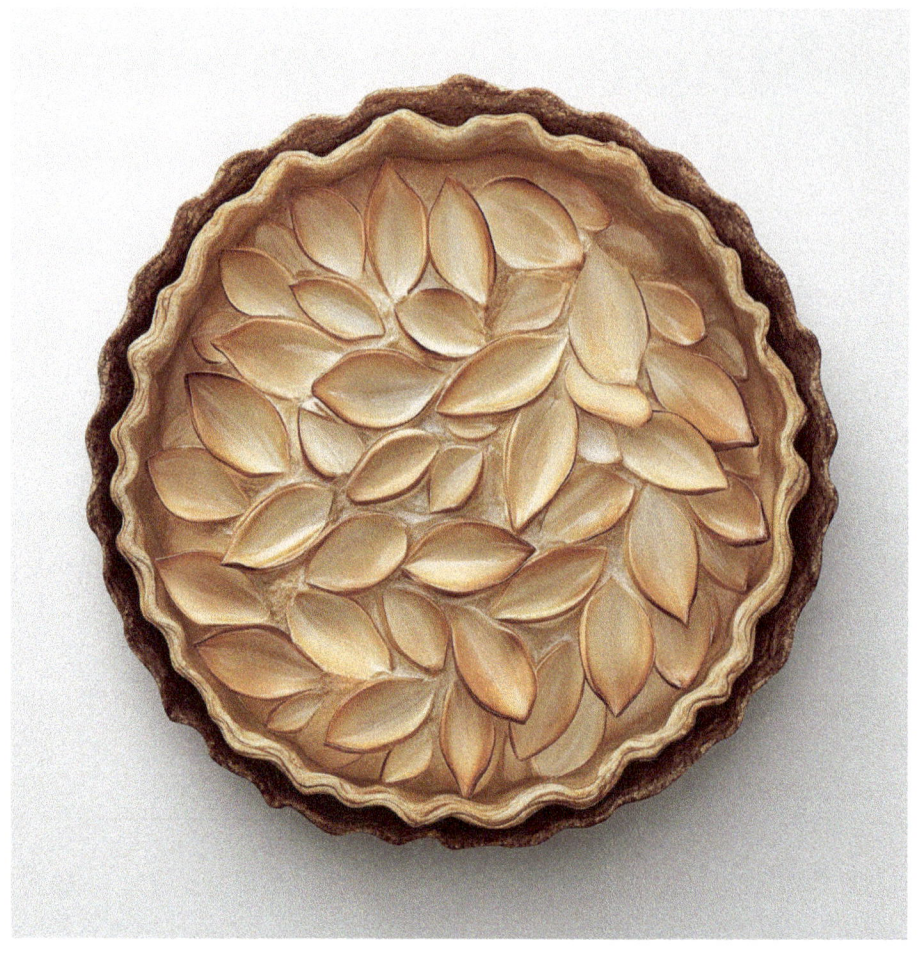

240

Almond Pastry

A Crust of Golden Charm
A crumble light, a golden blend,
Where almonds rich and butter mend.
A press, a roll, a careful turn,
A pastry crisp yet soft to burn.

With tarts to fill and fruits to lay,
A base for sweets to steal the day.
A touch of skill, a heart so free,
A crust that holds sweet memory.

—*Inspired by Robert Louis Stevenson*

Pastry - Almond

Make enough for 1 x 20-23 cm tart

Ingredients

200 g plain flour

20 g ground almonds

35 g icing sugar

125 g butter

1 egg yolk

Method

1. For the pastry, pulse the flour, almonds, sugar and butter in a food processor until they resemble fine breadcrumbs.

2. Add the egg yolk and one Tbsp of cold water, and pulse again.

3. As the pastry comes together, remove it from the food processor, roll it into a ball, wrap it in cling film, and place it in the fridge to rest for 20 minutes.

4. Use according to your recipe, wrap, freeze, and use another day.

Desert

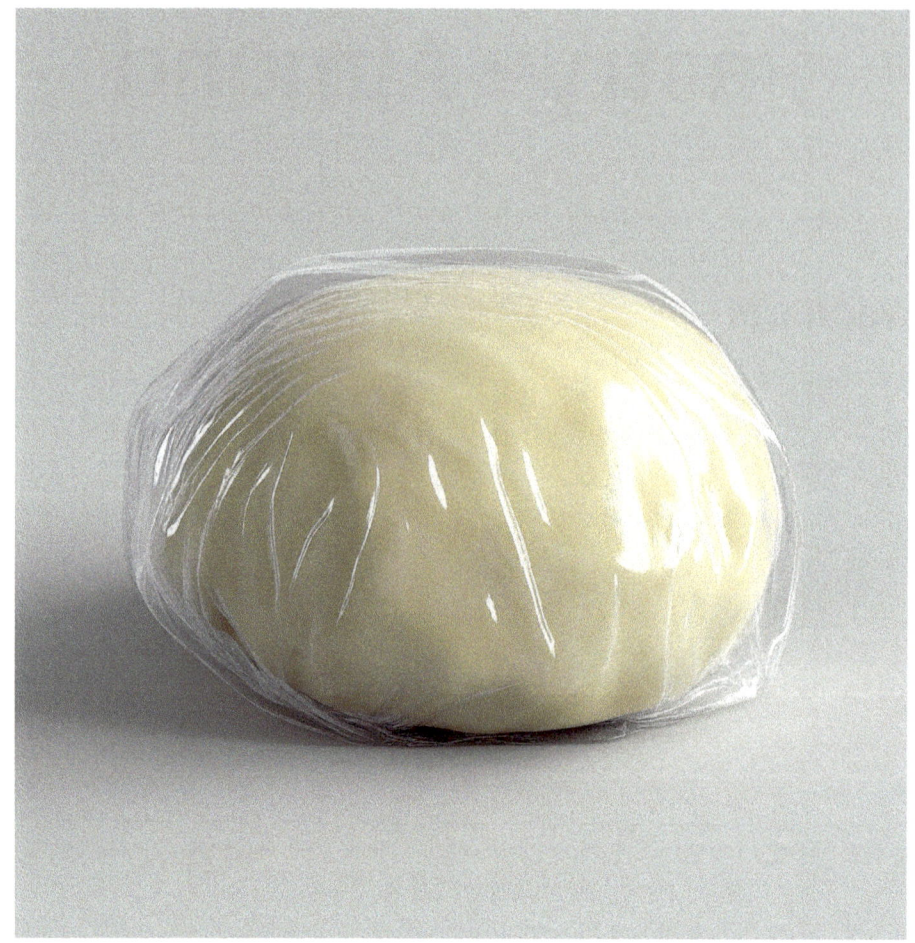

242

A Dough of Tender Care

The butter folds, the sugar sways,
A pastry made for golden days.
With hands so light and touch so true,
A base for tarts both old and new.

A roll so soft, a flake so fine,
A taste of love in every line.
A shell to hold the sweetest cheer,
A treat to cherish year by year.

—Inspired by John Buchan

Pastry - Sweet

This sweet pastry is suitable for all tarts and can be made without sugar if you want a good pastry for savoury tarts.

Makes 1 20 x 23 cm tart

Ingredients

150 g plain flour

80 g cold unsalted butter, cubed

30 g icing sugar

1 large egg yolk

3 Tbsp cold water

Method

1. Put the flour in a food processor and add the cold butter. Mix until it resembles breadcrumbs, then add the icing sugar. Pulse, and then add the egg yolk and water. Mix until it starts to come together to form a soft dough.

2. Put the mixture on a lightly floured surface. Bring the dough together to form a smooth pastry, being careful not to overwork it. Form into a slightly flattened disc, wrap in cling film, and chill for 20 minutes.

3. Roll out the pastry on a lightly floured work surface to about 3 mm (1/8) thick. Then, line a buttered tart tin, dish, or flan ring on a baking sheet 20-23 cm (8-9") diameter and 2.5 cm (1") deep. Trim the edges and keep the trimmings for decorations or latticework.

4. Prick the base of the pastry with a fork, and put the tin in the refrigerator to allow it to rest and chill for about 20 minutes.

5. Preheat the oven to 200°C.

6. Line the pastry with greaseproof paper, and pour in the baking beans. Bake blind for 15 minutes.

7. Remove the beans and paper (at this point, you can brush the bottom and sides with the egg white before returning to the oven; it does make it a little stronger), then return the pastry case to the oven for a further 3-5 minutes, until golden brown.

Desert

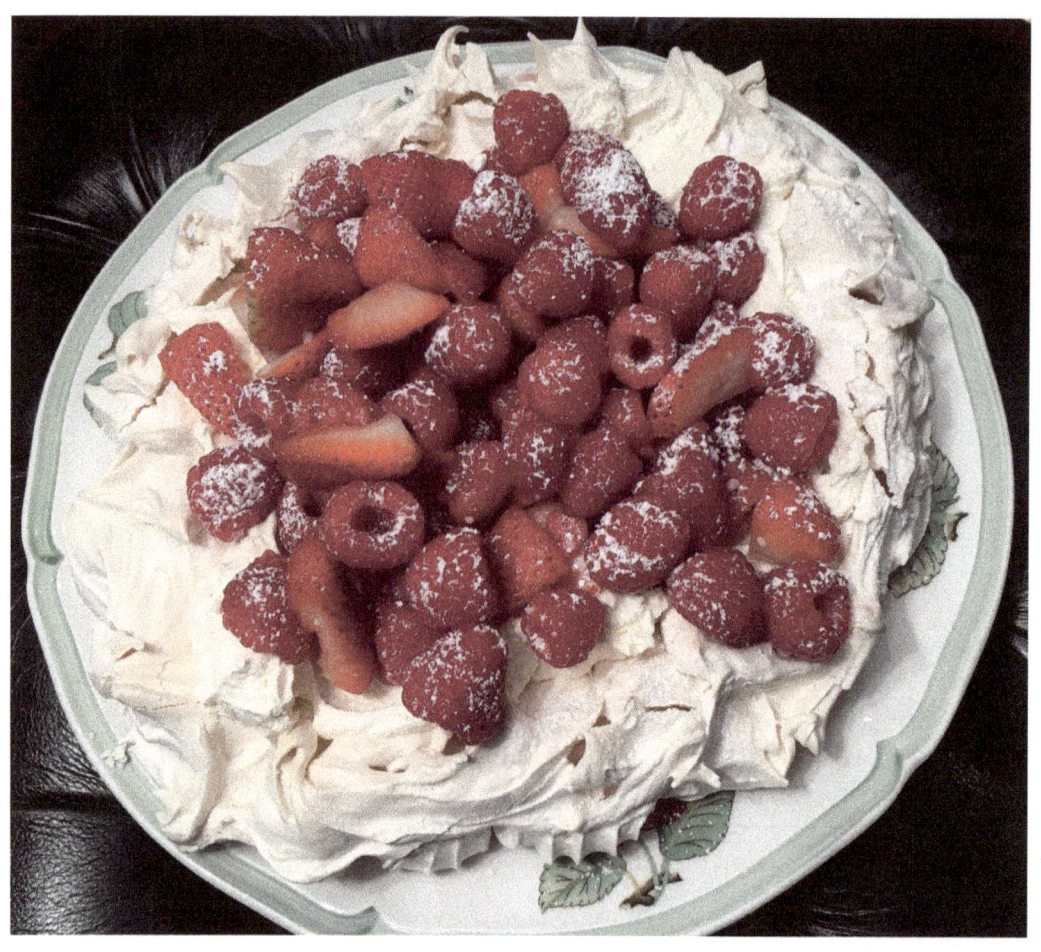

244

A Dance of Light and Cream

A shell so crisp, a heart so white,
A dish where fruit and sugar light.
The raspberries hum, the cream sways near,
A taste to bring the heart sincere.

A spoon, a bite, a dream so high,
A cloud of sweetness in the sky.
With berries bright and love so free,
A pavlova spun in memory.

—*Inspired by Robert Louis Stevenson*

Pavlova with Berries

Serves 10

Ingredients

For the meringue

1 level tsp cornflour
1 tsp of vanilla essence
1 tsp vinegar
4 egg whites (4 fluid oz)
225 g (8 oz) caster sugar

Or

30 ml of egg white to 50 g caster sugar
800 g mixed soft fruits, raspberries, strawberries and blackcurrants washed
1 tsp icing sugar sieved.

Method

1. Heat the oven to 150°C.
2. Line the baking tray with parchment paper, then draw a 23 cm/9" circle.
3. Blend the cornflour, vinegar and vanilla in a small basin.
4. Whisk the egg whites until stiff, then whisk in the caster sugar 1 Tbsp at a time. Finally, add the blended cornflour mixture.
5. Spread one-third of the meringue onto the baking tray within the drawn circle. Pipe the remainder around the edge (with a large star tube and piping bag).
6. Bake for 1½ hours or until firm (watch the colour of the meringue; if it becomes a light brown, immediately lower the heat). After 1 hour, turn off the heat and open the oven door slightly. Let the meringue cool completely.
7. Whip the cream to a soft peak, then spread it into the centre of the meringue.
8. Place the strawberries, raspberries, blackcurrants, or any fruit you choose over the cream, sprinkle with icing sugar, and serve.

Desert

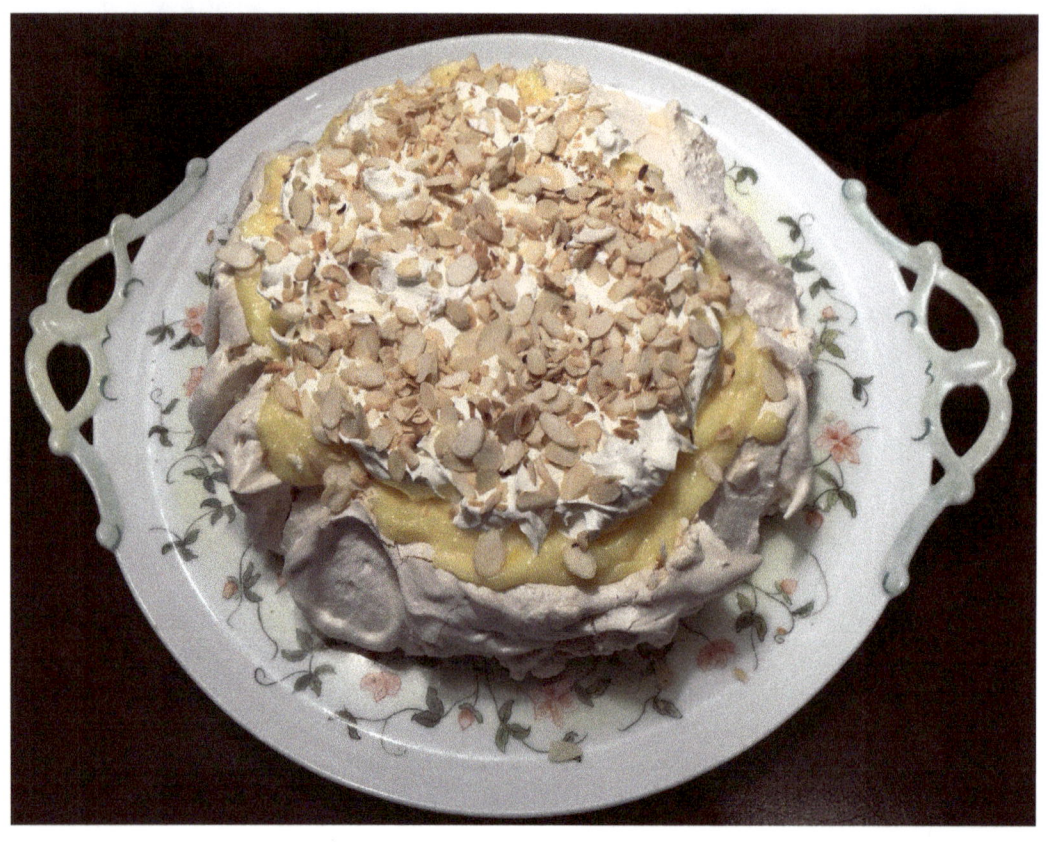

246

A Whisper of Citrus and Air

The meringue stands, the lemon flows,
A dish where airy sweetness glows.
The almonds crisp, the curd so bright,
A taste where tart and soft unite.

A spoonful light, a texture fine,
A bite where sugar's art aligns.
With golden zest and cream's soft cheer,
A taste to hold the heart sincere.

—*Inspired by Contemporary Scottish Poets*

Pavlova with Lemon Topping

Serves 10

Ingredients

6 egg whites

375 g caster sugar

2½ tsp cornflour

2 unwaxed lemons

325 g jar of homemade lemon curd

300 ml of double cream, whipped.

50 g toasted flaked almonds

Method

1. Heat the oven to 150°C.
2. Line the baking tray with parchment paper, then draw a 23 cm / 9" circle.
3. Beat the egg whites until satiny peaks form. Then whisk in the caster sugar one Tbsp at a time until the meringue is stiff and shiny.
4. Sprinkle the cornflour over the meringue, then grate in the zest of one lemon and add 2 tsp of lemon juice. Gently fold until everything is thoroughly mixed in.
5. Spread the meringue onto the baking tray within the drawn circle.
6. Bake for 1 hour or until firm (watch the colour of the meringue; if it becomes a light brown, immediately lower the heat). After 1 hour, turn off the heat and open the oven door slightly. Let the meringue cool completely.
7. Toast the flaked almonds by frying them in a dry pan over medium to high heat until they have started to colour. Shake the pan at regular intervals to prevent burning. When done, remove them to a cool plate to stop them from cooking.
8. Whip the cream until thick and airy, set to one side.
9. Put the lemon curd into a bowl and beat it with a wooden spoon to loosen it. Taste the lemon curd; if it is too sweet, add some lemon zest and a small amount of lemon juice.
10. Spread the lemon curd on top of the meringue base. Now top with the whipped cream. Sprinkle with the zest of the remaining lemon and finish by scattering the flaked almonds.

Desert

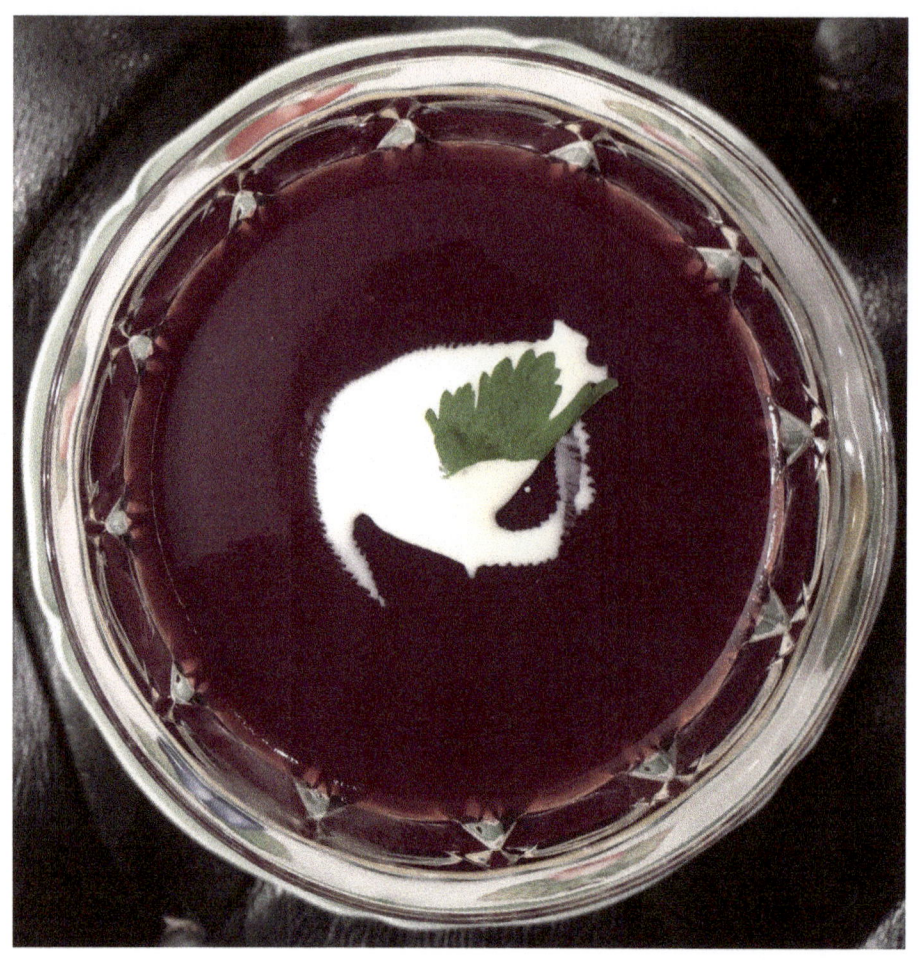

248

A Jewel of Deepest Red

A glass of wine, a sugar bright,
A jelly set in ruby light.
The cloves stand bold, the spice hums near,
A dish to bring both warmth and cheer.

A spoonful clear, a taste so wide,
A glow of fruit and depth inside.
With cream atop and time so free,
A dish of velvet mystery.

—*Inspired by Sir Walter Scott*

Port Wine Jelly

Serves 6

Ingredients

300 ml claret or red wine

100 g caster sugar

2 level Tbsp of red currant jelly

2.5 cm cinnamon stick

3 cloves

1 lemon rind and juice

4 sheets of gelatine (see packet instructions)

300 ml port

2-3 drops of red colouring (optional)

Whipped cream (optional)

Method

1. Soak gelatine in cold water as per instructions.

2. Combine red wine, sugar, red currant jelly, cinnamon stick, and cloves in a saucepan. Add thnly peeled lemon rind, strained lemon juice, and gelatine which has been softened in water. Simmer very gently for a few minutes and then add the port. Do not allow it to boil.

3. Strain through a piece of muslin and, if necessary, add a few drops of red colouring to improve the colour. Cool.

4. When almost cold, pour into small individual moulds rinsed with cold water. Chill until firm.

5. When ready to serve, turn out and decorate with whipped cream.

Desert

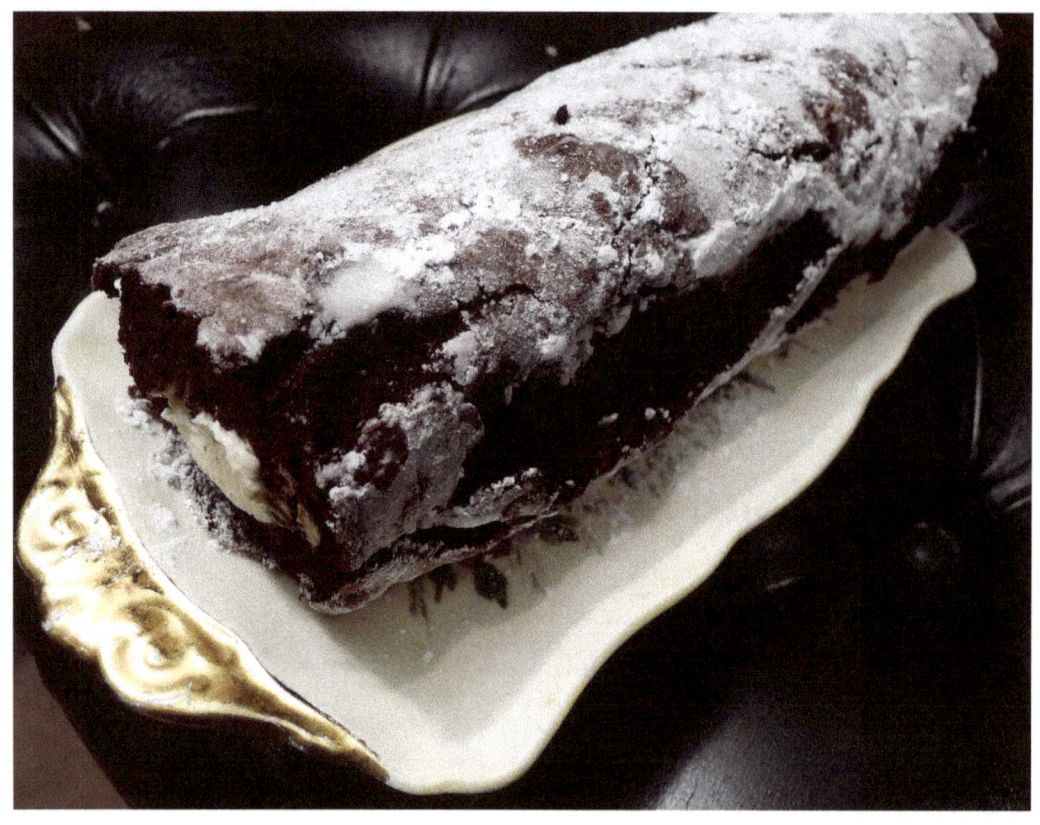

250

A Roll of Cocoa Dreams

The sponge is soft, the mousse so wide,
A roll of chocolate, deep inside.
With dust of sugar, silk so bright,
A treat where cocoa sings delight.

The knife glides smooth, the filling sways,
A dish of joy in cocoa's maze.
A taste so rich, a dream so free,
A log of chocolate ecstasy.

—*Inspired by Robert Burns*

Squidgy Chocolate Log

Serves 8

Ingredients

- 6 large eggs, separated. Keep the egg whites in a grease-free bowl
- 150 g caster sugar
- 50 g cocoa powder

For the chocolate mousse filling

- 100 g plain chocolate less than 40% cocoa solids
- 150 ml whipping cream

For the cream filling

- 225 ml double cream

To finish

- Dust with sifted icing sugar

Method

1. Preheat oven to 180°C.

2. Oil and line the base of a baking tray 29 x 18cm

3. Break the plain chocolate into pieces for the chocolate filling and place it in a basin. Gently heat over a saucepan of barely simmering water until the chocolate has melted. Remove from the heat and allow to cool.

4. Next, beat the whipped cream until it reaches a soft peak stage. Gently fold in the chocolate. Cover the bowl and chill in the refrigerator for about an hour.

5. Meanwhile, you can get on with the cake. First, place the egg yolks in a basin and whisk until the mixture thickens, then add the caster sugar and continue to whisk until the mixture thickens slightly. Be careful not to get it too thick.

6. Mix the cocoa powder into the egg yolk mixture, then beat the egg whites to the soft peak stage using a clean whisk and bowl. Next, carefully cut and fold the egg whites into the chocolate mixture gently and thoroughly, then pour the mixture into the prepared tin.

7. Bake the cake on the centre shelf for 20-30 minutes until springy and puffy. When the cake is cooked, remove it from the oven but leave it in the cake tin to cool (it will shrink quite a bit as it cools, but don't worry, that's normal)

8. When the cake is quite cold, turn it onto an oblong of greaseproof paper liberally dusted with icing sugar. Peel away the cake tin lining from the bottom of the cake (which is now facing upwards), then spread the chocolate mousse filling over the cake.

9. Next, whip the cream softly and spread it over the chocolate filling. Finally, gently roll up the cake to make a log shape.

This will serve 8 people, and although it is unlikely that there will be any left, you can cover any remaining cake with an upturned basin and keep it in the refrigerator. (Or freeze for a short time)

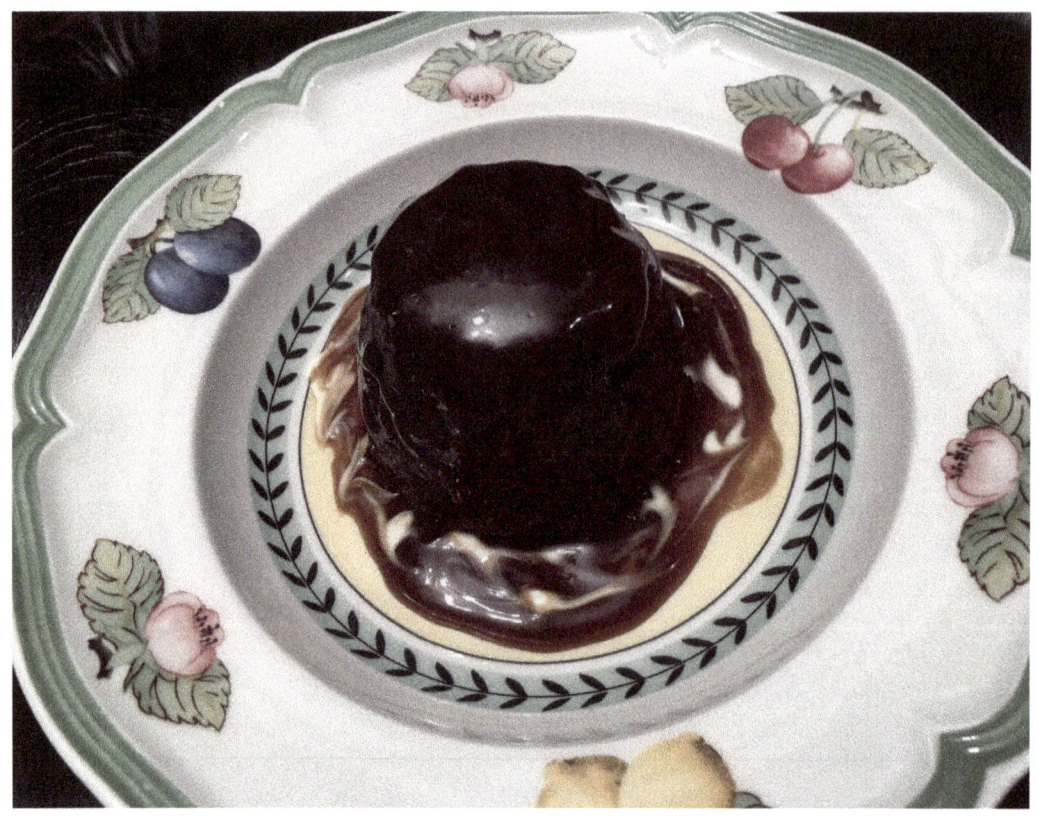

A Warm and Sugared Tale

The dates do melt, the butter sways,
A pudding rich in sugared maze.
The toffee flows, the sponge drinks deep,
A taste where golden comforts keep.

A spoon, a sigh, a warmth so wide,
A dish to bring both love and pride.
With cream so soft and sauce so bright,
A bite that turns the dark to light.

—*Inspired by Robert Burns*

Sticky Toffee Pudding

Serve 7 little puddings

Prep about 1 hour

Cook 20-25 minutes

(Can be made 1-2 days ahead and left to soak up the sauce)

(If you don't want to eat the pudding all at once, freeze a few in an oven-proof dish with some of the sauce. Thaw for a few hours and reheat as in step 5)

Ingredients

For the Puddings

225 g whole dates, preferably Medjool

175 ml boiling water

1 tsp vanilla extract

175 g self-raising flour, plus 1 Tbsp extra

1 tsp bicarbonate of soda

2 eggs

85 g butter, softened, plus extra for greasing

140 g Demerara sugar

2 Tbsp black treacle

100 ml milk

Cream or custard to serve (optional)

For the toffee sauce (make double the quantity if you love sauce, half for the pudding and half to hand round)

175 g light muscovado sugar

150 g butter, cut into pieces

225 ml double cream

1 Tbsp black treacle

Method

1. Heat the oven to 180°C.
2. Stone and chop the dates quite small. Put them in a bowl, then pour the boiling water over them. Leave for about 30 minutes, until cool and well soaked, then mash with a fork. Stir in the vanilla extract. Butter and flour seven mini pudding tins (each about 200ml) and sit them on a baking sheet.

3. While the dates are soaking, make the puddings. Mix the flour and bicarbonate of soda and beat the eggs in a separate bowl. Beat the butter and sugar in a large bowl for a few minutes until slightly creamy (the mixture will be grainy from the sugar).

4. Add the eggs a little at a time, beating well between additions. Beat in the black treacle, gently fold in one-third of the flour using a large metal spoon, then half the milk, and be careful not to overbeat. Repeat until all the flour and milk is used.

5. Stir the soaked dates into the pudding batter. The mix may look slightly curdled at this point and look like a soft, thick batter. Spoon it evenly between the tins and bake for 20-25 minutes, until risen and firm.

6. Meanwhile, put the sugar and butter for the sauce in a medium saucepan with half the cream. Bring to a boil over medium heat, stirring all the time, until the sugar has completely dissolved.

7. Stir in the black treacle, turn up the heat slightly, and let the mixture bubble away for 2-3 minutes until it is rich toffee, stirring occasionally to ensure it doesn't burn. Take the pan off the heat and beat in the rest of the cream.

8. Remove the puddings from the oven. Leave in tins for a few minutes, and then loosen them well from the sides of the tins with a small palette knife before turning them out.

9. You can now serve them with the sauce drizzled over, but they'll be even stickier if left coated for a day or two. To do this, pour half the sauce into one oven-proof serving dish. Sit the upturned puddings on the sauce, and then pour the rest of the sauce over them. Cover with a loose tent of foil so that the sauce doesn't smudge (no need to chill)

10. When ready to serve, heat oven to 160°C. Warm the puddings through, still covered, for 15-20 minutes or until the sauce is bubbling. Serve them on their own or with cream or custard.

It should not be eaten piping hot but warm. Once the sponge has been topped with a sauce glaze, it should stand for 30 minutes to reach its optimum temperature.

Flint Family Cookbook

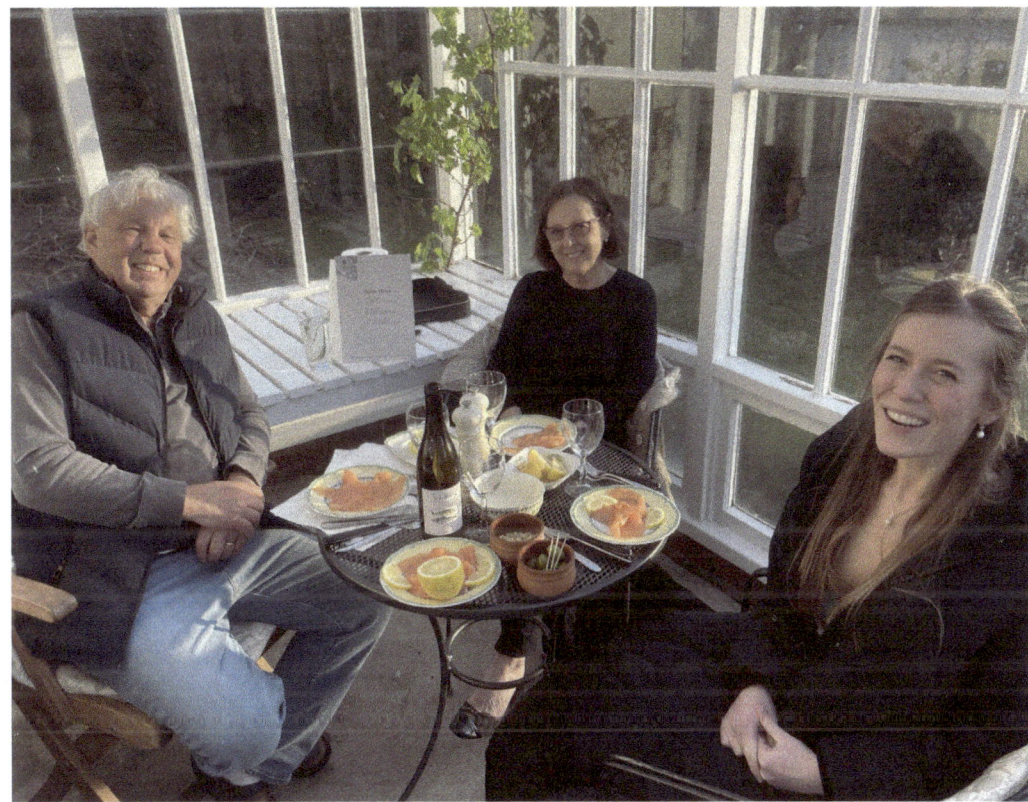

Desert

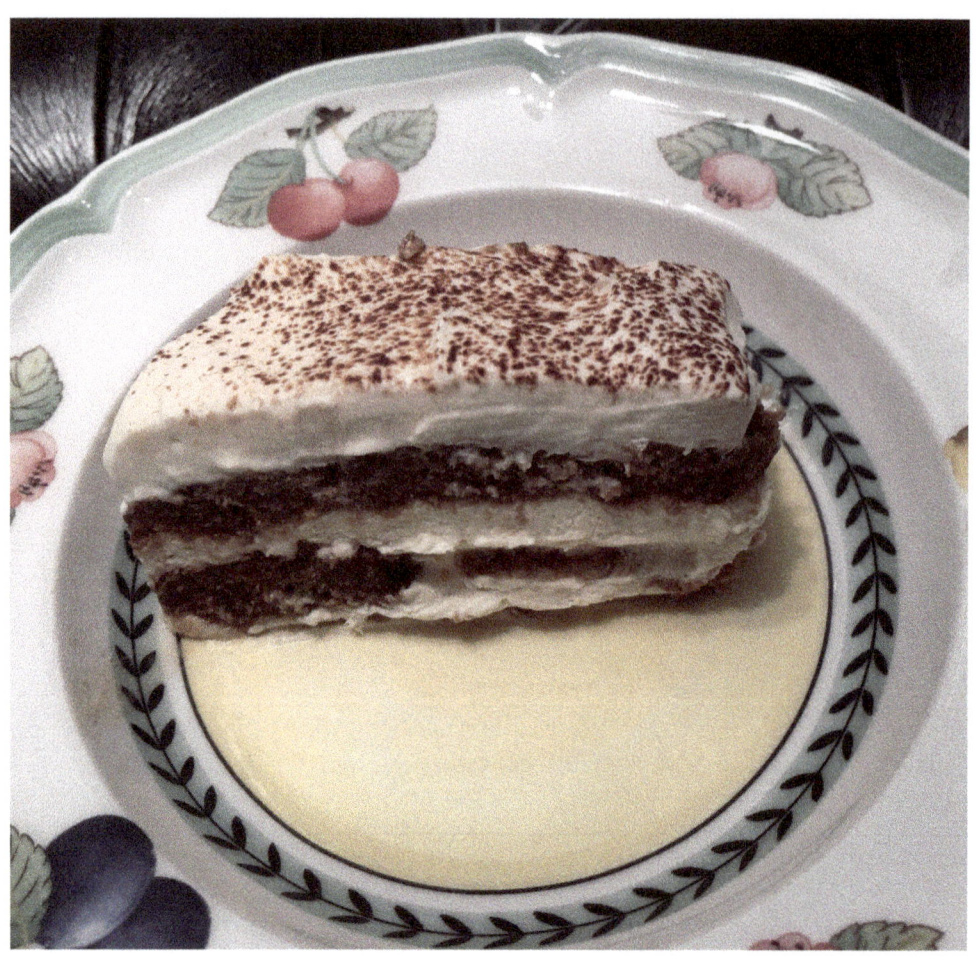

A Sip of Time and Cocoa

A layer deep, a coffee bright,
A dish where time and cream unite.
The sponge drinks slow, the cocoa sways,
A bite that lingers past the days.

A moment rich, a dream so wide,
A plate of love, a taste with pride.
A spoonful bold, a sigh so free,
A dish of whispered luxury.

—*Inspired by Robert Louis Stevenson*

Tiramisu

Serves 12

Ingredients

2 egg yolks

3 Tbsp (45 ml) caster sugar

2 tsp (10 ml) vanilla essence

700 g mascarpone cheese or a mix of full-fat soft cheese and mascarpone

284 ml whipping cream

2 Tbsp (30 ml) icing sugar)

250 ml strong black coffee

250 ml Tia Maria

250 g Savoiardi (lady's fingers) biscuits

Cocoa powder to dust

Method

1. Line the base and sides of a 23 cm spring-release tin with non-stick baking parchment. Beat the egg yolks with the caster sugar until pale and thick, then add the vanilla essence and mascarpone cheese to the egg mixture and whisk until evenly combined.

2. Lightly whip the cream with the icing sugar and fold gently into the mascarpone mixture.

3. Mix the coffee and Tia Maria. Dip each Savoiardi, one by one, in the coffee mixture, then line the base of the tin.

4. Spoon a third of the mascarpone mixture over the base, then repeat the dipping process for the remainder of the biscuits and arrange them on top of the mascarpone layer. Spoon the second third of the mascarpone mixture over the sponge fingers and chill overnight. Cover and store the remaining mascarpone mixture in the fridge.

5. Remove the Tiramisu from the fridge. Remove the tin from around the sides, place a plate over the top of the Tiramisu, turn upside down, lift off the base and parchment paper, and spread the remaining mascarpone mixture over the top of the cake. Keep chilled until required, up to 2 hours.

6. Dust the top liberally with cocoa powder and cut into wedges.

Desert

258

Cake

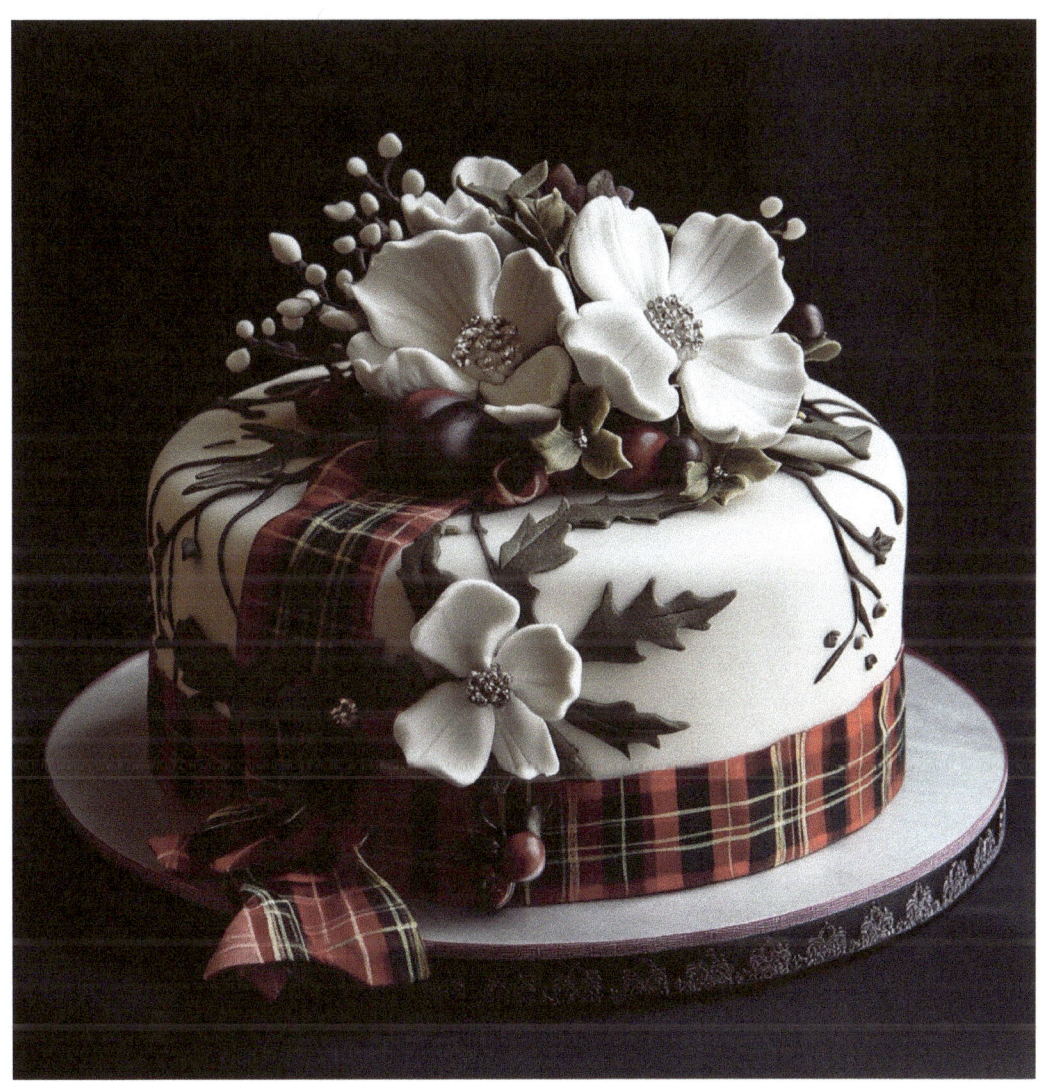

Cake

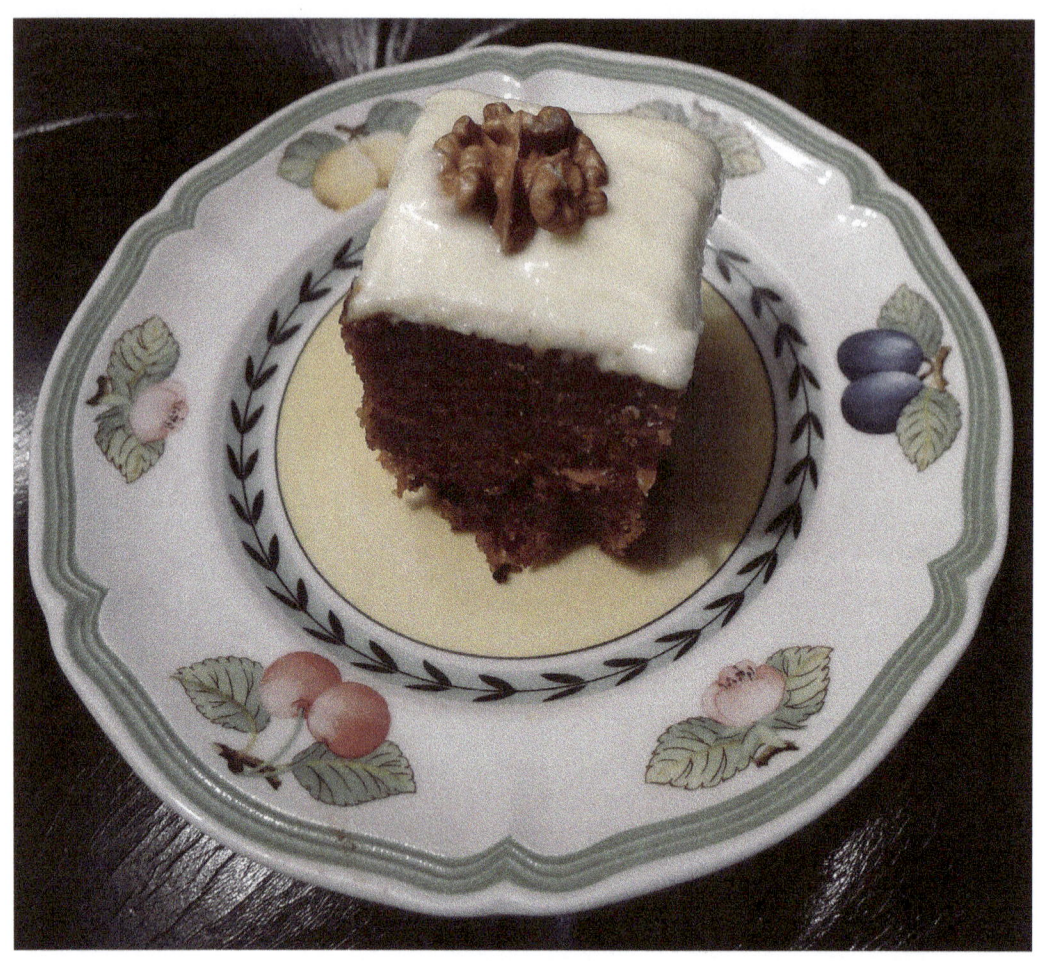

A Slice of Spice and Cheer

*A golden crumb, a hint of spice,
A bite so soft, a touch so nice.
With walnuts bold and sugar deep,
A cake the heart shall always keep.*

*The frosting swirls, so rich, so bright,
A velvet touch, a pure delight.
So take a fork, embrace the cheer,
A taste that lingers year by year.*
—Inspired by Robert Burns

Carrot Cake

Serves 10

Ingredients

200 g plain flour
2 tsp of bicarbonate of soda
1 tsp cinnamon
Pinch of grated nutmeg
½ tsp salt
400 g soft brown sugar
350 ml vegetable oil
4 large eggs, beaten
400 g grated carrots
275 g chopped walnuts

Butter for greasing

For the frosting
100 g cream cheese (Philadelphia)
40 g butter
200 g icing sugar
3 drops of vanilla essence
10 half walnuts for decoration

Method

1. Preheat the oven to 180°C.
2. Sift the flour, bicarbonate, cinnamon, nutmeg and salt together in a large bowl.
3. Mix the sugar and oil together in another bowl, then add the eggs. Make a well in the flour, stir in the liquid, then the carrots and the walnuts.
4. Grease an 18 cm square cake tin. Line the sides and base with greaseproof paper. Spoon in the cake mixture and bake for 1¼ hours or until the skewer comes out cleanly.
5. Leave the cake to cool in the tin, and then turn out onto a wire rack. When cold, wrap it in foil and leave for a day.
6. To make the frosting: mash the cheese, butter, sugar, and vanilla essence together. Spread over the top of the cake and serve cut into square.

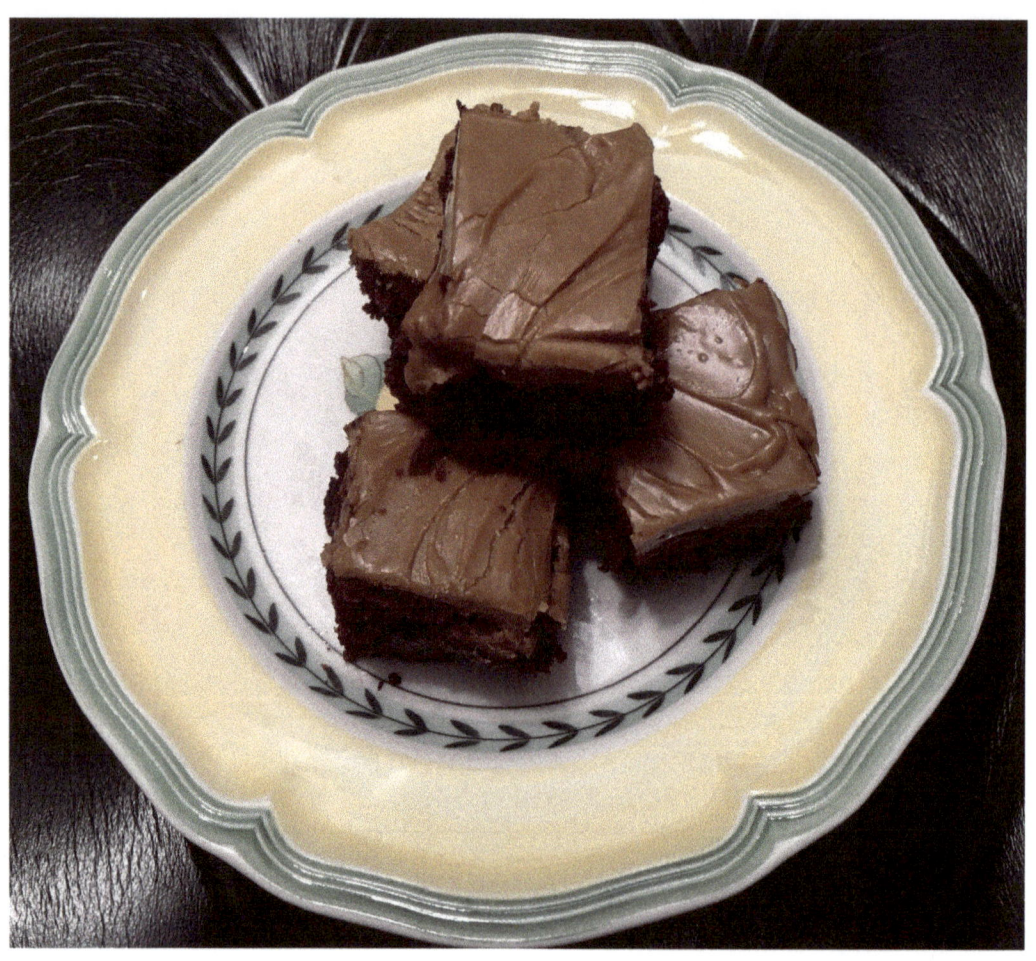

A Bite of Cocoa Bliss

A crackled top, a centre sweet,
Where chocolate swirls in dark retreat.
The walnuts hum, the cocoa sings,
A dish where joy in richness clings.

A bite, a pause, a dream so deep,
A taste that chocolate lovers keep.
With fudge so bold and crumbs so wide,
A brownie's love will never hide.

—Inspired by Robert Louis Stevenson

Chocolate Chip Brownies

Makes 15

Preparation: 15 minutes

Cooking: 25–30 minutes, plus 20 minutes cooling

Ingredients

300 g plain chocolate 70%

250 g butter, cubed

5 medium eggs beaten

350 g golden caster sugar

200 g plain flour

100 g plain chocolate chips

50 g walnuts, chopped

Vanilla ice cream and dark chocolate sauce to serve

Method

1. Preheat oven to 180°C.
2. Melt the chocolate in a heat proof bowl over a pan of simmering water. Cool.
3. Grease and base-line a 20cm x 30cm rectangular cake tin with baking parchment.
4. Beat the butter until light and fluffy, add the sugar and beat well, add the eggs a little at a time, then pour in the cooled chocolate mixture. Add a pinch of salt and sift in the flour. Beat until blended and then stir in the chocolate chips and walnuts.
5. Pour into the tin and bake for 25-30 minutes.
6. The outside will looked cracked whilst the inside will feel firm but gooey, don't be tempted to overcook the brownie.
7. Allow to cool in the tin for 20 minutes. Cut into squares and serve.

They can be covered with fudge icing, or served with ice cream and chocolate sauce!

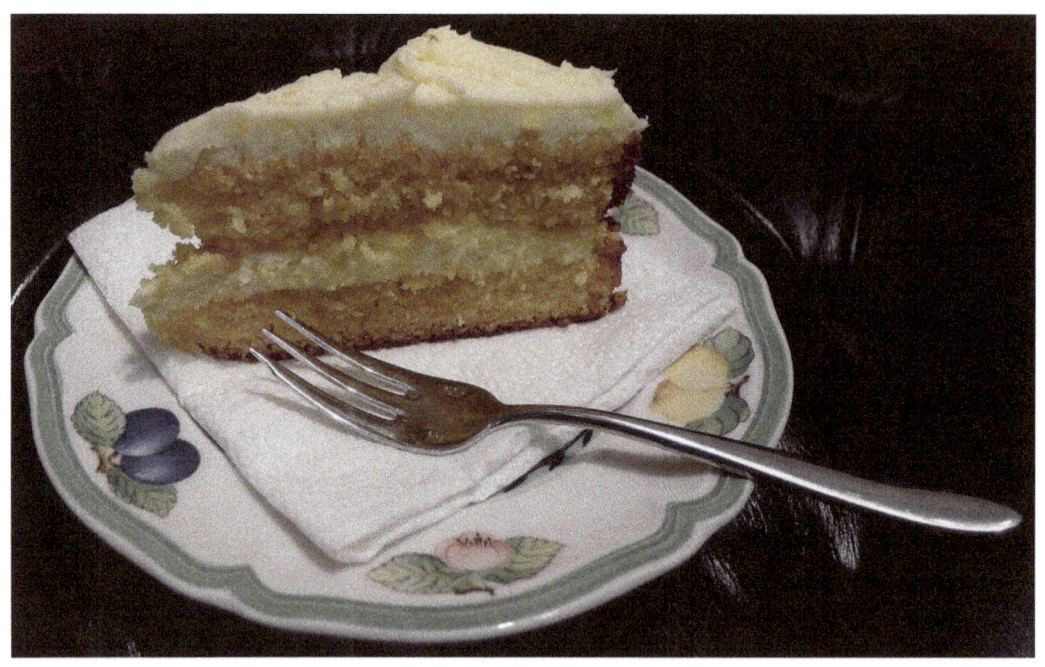

A Citrus Dream

The fruit is boiled, the zest runs bright,
A cake of gold, both soft and light.
The almonds hum, the sugar sways,
A bite that holds the sun's own rays.

With sweetness pure and orange free,
A taste of warmth and memory.
A slice so soft, a joy untold,
A dish of citrus spun in gold.

—*Inspired by Contemporary Scottish Poets*

No Flour Clementine Cake

Serves 8-10

Ingredients

320 g clementines (approx 3-4 medium size ones)

6 large eggs

225 g caster sugar

250 g ground almonds

1 tsp baking powder

Filling

175 g butter, 300 g icing sugar (sieve)

2 Tbsp orange pulp

Method

1. Put the clementines in a pan with some cold water, bring to the boil and cook for 2 hours.

2. Drain and when cool, cut each clementine in half and remove the pips.

3. Dump the clementines-skins, pith, fruit and all. Blitz in a food processor.

4. Preheat the oven to 190°C. Butter and line a 21 cm spring form tin.

5. Beat the eggs in a bowl for 3 minutes on full with an electric mixer; add all the sugar, ground almonds and baking powder, mix until everything is incorporated.

6. Remove 2 tablespoons of pulped orange for the butter cream. Add the remaining pulp oranges to the mixture.

7. Pour the cake mixture into the prepared tin and bake for 40 minutes, cover with foil and continue to bake for a further 20 minutes until a skewer comes out clean. Remove from the oven and leave to cool, on a rack, but in the tin.

8. When the cake is cold remove from the tin. It is even better to eat a day after it is made.

This cake can be made with an equal weight of oranges, and with lemons, in which case increase the sugar to 250 g.

Filling

1. Beat the butter until light and fully.

2. Add the orange pulp, mix slowly, and add the icing sugar a little at a time. When all the icing sugar is fully added give it a really good beating to make it lovely light and fluffy.

3. Cut the cake in half; add half of the filling to the centre and the rest to the top.

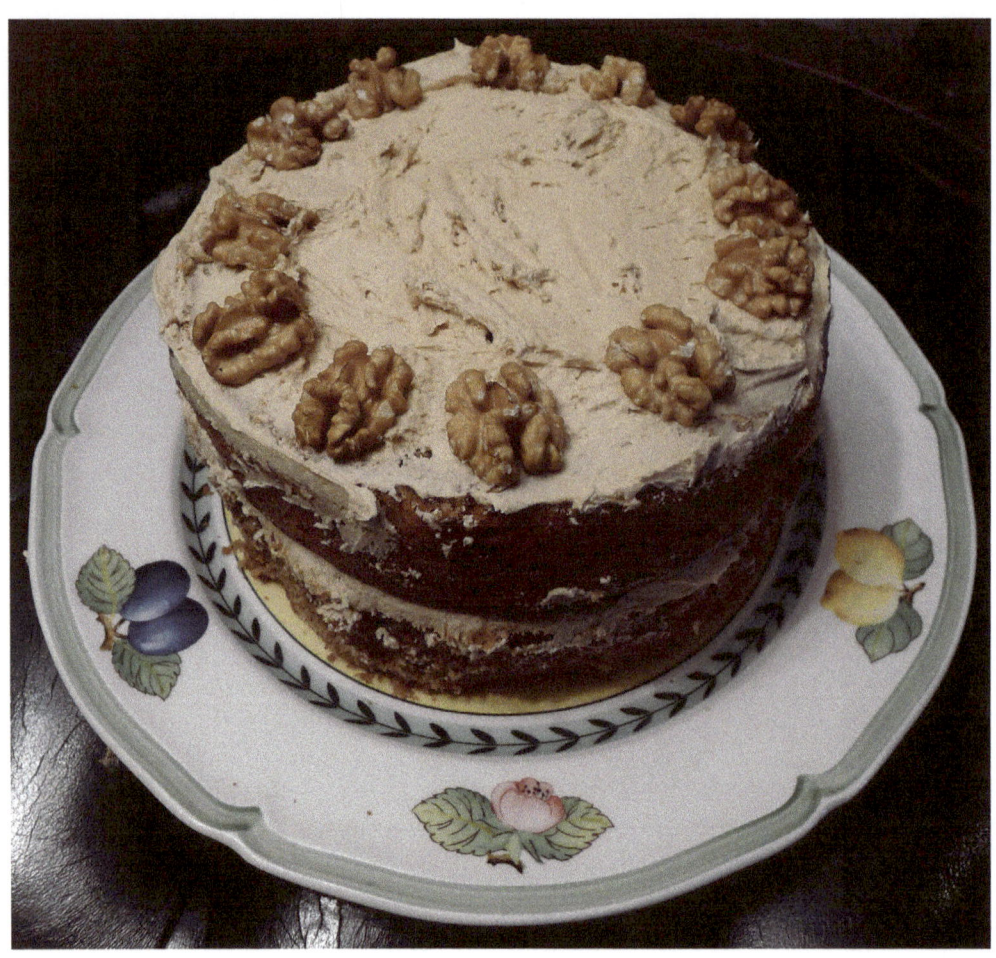

A Cup and Crumb Delight

The coffee swirls, the walnuts toast,
A cake where flavour lingers most.
With butter rich and sponge so light,
A bite of morning's pure delight.
The icing smooth, the layers bold,
A tale of warmth and hands that hold.
A cake to share, a plate so wide,
A taste that lifts both heart and pride.

—*Inspired by John Buchan*

Coffee and Walnut Cake

Preparation: 40 minutes, plus cooling. Cooking 23-28 minutes. Serves 12

Ingredients

For the coffee sponge

- 225 g unsalted butter, softened, plus extra for greasing
- 225 g golden caster sugar
- 4 medium eggs, beaten
- 1 Tbsp espresso coffee (or 2 Tbsp instant espresso mixed with 1 Tbsp of boiling water)
- 225 g self raising flour
- 1 tsp baking powder
- 75 g walnut halves, finely chopped, plus 25 g for decoration.

For the filling and coffee icing

- 250 g of sieved icing sugar
- 125 g of butter
- 2 Tbsp of espresso coffee mixed with 1 Tbsp of boiling water.

Method

1. Preheat oven to 180°C /Gas 4.
2. Grease and line the base of 2 cake tins with non stick parchment. (2 x 20 cm loose bottom cake tins)
3. Place the butter in a food mixer and beat until light and fluffy. Add the sugar and beat again until lighter. Add a quarter of the beaten egg and beat on full speed, then add the rest gradually, beating well after each addition. (If it curdles add 2 Tbsp of flour from the 225 g flour now)
4. Add the espresso coffee and whisk in. Turn off the mixer, sift in the flour and baking powder, gently, and add the chopped walnuts. Fold everything through until no pockets of flour remain.
5. Divide the cake mixture between the two cake tins, then place on the middle shelf of the oven for 23-28 minutes, or until a skewer inserted in the cake comes out clean.
6. Allow to cool for 15 minutes, remove the cake from the tins and place onto a wired rack to prevent the cake from becoming to soggy.

For the coffee icing

1. Cream the butter; slowly add the icing sugar then finally the coffee.
2. When the cake is cold, divide the icing, and put half on the top and the rest in the middle.
3. Decorate with walnut halves and serve.

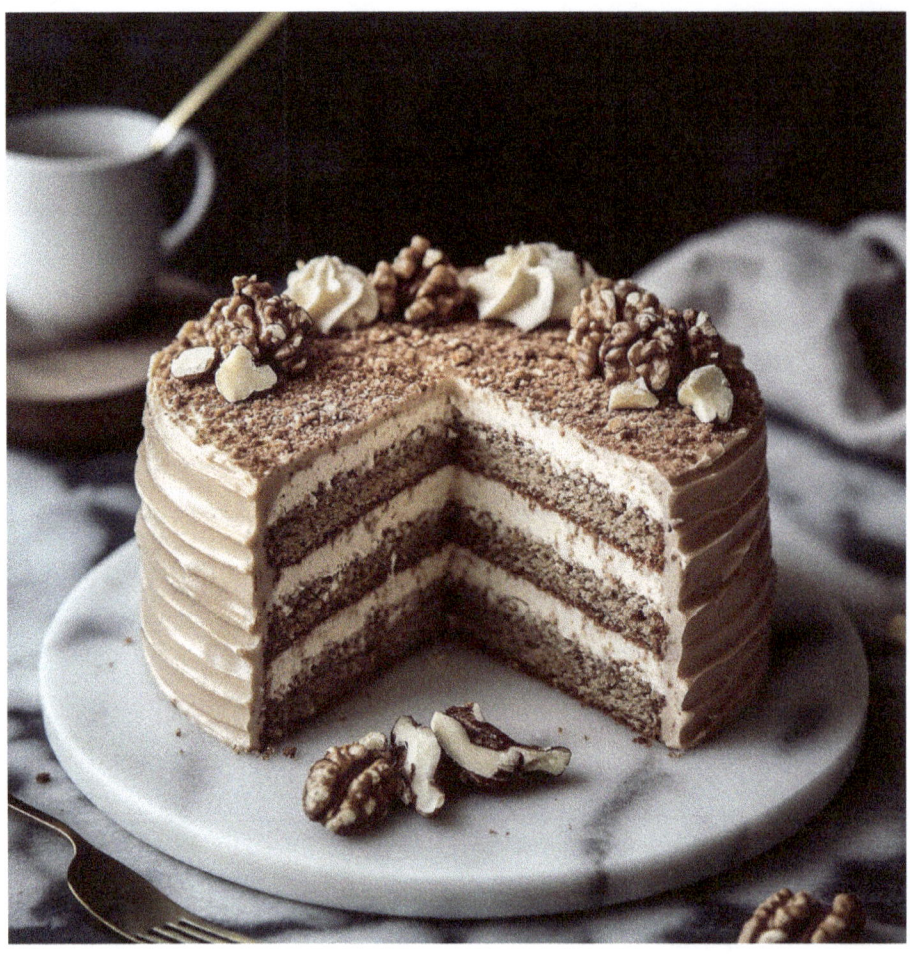

268

A Brew of Sweet Indulgence

The butter sways, the sugar glows,
A hint of coffee softly flows.
With almonds light and walnuts deep,
A golden sponge where flavors keep.

The icing swirls in layers high,
A touch of cream, a soft supply.
A slice to pair with morning's light,
A taste of warmth in each delight.

—*Inspired by Robert Louis Stevenson*

Coffee and Walnut Cake with Almonds

Serves 10

Ingredients

350 g butter

350 g golden caster sugar

140 g walnut pieces roughly ground (blitz in a food processor)

6 medium eggs

250 g self-raising flour, sifted

1½ level tsp baking powder

100 g ground almonds

3 tsp of espresso coffee granules, dissolved in 1 Tbsp hot water

For the filling and icing

300 g soften butter

600 g sifted icing sugar

3 tsp of espresso coffee granules, dissolved in 1 Tbsp of hot water

75 g walnut halves

Optional - Grated chocolate for decorating the top of the cake

If not putting icing around the sides cut the filling down to 400 g icing sugar and 200 g butter.

Method

1. Heat the oven 150°C
2. Butter 2 20 cm wide x 5 cm deep cake tins and line with a circle of baking paper.
3. Make the sponge. Whip the butter until light in colour. Then cream the butter and sugar until pale, in a mixer.
4. Stir in the ground walnuts, and then add the eggs slowly, a little at a time. Then fold in the flour mixed with the baking powder, ground almonds and coffee.
5. When well mixed, divide between the 2 tins and bake for 45 minutes or until the cake feels firm to touch. If you stick a skewer in to the cake it should come out clean. Turn the cakes out onto a rack to cool completely. If the cakes starts to burn on top cover with a sheet of greaseproof paper.
6. Make the icing by beating the butter, then slowly add the icing sugar until very light and pale, then add the coffee. Place a tea towel over the mixture so the icing sugar does not fly everywhere.
7. Spread ⅓ of the filling onto one cake. Place the next ⅓ of the remaining filling on the top and finally the last ⅓ on the sides.
8. Place the walnuts on the top. Dust with a little icing sugar

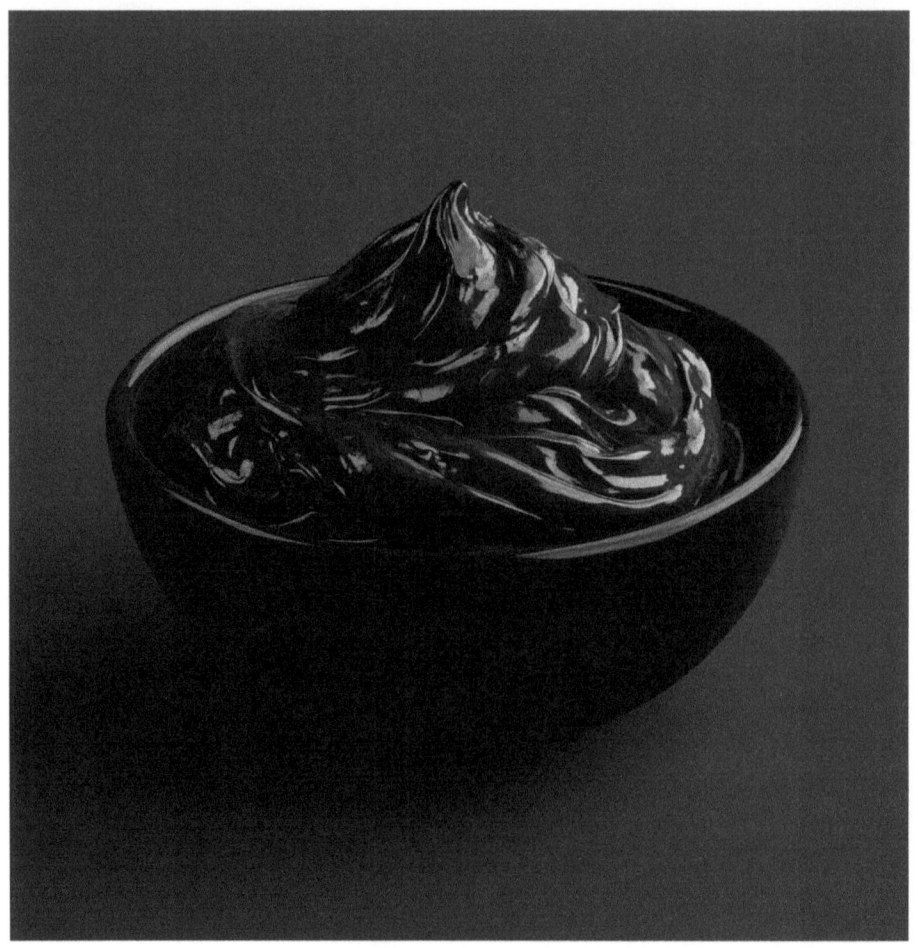

270

A Stream of Sugar's Song

A pot of gold, a melting stream,
A glaze of butter, smooth as dream.
The sugar sways, the richness flows,
A touch of cocoa, warm and close.

A spoon, a spread, a cake made bright,
A taste of pure and sweet delight.
A moment soft, a glaze so true,
A finish fine for treats anew.

—*Inspired by Robert Louis Stevenson*

Fudge Icing

Makes enough to ice a 20 cm square cake

Ingredients

125 g dark brown musacovado sugar

75 g unsalted butter

3 Tbsp single or double cream

125 g icing sugar, sifted

Method

1. Press any lumps out of the musacovado sugar, then put it in a small, heavy-based pan with the butter. Set over low heat and stir until melted and smooth, then bring to the boil and simmer for 1 minute.

2. Stir in the cream and simmer for one minute, stirring constantly so the mixture doesn't catch on the base of the pan. Remove from the heat and add the icing sugar, then beat well with a wooden spoon until the mixture is smooth and thick.

3. Spread the icing on the top of the turned out brownie. Leave to set before cutting into squares.

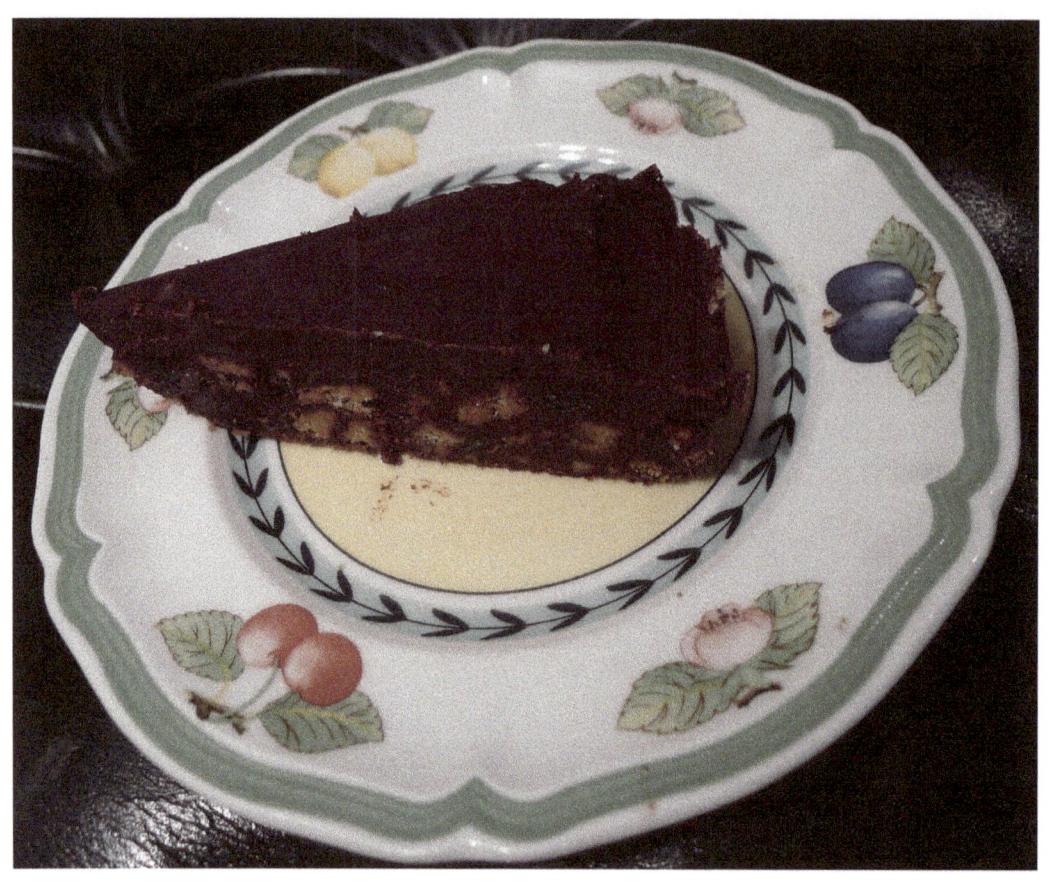

A Simple, Sweet Indulgence

A mix of crisp, a swirl of sweet,
A treat where chocolate dreams do meet.
The nuts hum low, the fruit stands bright,
A bite where joy takes pure delight.

No oven hums, no heat, no wait,
A cake so rich, so bold in fate.
A spoon, a square, a joy so free,
A plate of simple luxury.

—*Inspired by Contemporary Scottish Poets*

No Cook Chocolate Cake

18 squares

Ingredients

250 g digestive biscuits broken into small bits by hand

60 g walnuts, broken

75 g raisins, chopped

150 g plain chocolate

150 g milk chocolate

150 g syrup

100 g butter

200 g soft apricots, chopped

75 g cherries halved

75 g sultanas

Method

1. Grease a 15-18 cm plain or fluted deep flan ring
2. Mix the biscuits, walnuts, raisins, cherries, apricots, walnuts and sultanas together.
3. Melt the chocolate, butter and syrup together. Add to the rest of the ingredients. Mix well and press into the flan ring. Chill overnight or until thoroughly set.
4. Remove the ring carefully.
5. Cut into squares and serve

Cake

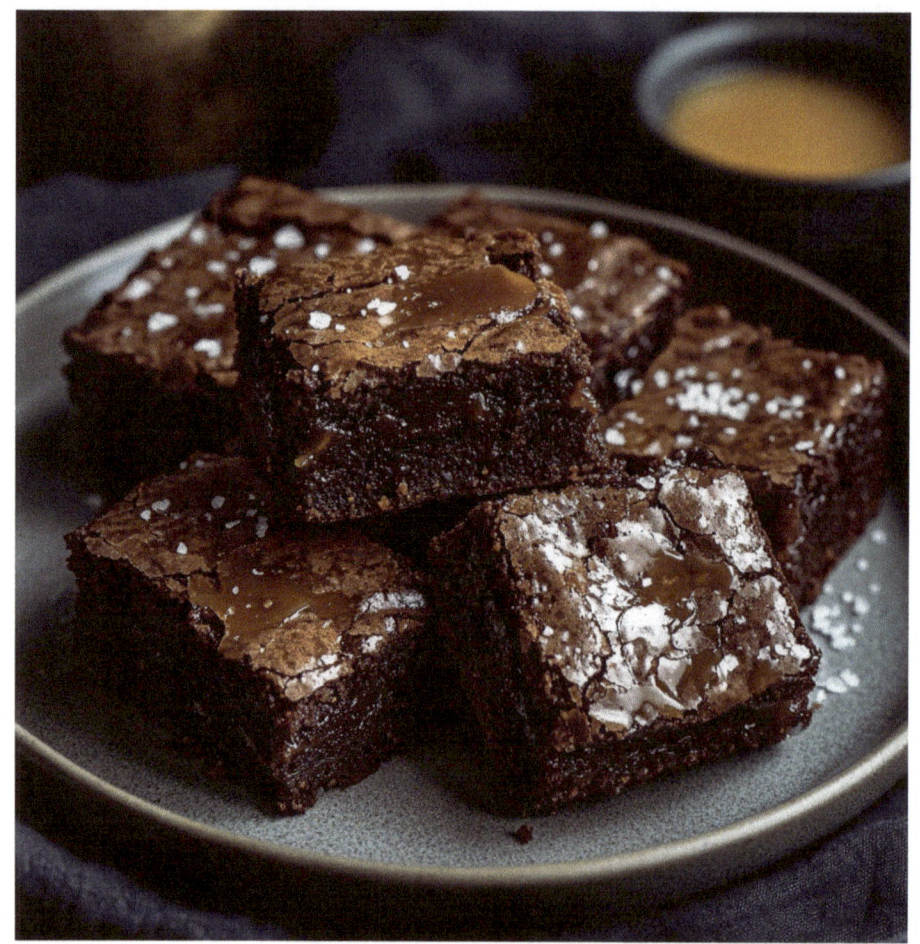

A Dance of Sweet and Bold

The chocolate melts, the caramel sighs,
A bite of gold 'neath cocoa skies.
The salt stands bright, the sugar sings,
A dish where depth and sweetness clings.

A moment soft, a taste so deep,
A bite the soul will always keep.
A brownie rich, both smooth and wide,
A feast of flavour, pure and tried.

—*Inspired by Robert Burns*

Salted Caramel Brownies

16 squares

Ingredients

220 g butter, plus a little extra for greasing

100 g chocolate, 70% cocoa solids

100 g chocolate, 50% cocoa solids

379 g can Carnation caramel

1 tsp flaky sea salt

200 g golden caster sugar

4 medium eggs, lightly beaten

130 g plain flour

50 g cocoa powder

Method

1. Heat the oven to 160°C.

2. Grease then line a 23cm square traybake tin with baking parchment. Break the chocolate in a pan and place over a pan of barely simmering water, once melted allow to cool.

3. Beat the sugar and butter in a bowl, until light in colour. Add the eggs a little at a time. Pour in the cooled melted chocolate and followed by the caramel, mix well.

4. Sift the flour and cocoa powder together in a bowl. Then fold the flour into the chocolate mixture. Add the salt. Beat briefly until smooth.

5. Pour the brownie batter into the tin. Bake in the oven for 25-30 minutes until risen all the way to the middle with a firm crust on top. When ready, the brownie will jiggle just a little when you shake it.

6. Let it cool completely in the tin, then cut into squares.

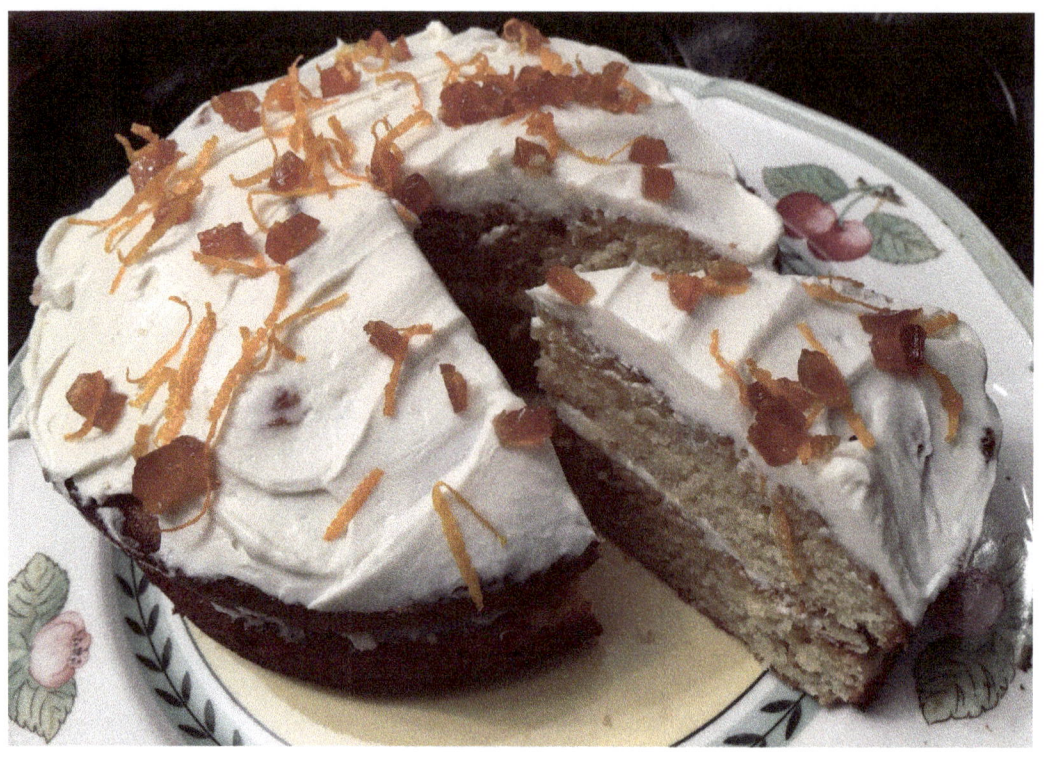

A Cake of Tang and Gold

The zest stands bright, the sponge sways light,
A citrus bite, a pure delight.
The marmalade hums, the sugar flows,
A taste where warmth and sharpness grows.

With syrup rich and golden cheer,
A slice to bring the heart sincere.
A cake where orange sings so free,
A dish of zest and history.

—*Inspired by John Buchan*

Seville Orange Marmalade Cake

Serves 8

Ingredients

125 g unsalted butter, softened, plus extra for greasing

200 g caster sugar

3 large eggs

100 ml single cream

250 g ground almonds

125 g plain flour

1 tsp baking powder

½ tsp salt

1 orange, zest

3 Tbsp Seville orange marmalade (no peel)

Orange syrup

1 small orange, juice

2 Tbsp Seville orange marmalade (no peel)

Mascarpone Filling

150 g mascarpone

125 g Greek yogurt

4 Tbsp icing sugar

2 Tbsp Seville orange marmalade (no peel)

Thinly slices of zest of an orange

Chopped marmalade peel.

Method

1. Preheat the oven to 180°C.

2. Grease and line the base of 2 x 20 cm cake tins with baking parchment. Using handheld electric beaters, or in a freestanding mixer, beat the butter and sugar together for 5 minutes until light and fluffy.

3. Beat in the eggs one at a time, then the cream, followed by the ground almonds. Fold in the flour, baking powder and salt, then stir thought the orange zest and marmalade until you have a smooth batter.

4. Divide evenly between the cake tins and bake for 20-25 minutes until a skewer inserted into the centre of the cakes comes out clean. Set on a wire rack to cool in the tins.

5. Once cool, make the syrup put the orange juice and marmalade in a small saucepan over a low heat, stirring until the marmalade has dissolved. Prick holes all over the cakes with a toothpick and pour the syrup evenly over the tops.

6. When you are ready to assemble the cake, make the frosting. Using handheld electric beater, mix all the ingredients, apart from 1tsp orange zest, together for 1 minute until combined.

7. Remove the cakes from their tins and discard the baking parchment. Put one cake onto a plate onto a plate or cake stand and spread with half the frosting. Sit the second cake on top, spread on the remaining frosting and scatter over the reserved orange zest.

Cake

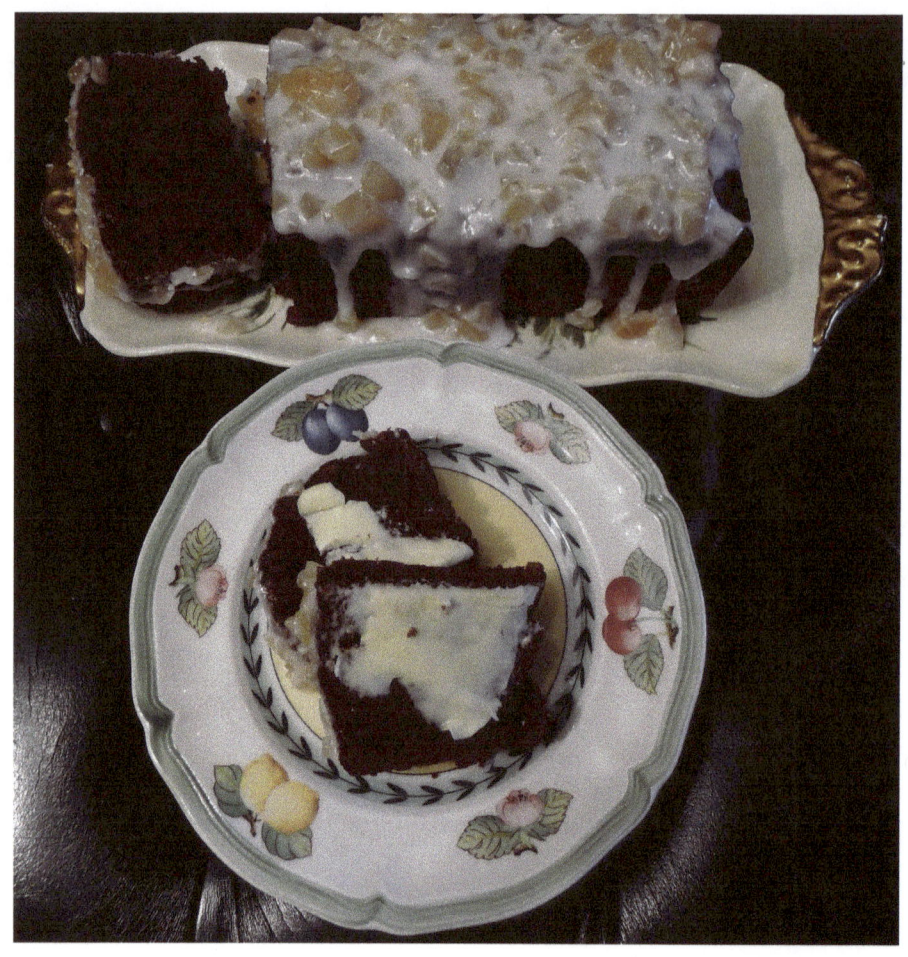

A Slice of Spice and Time

*The treacle sways, the spices glow,
A cake where warming whispers flow.
The ginger hums, the butter sighs,
A dish where winter's comfort lies.*

*A slice so soft, a taste so wide,
A plate of warmth and love inside.
With cream or tea, the time stands still,
A treat that bends to heart's own will.*

—*Inspired by Robert Burns*

Sticky Gingerbread

Serves 10

Ingredients

100 g golden syrup

100 g black treacle

75 g unsalted butter

75 g light soft brown or muscovado sugar

150 g plain flour

1 tsp ground ginger

½ tsp ground mixed spice

½ tsp ground cinnamon

1 egg, slightly beaten

75 ml milk

Finely grated zest of 1 lemon

½ tsp of bicarbonate of soda

75-100 g finely chopped preserved stem ginger in syrup drained

To finish, optional

50 g icing sugar, sifted

1 Tbsp of lemon juice or water

50 g whole stem ginger (2 pieces)

Equipment

1 L loaf tin, approx 20 x 10 cm, lightly greased, lined with parchment paper.

Method

1. Preheat the oven to 160°C.
2. Put the golden syrup, treacle, butter and sugar into a small saucepan. Place over a gentle heat and stir until the butter has melted and the ingredients are evenly blended. Set aside to cool.
3. Sift in the flour, ground ginger, mixed spice and cinnamon into a medium mixing bowl. Make a well in the centre and add the cooled treacle mixture, egg, milk and lemon zest.
4. Using a wooden spoon, beat well until the mixture is smooth and glossy. Then add the chopped ginger.
5. Dissolve the bicarbonate of soda in 1 Tbsp hot water. Add to the mixture with the chopped ginger and mix thoroughly to create a pourable batter.
6. Pour into the prepared tin and bake in the oven for 50-60 minutes, or until the cake is firm to touch and a skewer inserted into the centre comes out clean. Leave in the tin for 10 minutes before turning the cake out onto a wire rack to cool.
7. When cold, if you wish, mix the icing sugar with the lemon juice or water and drizzle over the cake, then top with silvers of stem ginger.

This cake will store well up to a week. The cake is very good sliced and buttered!

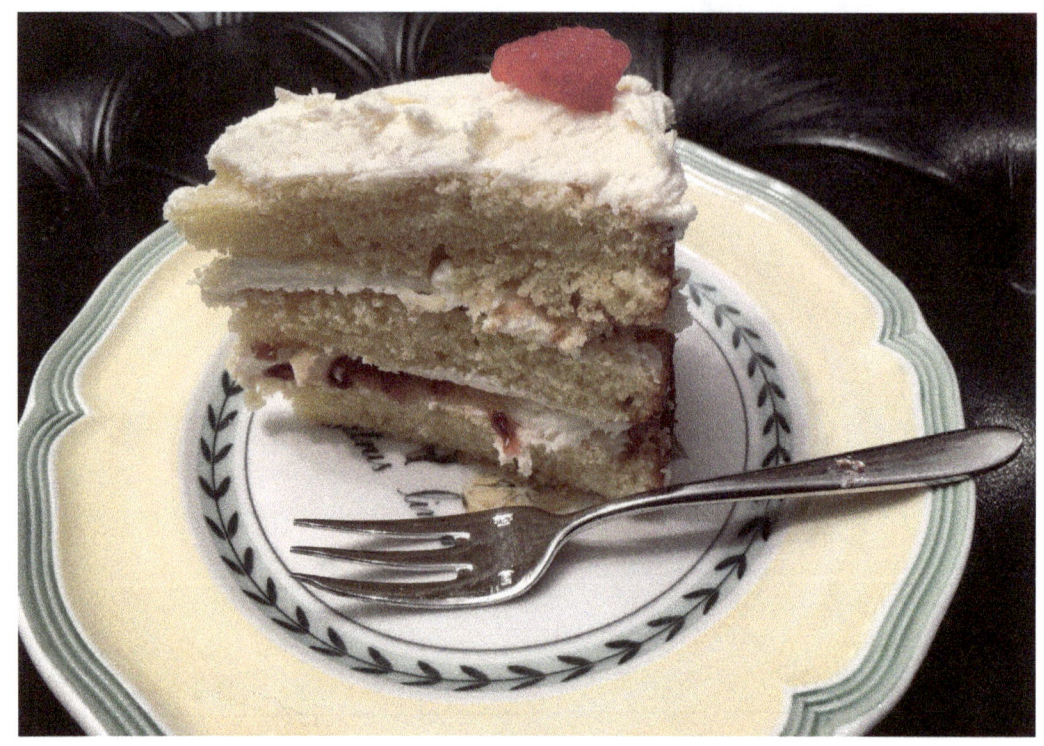

A Cake of Light and Love

A sponge so soft, a cream so white,
A jam so sweet, a pure delight.
The butter folds, the sugar sways,
A dish to mark the brightest days.

With hands that bake and hearts that cheer,
A cake to bring all souls sincere.
A slice, a sigh, a taste so free,
A love of baking's history.

—*Inspired by Robert Louis Stevenson*

Victoria Sponge Cake

Serves 10

Ingredients

225 g butter cut into small pieces and softened

225 g caster or vanilla sugar (or 1 tsp of vanilla essence)

4 eggs, lightly beaten, room temperature

225 g self raising flour

2 tsp baking powder

Method

1. Preheat the oven to 160°C.

2. 2 x 20 cm sandwich tins, lightly greased and base lined with baking parchment.

3. Sift the flour into a bowl and set aside.

4. In a large mixing bowl, using a hand held mixer beat the butter until light in colour. Add the caster sugar and continue to beat until the mixture is very light and creamy. The lighter the fluffier the butter and sugar mix is, the easier it will be to blend in the eggs, which in turn helps to prevent the mixture curdling.

5. Break the eggs into a small bowl and beat lightly with a fork until broken. Add the eggs, a little at a time beating well after each addition, adding the eggs when cold or too quickly can cause the mixture to curdle. Add 1 Tbsp of the flour towards the end of adding the eggs if you are worried about the mixture curdling, this will stabilise the mixture. Beat in the vanilla extract.

6. Sift in the rest of the flour, and baking powder, half at a time, and use a large metal spoon to carefully fold it in using a figure of 8 motion. The mixture should drop off the spoon easily when tapped against the side of the bowl. If it doesn't then add 1-2 Tbsp of hot water to loosen the mixture.

7. Divide the mixture equally between the prepared sandwich tins, spreading it out lightly and evenly with the back of the spoon. Bake in the centre of the oven for about 25 minutes or until the cakes are lightly golden and spring back into shape when gently pressed in the centre with a finger.

8. Leave them in the tin for a couple of minutes before turning them out onto a wire rack to cool completely.

9. When cold, spread one cake with the jam, then whip the double cream, spread this over the jam. Put the other half on top .Mix the icing sugar with the lemon juice spread over the top.

The cake will keep for 2-3 days in an airtight tin.

Butter Cream Filling

Ingredients

½ pint double cream, lightly whipped
3-4 Tbsp of soft set raspberry jam
30 g icing sugar, sifted
1 tsp lemon juice

Or

150 g butter
300 g icing sugar sieved
1 tsp vanilla essence

Method

1. Place the butter in a mixing bowl and, beat until creamy. Incorporate the icing sugar in three lots, beating well after each addition. When it is all added, the mixture should be a light creamy. Finally mix in the vanilla extract.

Put a tea towel over the machine to stop the icing sugar from bowing out of the bowl.

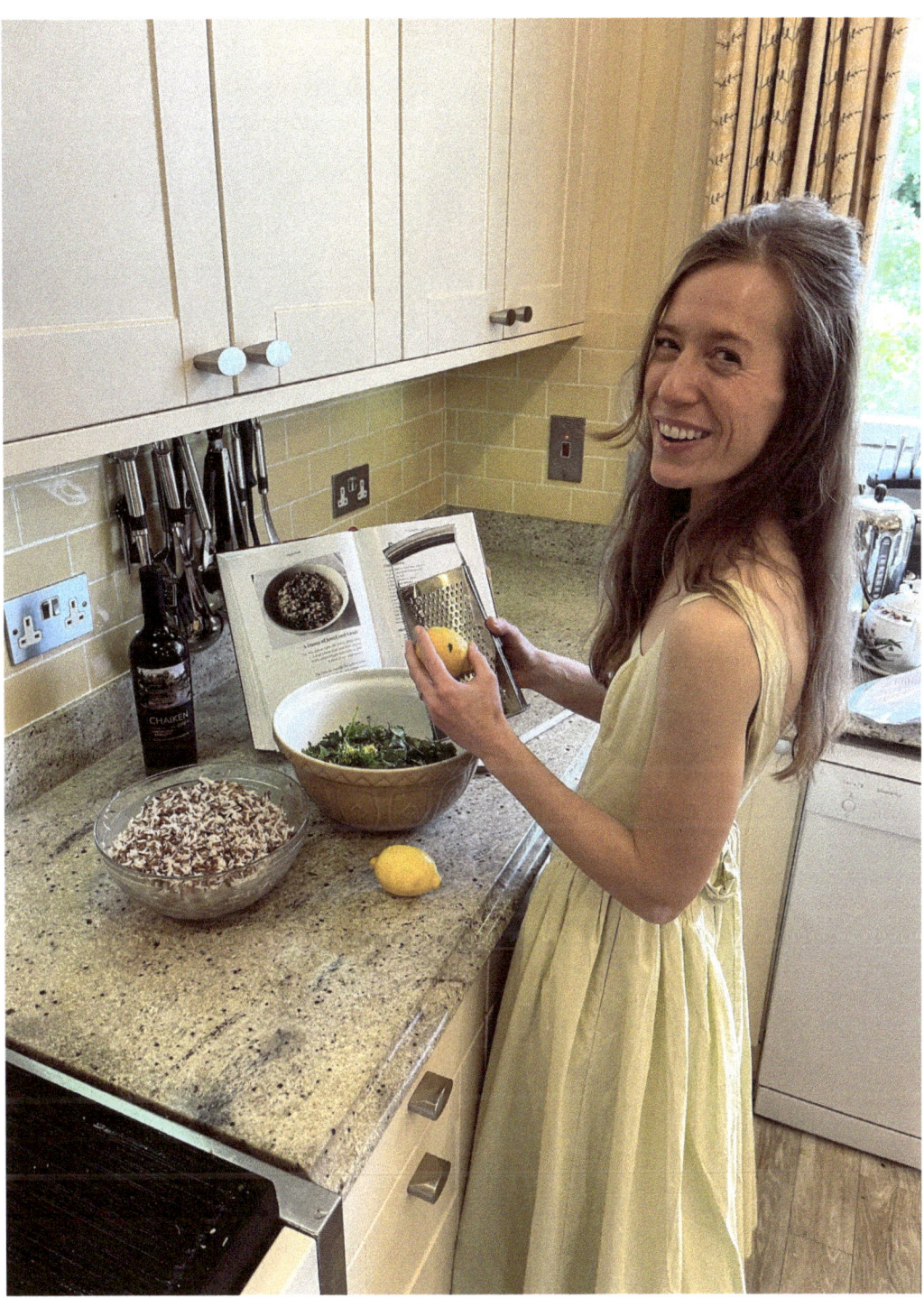

Cake

Flint Family Cookbook

Biscuits

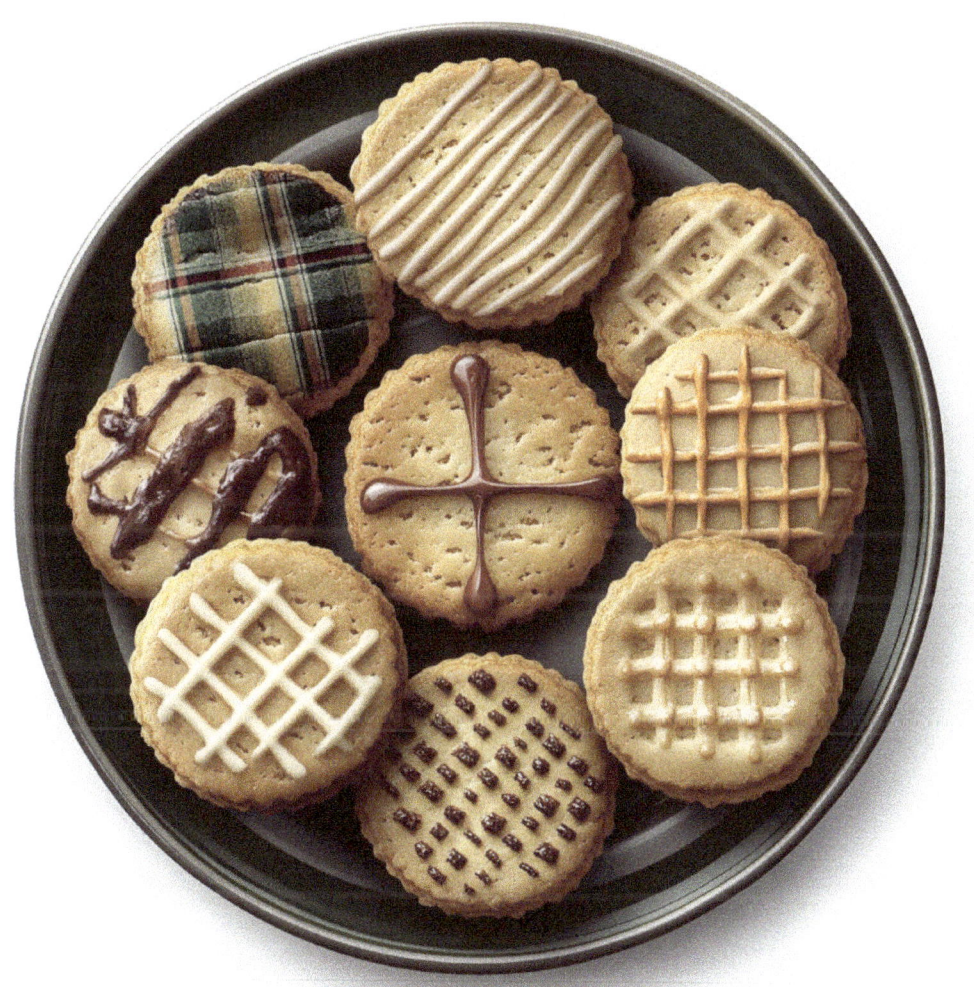

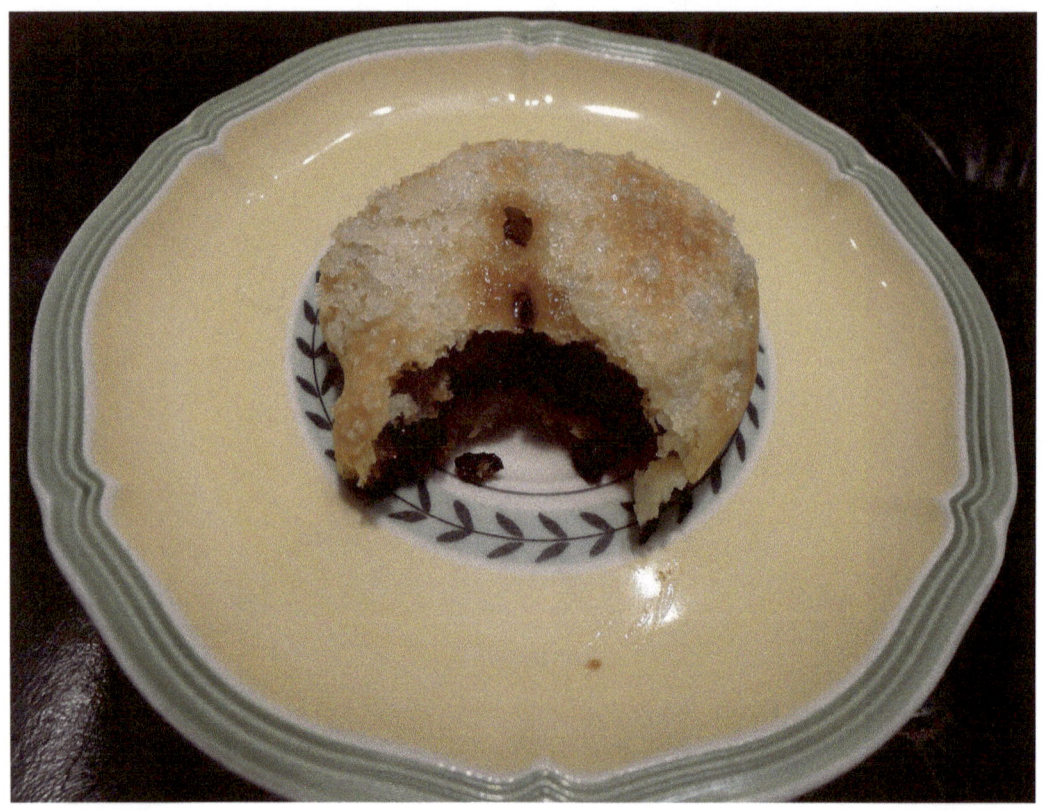

A Pastry's Secret

A golden fold, a hidden sweet,
A tale of currants, dark and neat.
The sugar glows, the pastry sways,
A treat from long and cherished days.

With butter rich and spice so deep,
A taste of warmth the heart shall keep.
A bite, a pause, a moment free,
A pastry kissed by history.

—*Inspired by Robert Louis Stevenson*

Eccles Cakes

Makes 6

Ingredients

320 g packet of puff frozen pastry

Filling
80 g softened butter
80 g Demerara sugar
100 g currants
50 g raisins
100 g sultanas

For the glaze
Water
Granulated sugar

Method

1. Roll out the pastry on a lightly floured work surface and cut into 6 squares.

2. Cream the butter and brown sugar together.

3. Fold in the rest of the ingredients; divide the mixture between each of the pastry squares. Dampen around the outer edges and draw up the pastry edges together and reshape into a round shape.

4. Turn it over and lightly press down. Make a very small sharp cut on the top.

5. Allow the cakes to rest on a baking tray in the fridge for about 10 minutes.

6. Brush the surface with water and sprinkle with sugar.

7. Bake in the oven at 180°C for about 10 minutes until s light brown. Leave to cool on a wire rack.

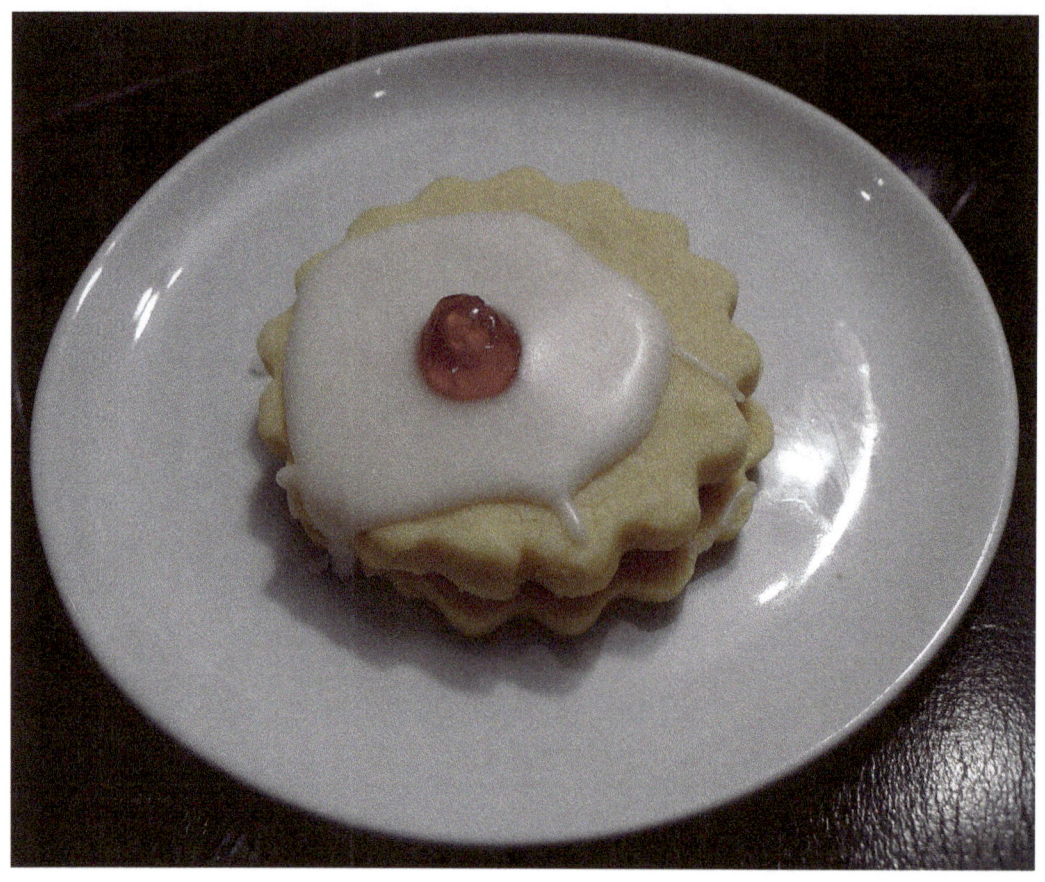

A Regal Delight

A biscuit light, a centre bright,
With jam that sings in soft delight.
The icing shines, the cherry sways,
A treat of childhood's golden days.

A crunch, a sweet, a flavour grand,
A taste made fine by careful hand.
With sugar's kiss and butter's cheer,
A joy to bring the heart sincere.

—*Inspired by John Buchan*

Empire Biscuits

Makes 14 biscuits (depending on the thickness of the biscuits)

Ingredients

250 g plain flour, extra for dusting

125 g icing sugar

125 g cornflour

250 g soft unsalted butter

100 g raspberry jam

7 glace cherries cut in half

Icing

175 g icing sugar

1 Tbsp of lemon juice (optional)

Method

1. Preheat the oven to 180°C.
2. Put the flour, icing sugar, and cornflour in a large bowl and rub in the butter with your fingers until it forms a dough (or put it in a food processor and blitz until it comes together). Depending on the softness of the butter, 1 tablespoon of cold water may be needed to bring it together.
3. Put on a floured surface and roll with a floured rolling pin until about 6mm thick. Use a 4-5 cm cutter to cut 28 circles.
4. Put on trays and bake for 10-12 minutes. Take them out just before they turn golden brown. Cool on a rack.
5. To make the icing, sift the icing sugar into a bowl, add 1 Tbsp water or lemon juice and stir until thick and glossy.
6. Sandwich jam between the undersides of the two biscuits. Then top with the icing and half a glace cherry.

Biscuits

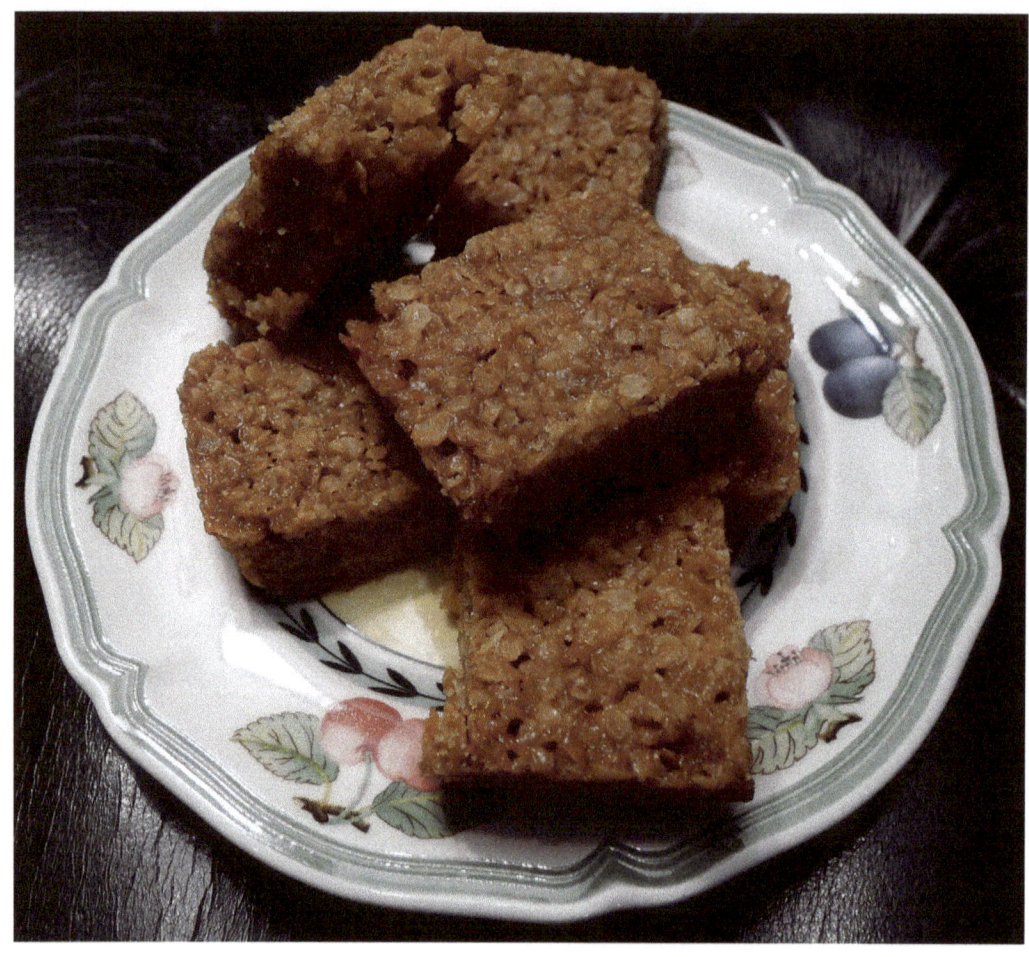

A Hearthside Treat

Oats and syrup, rich and deep,
A bite where golden comforts keep.
The butter melts, the kitchen glows,
A scent that lingers, soft and slow.

A square of warmth, both firm and sweet,
A humble gift, a homely treat.
With hands held high, the tray passed round,
A taste of joy, a love profound.

—Inspired by Robert Burns

Flapjacks

20 squares

Ingredients

225 g butter (plus butter to grease the dish)

225 g demerara sugar

75 g (3 oz) golden syrup

275 g (10 oz) rolled oats

Method

1. Grease a 20 cm square cake tin.

2. Melt the butter with the sugar and syrup, and heat gently until the sugar has melted.

3. Remove from the heat and add the oats. Mix well, turn the mixture into the prepared tin and press down well.

4. Bake the flapjacks in the oven at 160°C for 16-18 minutes until golden brown.

5. The cooked mixture will set as it cools. If it is overcooked, it will become quite hard and difficult to cut into squares.

6. After about 20 minutes, mark the flapjacks into squares with a sharp knife and loosen around the edges. When firm, remove them from the tin and break them into squares.

The flapjacks may be stored in an airtight container for up to a week.

Biscuits

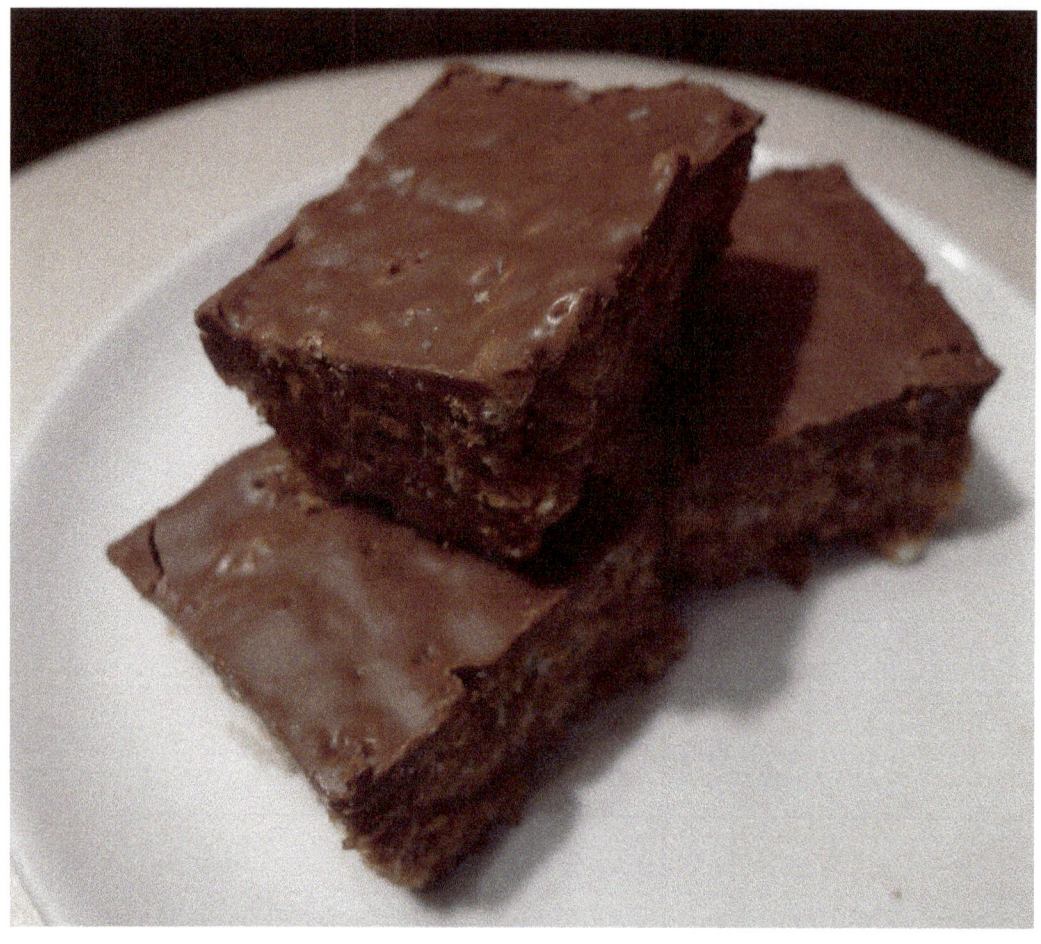

A Mischief of Sweetness

A swirl of chocolate, crisp below,
A childhood treat, a simple glow.
The caramel hums, the cocoa sways,
A memory made in golden days.

With hands that press and tongues that wait,
A square of joy upon the plate.
So take a bite, embrace the cheer,
A taste that lingers, bright and clear.

—*Inspired by Contemporary Scottish Poets*

Mars Bar Slices

16 squares

Ingredients

3 Mars bars
3 Tbsp of golden syrup
90 g butter
75 g Rice Krispies

For the Topping
200 g milk chocolate

Method

1. Grease and line the base of an oblong tin, 24 x 17 x 4 cm
2. Melt the Mars bars, butter and syrup over low heat.
3. Add the Rice Krispies and stir gently until coated.
4. Press into a greased and lined oblong tin and leave to set.
5. Top with melted chocolate, leave to set and cut into squares.

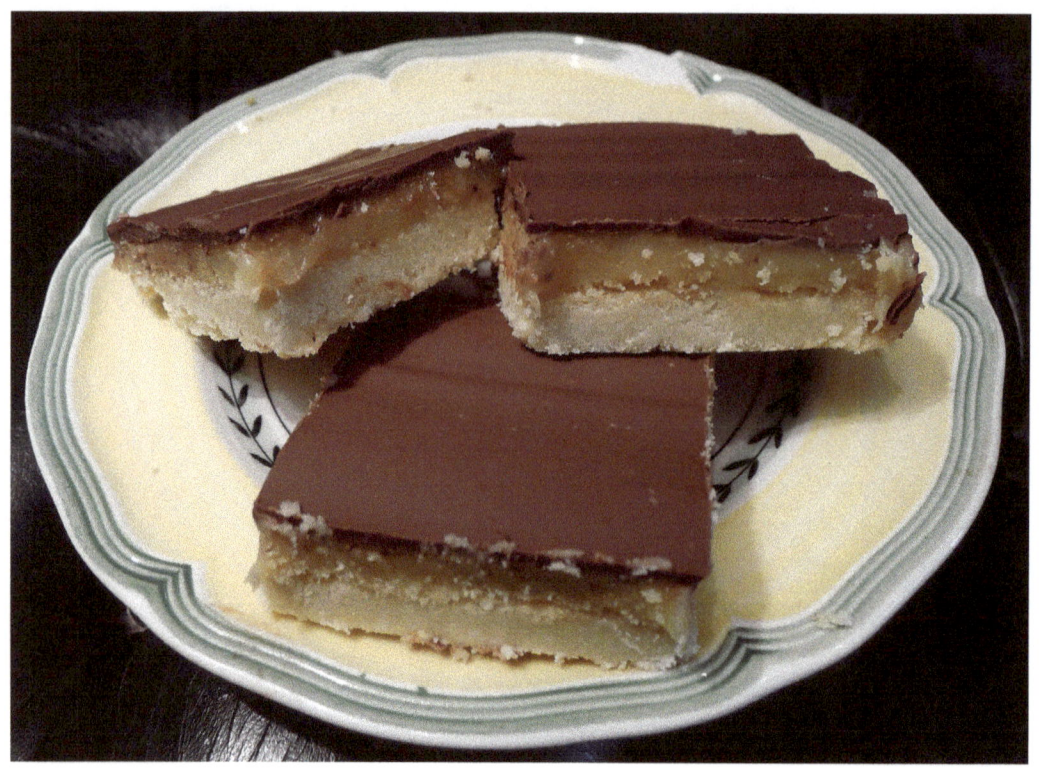

A Bite of Fortune

A layer crisp, a golden pour,
A bite that begs for one slice more.
The butter hums, the sugar sings,
A treat where wealth in sweetness clings.

With caramel rich and chocolate high,
A feast to bring both cheer and sigh.
A taste so bold, so fine, so bright,
A dish of pure and sweet delight.

—*Inspired by Robert Louis Stevenson*

Millionaire's Shortbread

30 squares

Ingredients – Shortbread

1 tray bake tin 25 x 30 x 5 cm, greased and lined with butter

220 g unsalted butter, softened

30 g icing sugar

80 g caster sugar

30 g cornflour

300 g plain flour

Method

1. Heat the oven to 160°C.
2. Put the soft butter into a mixing bowl and beat with an electric mixer until light and creamy.
3. Sift the icing sugar into the bowl and beat in (if using an electric mixer, use a low speed to start). Beat in the caster sugar.
4. Scrape down the sides of the bowl, and then speed beat thoroughly for a couple of minutes until the mixture is light and fluffy.
5. Sift the cornflour into the bowl and beat in. Sift the flour, a little at a time, into the bowl and mix on the lowest setting to make a crumbly mixture.
6. Tip into the prepared tin and spread evenly. Gently press out the mixture into the corners of the tin, too. Prick all over with a fork.
7. Place in the heated oven and bake for about 35 minutes until pale golden.
8. Remove from the oven and allows to cool on a heatproof surface.

Toffee Layer

Ingredients

225 g unsalted butter, diced

115 g caster sugar

4 Tbsp of golden syrup

379 g condensed milk

For the topping

200 g milk chocolate (40-50% cocoa solids)

Method

1. Leave the shortbread in the tin until completely cold.

2. Put the diced butter, sugar, syrup, and condensed milk into a medium-sized heavy-based pan to make the toffee layer. Set over low heat and stir frequently with a wooden spoon until the butter melts.

3. Bring to a boil, stirring constantly to prevent the mixture from catching on the base of the pan, for 3-5 minutes until it turns golden (don't let the mixture turn to a dark caramel colour, or it will set too hard to cut).

4. Pour the toffee mixture over the cold shortbread and spread it evenly. Leave until cold.

5. Put the chocolate in a heatproof bowl, set the bowl over a pan of simmering water and melt gently, stirring occasionally.

6. Spread the chocolate evenly over the toffee.

7. Leave in a cool place—not the fridge—to set, then use a sharp knife to cut into 30 fingers.

8. Store in an airtight container and eat within 5 days.

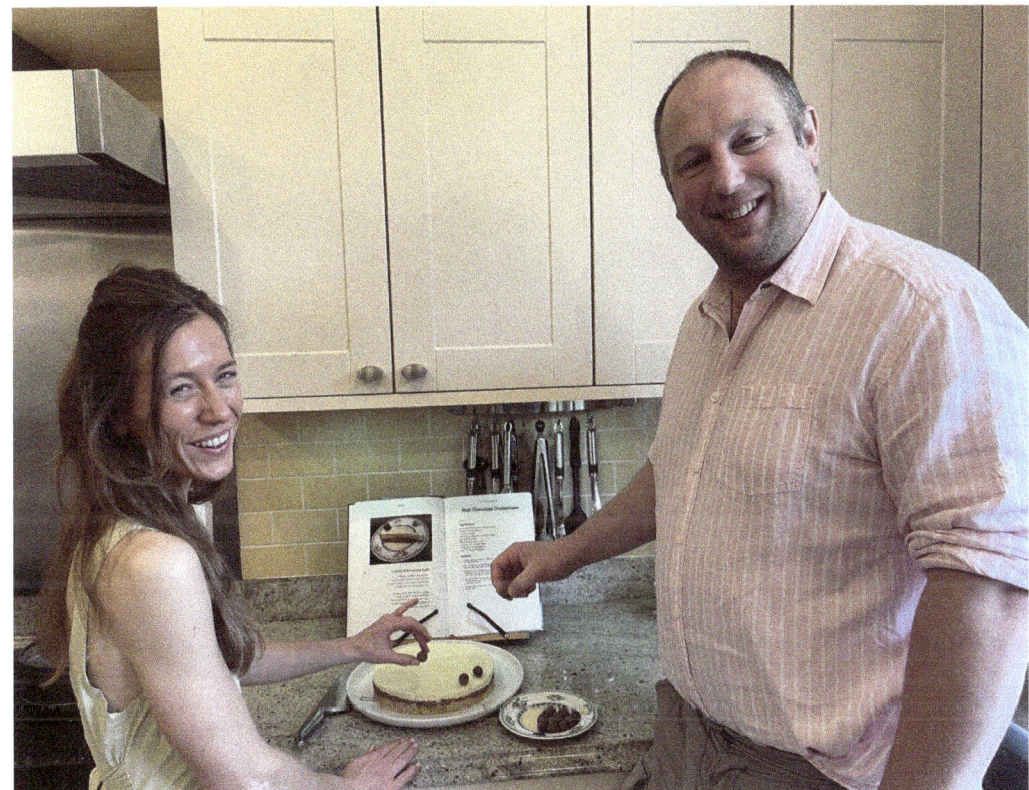

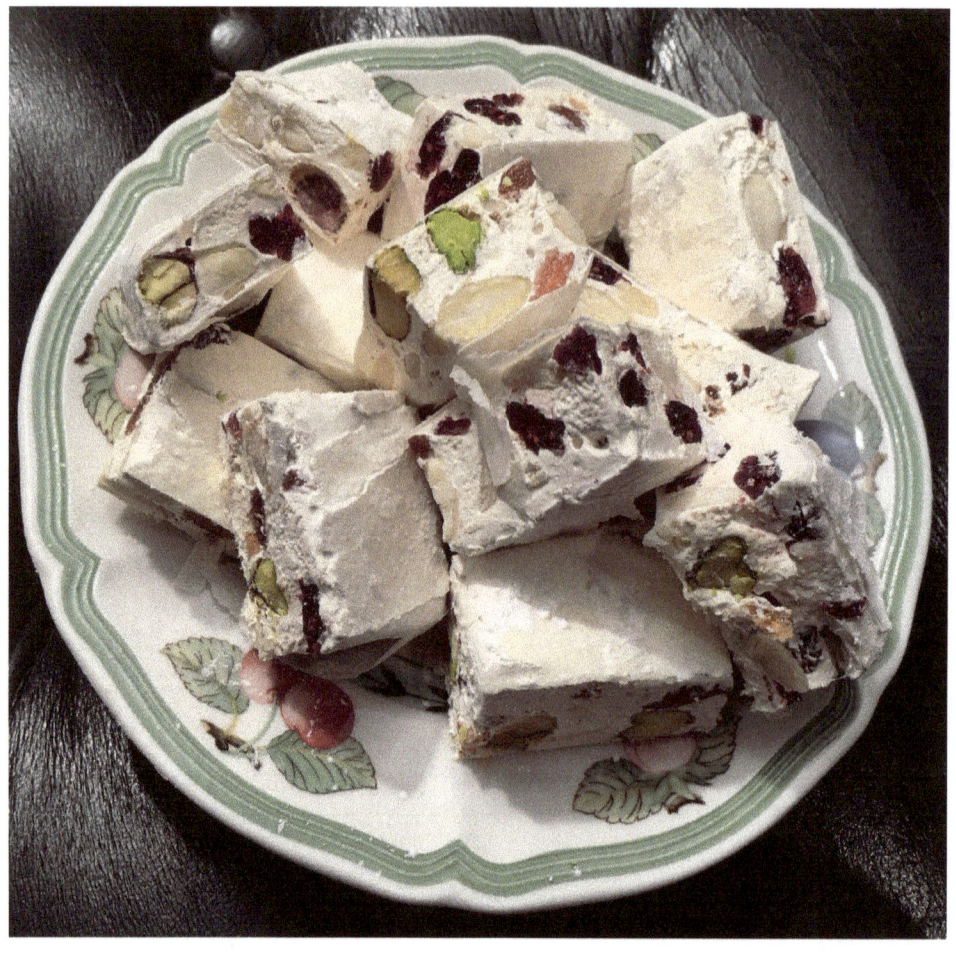

A Dance of Nut and Sweet

A sticky touch, a nut's embrace,
A treat so light, yet rich in place.
With almonds crisp and cherries bright,
A taste that lingers soft and light.

A bite of cheer, a feast so free,
A candy spun through history.
With hands that shape and hearts that share,
A joy that floats upon the air.

—*Inspired by Contemporary Scottish Poets*

Nougat

36 squares

Ingredients

175 g pistachio Kernels
100 g blanched almonds
100 g dried cranberries
50 g cherries halved
275 g granulated sugar

150 g runny honey
1 Tbsp liquid glucose (lightly grease spoon with oil before measuring)
2 large egg whites
Edible rice paper or 15 g icing sugar

Method

1. Preheat the oven to 110°C.

2. Spread nuts, cranberries, and cherries on a baking tray and put in the oven to warm.

3. Line the sides and base of a 20 cm square cake tin with parchment, leaving excess to hang over the sides. Next, line the base of the tin with a square of rice paper trimmed to fit. If you don't have rice paper, dust it with cornflour.

4. Heat the sugar, honey, glucose, and 75 ml water in a medium pan over low heat. Once the sugar dissolves, turn up the heat and boil until the temperature reaches 157°C on a sugar thermometer.

5. Just before the mixture reaches this temperature, beat egg whites in a freestanding mixer to stiff peaks. With the motor running and the honey mixture at 157°C, carefully and slowly pour the hot liquid into the egg bowl trying not to get it on the whisk.

6. Continue whisking for 10-15 minutes or until the outside of the bowl feels warm (not hot) and the mixture is thick, elastic and coming away from the sides of the bowl.

7. Pop the nuts and berries in a jug and pour the mixture into it. When mixed through, quickly spread the mixture in the prepared tin with a wet spatula. Press a layer of rice paper on top, dust it with cornflour, and top it with baking parchment.

8. Leave to set overnight at room temperature. Using the excess parchment, lift the nougat out on a board. Trim edges to neaten, and then cut into 3cm squares.

Keep the nougat in an airtight container at a cool temperature for up to two weeks.

Biscuits

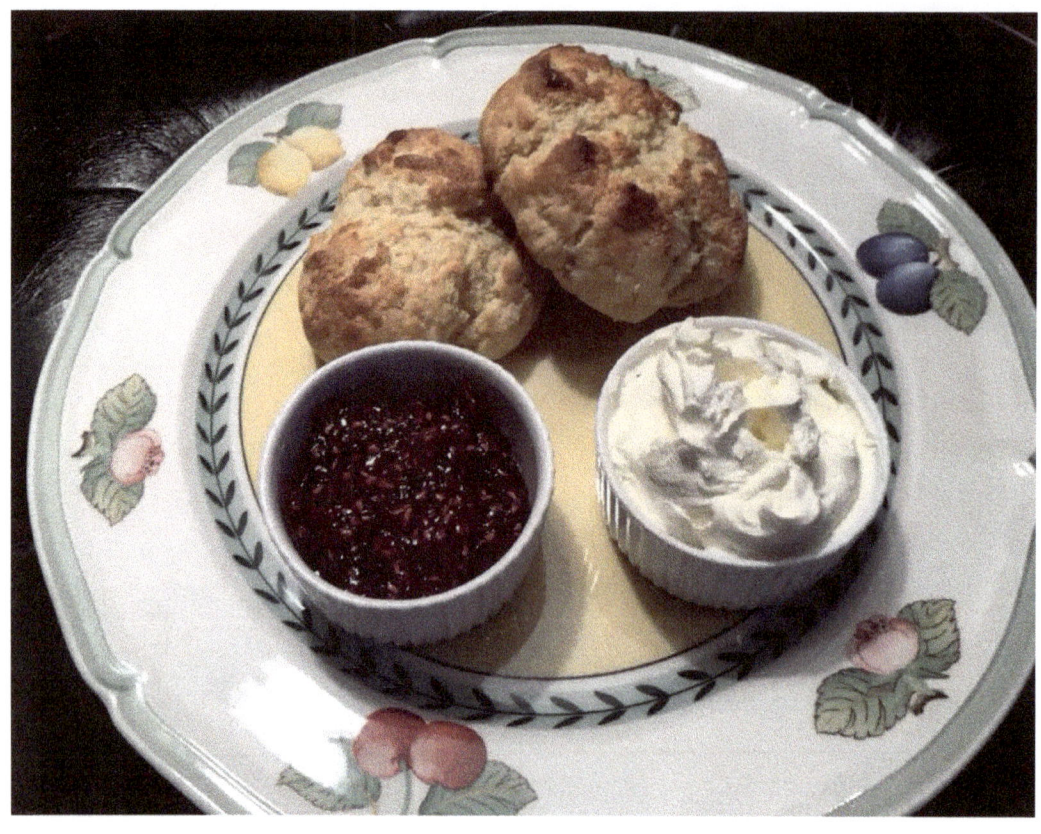

A Bite of Cream and Cheer

The butter folds, the dough turns light,
A scone that rises soft and bright.
With jam so red and cream so wide,
A taste where simple joys abide.

The oven hums, the tray stands near,
A smell to bring both warmth and cheer.
So break, so share, so sip with tea,
A treat of Scottish harmony.

—*Inspired by Robert Burns*

Scones

Makes 6

Ingredients

250 g self-raising flour, sieved, plus extra flour for dusting

1 heaped tsp baking powder, sieve

A pinch of salt

40 g unsalted butter, cubed

75-100 ml buttermilk, plus extra for glazing

1 large egg

25 g caster sugar

To serve
Clotted cream
Raspberry or strawberry jam

Method

1. Preheat the oven to 200°C.
2. Lightly grease a baking sheet and dust it with a bit of flour.
3. Sieve the flour, baking powder and salt into a mixing bowl. Stir in the butter cubes until they are coated with flour, then start rubbing them in with your fingertips until the mixture looks like fine bread crumbs. Add the sugar and mix into the flour.
4. Beat the egg and place it in a measuring jug. Pour enough milk to make the liquid up to 100ml; set the rest aside for glazing the scones.
5. Gradually add the egg and milk to the dry ingredients, stirring it with a blunt knife until you have a soft, slightly sticky dough that is not so wet that it is too sticky to pick up.
6. Lightly dust the work surface with flour. Scoop the dough out and pat it out until it is about 2cm thick. Stamp out with a 1½" cutter, brush with the remaining milk, and sprinkle on caster sugar. (Do not twist the cutter, or the scone will rise unevenly.)
7. Pop into the oven for 8-12 minutes until well risen and golden. Pat under the scone; it should sound like a drum. Place on a wire rack to cool slightly, cut in half and serve warm with cream and jam.

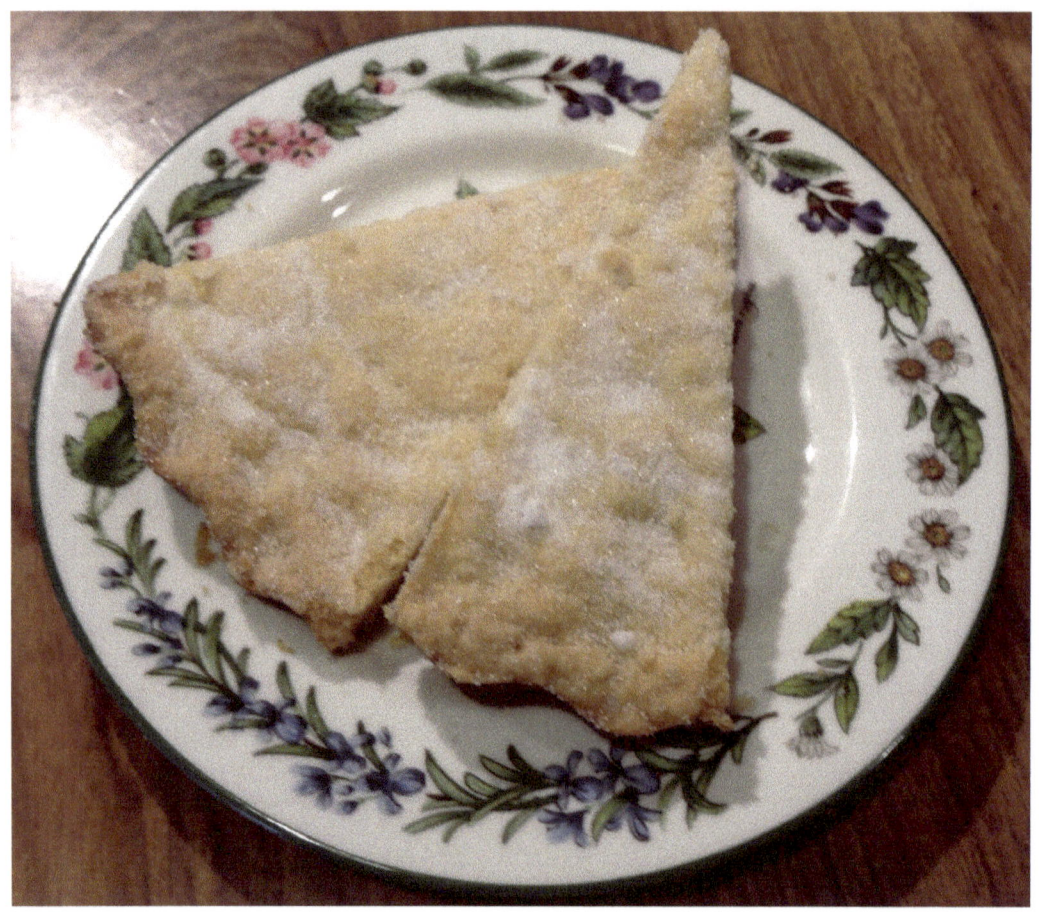

A Classic and True Delight

A biscuit firm, yet soft in hand,
A simple joy, both pure and grand.
The butter lingers, light yet deep,
A taste of home the heart shall keep.

With sugar dusted, crisp yet fine,
A treat of time, a gift divine.
So take a square, embrace the cheer,
A taste that stands through every year.

—*Inspired by Robert Burns*

Shortbread

Serves 24

Ingredients

1 tray bake tin 20.5 x 25 x 5 cm, greased with butter.

220 g unsalted butter, softened

30 g icing sugar

80 g caster sugar, plus extra for sprinkling

30 g cornflour

300 g plain flour

Method

1. Heat the oven to 160°C.
2. Put the soft butter into a mixing bowl and beat with an electric mixer until light and creamy.
3. Sift the icing sugar into the bowl and beat it in (if using an electric mixer, use a low speed to start). Beat in the caster sugar.
4. Scrape down the sides of the bowl, and then speed beat thoroughly for a couple of minutes until the mixture is light and fluffy.
5. Sift the cornflour into the bowl and beat in. Sift the flour, a little at a time, into the bowl and mix on the lowest setting to make a crumbly mixture.
6. Tip into the prepared tin and spread evenly. Gently press out the mixture into the corners of the tin, too. Prick all over with a fork.
7. Place in the heated oven and bake for about 35 minutes until pale golden.
8. Remove the tin from the oven and set it on a heatproof surface. Using a sharp knife, cut into 24 squares, then sprinkle with sugar.
9. Leave to cool completely before removing from the tin. Store the fingers and ears in an airtight container within a week.

Biscuits

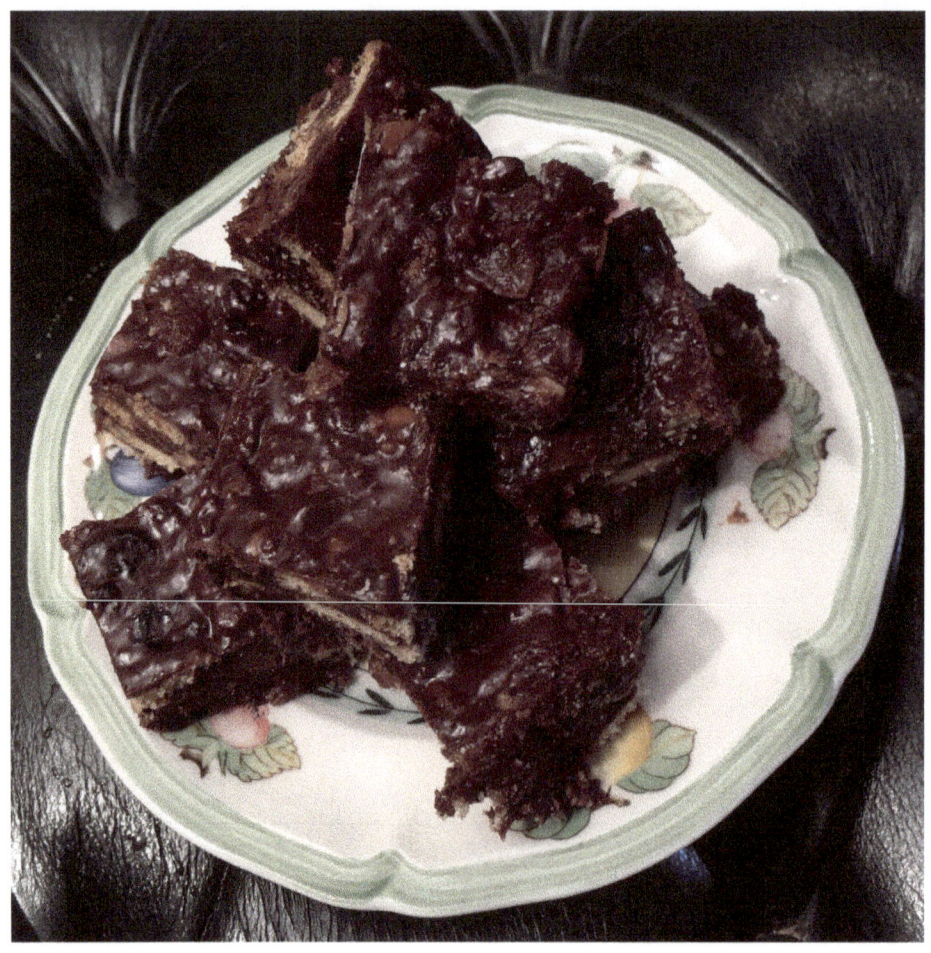

304

A Layered Memory

A mix of crisp, a swirl of sweet,
A treat where cocoa and biscuit meet.
The raisins hum, the orange sighs,
A plate of joy for eager eyes.

A crunch, a melt, a moment bright,
A square of pure and sweet delight.
With tea in hand and stories spun,
A taste where time and comfort run.

—*Inspired by Robert Louis Stevenson*

Tiffin

16 squares

Ingredients

50 g raisins

75 g chopped dates

1 Tbsp brandy

200 g bar plain chocolate

150 g butter

3 Tbsp golden syrup

250 g digestive biscuits, roughly crushed

Zest of ½ large orange

For the topping

150 g dark chocolate, at least 70% cocoa solids

Method

1. Grease and baseline a 20 cm round tin with a depth of 4 cm.

2. Put the raisins, dates and brandy in a bowl and leave to soak for 30 minutes.

3. Melt the plain chocolate, 125 g butter and golden syrup in a pan over a gentle heat.

4. Add the biscuits, orange zest, raisins, dates and any remaining brandy. Mix well, spoon into the tin, level the surface, then cool and chill for 1 hour.

5. Melt the dark chocolate in a pan with the remaining butter to make the topping. Pour over the biscuit layer and chill overnight.

The cake can be kept in the fridge in an airtight container for five days.

Biscuits

Flint Family Cookbook

Jam

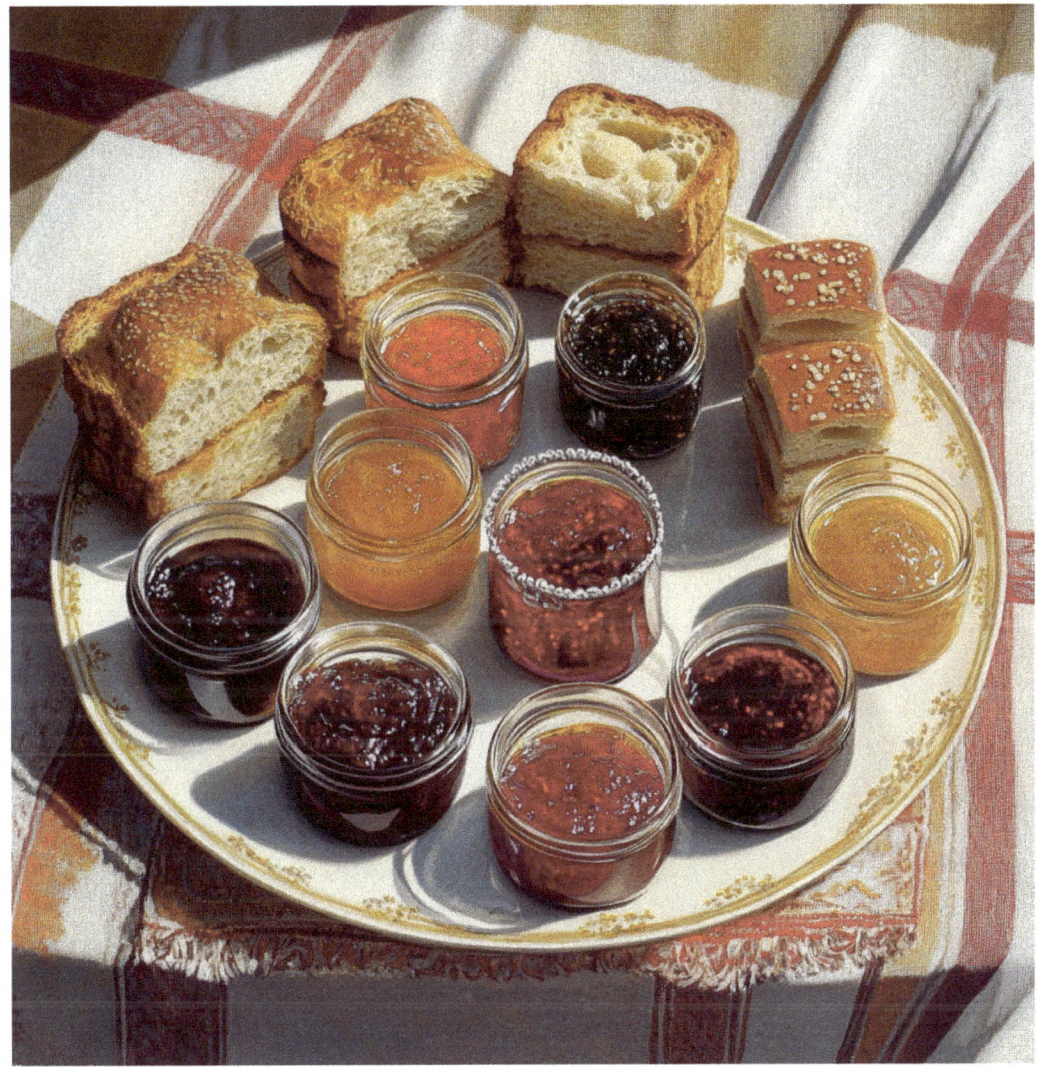

Jam

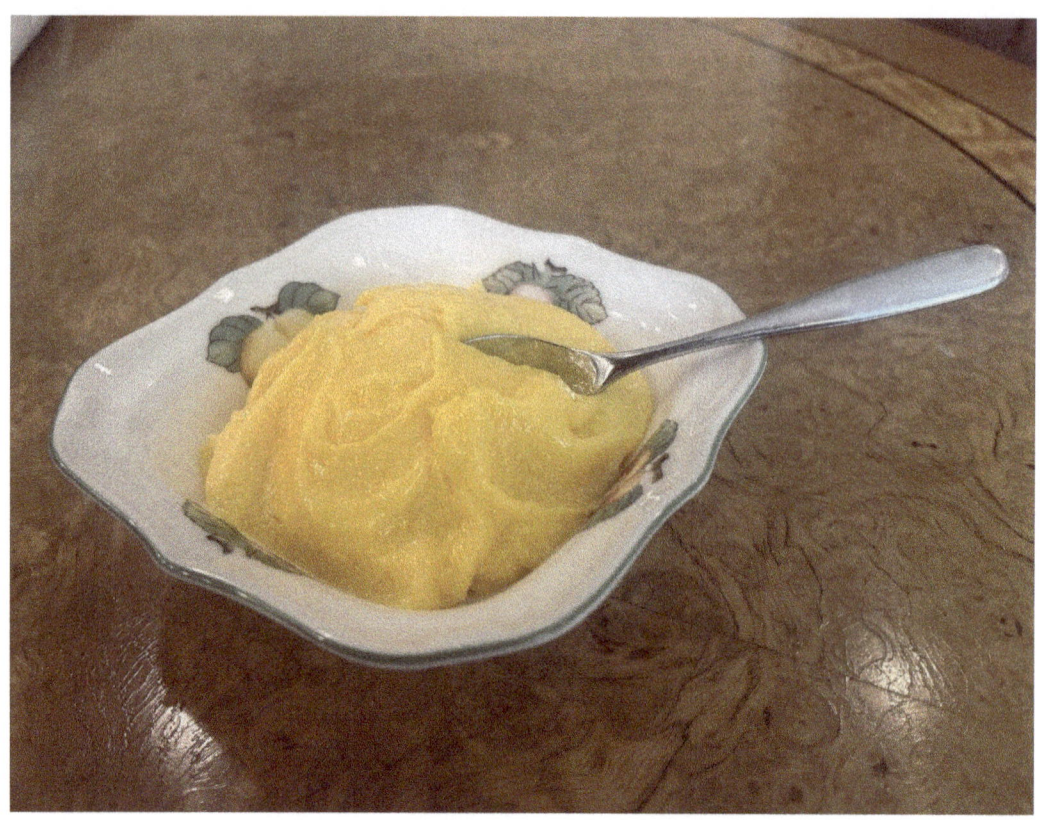

A Spoon of Sunshine

A golden swirl, so bright, so sweet,
A taste where sun and sugar meet.
The butter hums, the citrus sings,
A curd of light on golden wings.

Spread thick on toast or sponge so fair,
A bite of warmth, beyond compare.
A jar of cheer, a spoon so free,
A taste of joy for you and me.

—Inspired by Robert Louis Stevenson

Fresh Lemon Curd

Makes approximately ¾ pint

Ingredients

2 large lemons, grated rind and juice
150 g caster sugar
4 large eggs
100 g unsalted butter

Method

1. Place the grated lemon rind and sugar in a bowl. Whisk the lemon juice with the eggs in another bowl, and then pour this mixture over the sugar.

2. Add the butter cut into little pieces, and place the bowl over a pan of barely simmering water.

3. Stir frequently till thickened, about 25 minutes. When cool, use the curd for sponges, toast, etc.

Store in a screw top lid jar, keep in the fridge and is best eaten within a week to ten days.

Jam

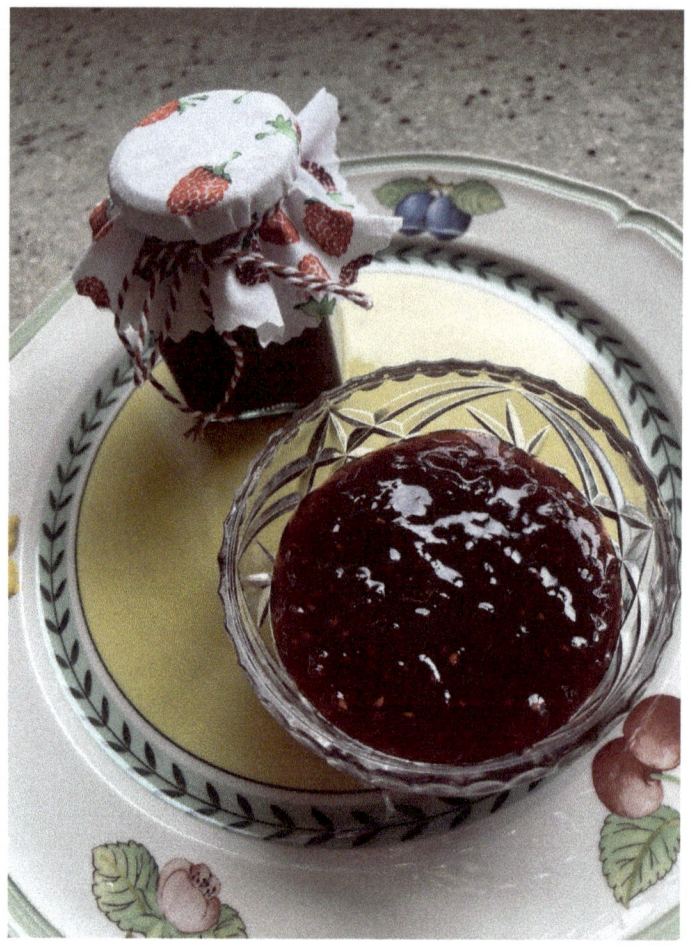

A Jar of Summer's Glow

The berries burst, the sugar sways,
A pot of light from summer's days.
The crimson swirls, the sweetness hums,
A taste where warmth and sunlight runs.

A spoon, a spread, a treat so bright,
A jam that holds the morning light.
Upon the toast, upon the scone,
A fruit-filled love, a gift well-known.

—*Inspired by Robert Burns*

Raspberry Jam

Makes about 3 kg

Ingredients

1.8 kg (4 lb) raspberries, washed

1.8 kg (4 lb) granular sugar

1 tsp lemon juice

Knob of butter

Sterilised jars

Method

1. Place the raspberries in a preserving pan and simmer very gently in their juice for about 15 minutes, stirring carefully from time to time, until the fruit is really soft.

2. Remove the pan from the heat and add the sugar, stirring until dissolved, then add the knob of butter and boil rapidly for about 15 minutes. (Do not overcook, or it will set too firmly.)

3. Test for a set when the temperature reaches 104°C. The jam will start to congeal on the edge of a wooden spoon. When the jam has reached the setting point remove from the heat and remove any surface scum with a slotted spoon. Allow to cool for 15 minutes before pouring into sterilised glass jars.

4. Warm the jars before pouring in the jam.

5. Leave to stand for 15 minutes: pot and cover.

For food safety, sterilised jars must be used.

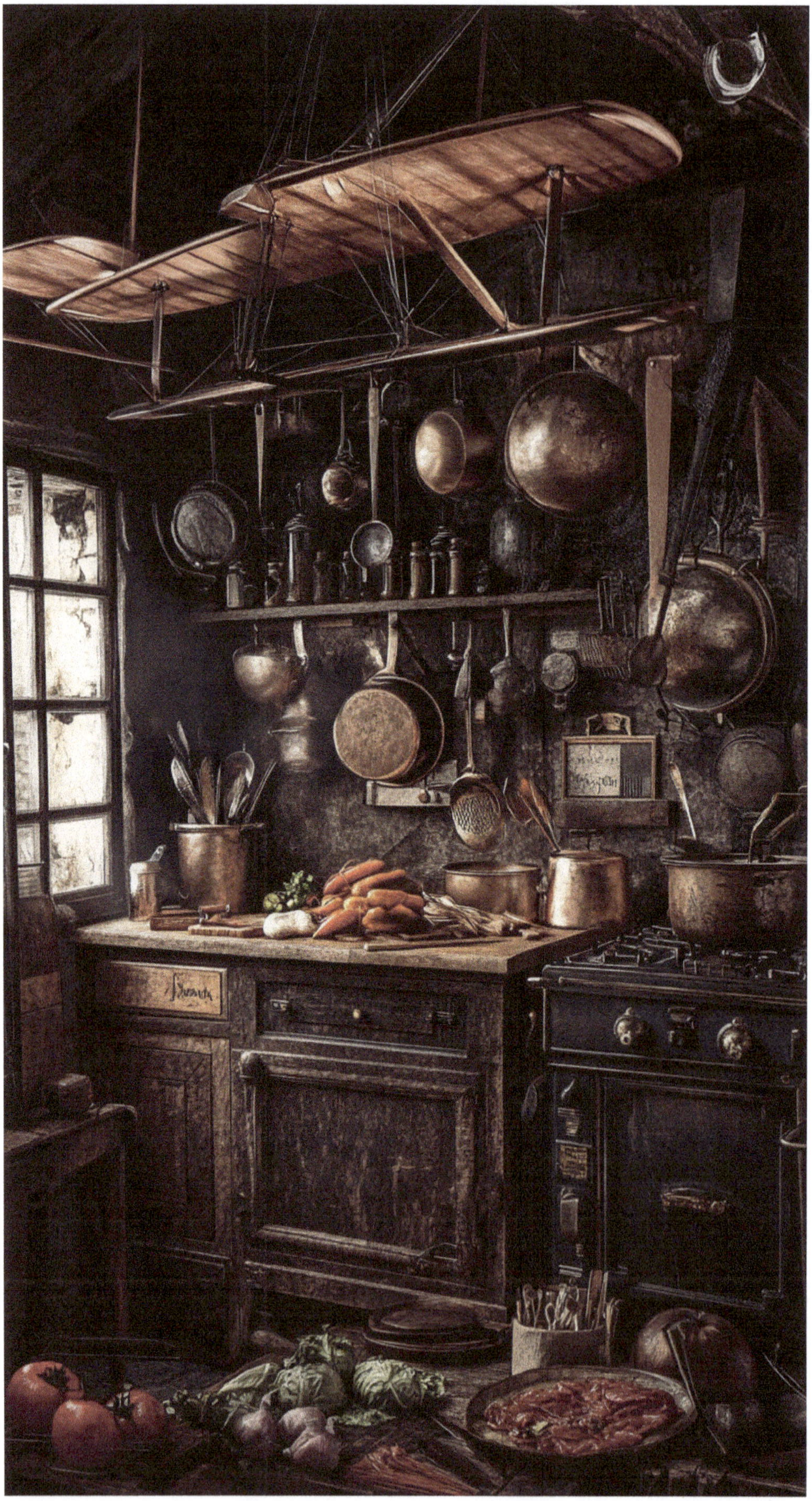

A Tribute

O noble heart, whose wisdom shines so bright,
In thee doth blend both art and reason's might.
With hand most kind and vision keenly true,
Thou gav'st to time what time might else undo.

Through thee, dear Barry, long shall mem'ries last,
A feast of love from present to the past.
For tradition and craft, thou didst entwine,
And wove a legacy both rich and fine.

Thus, take our thanks, in word and heart so deep,
Thy gift we cherish, and forever keep.

—*Inspired by William Shakespeare*

To Mum,

On the occasion of Suzanne's 70th birthday – a special milestone – we pay our tribute to a wonderful mother, wife and masterful chef with this recipe cookbook created from the favourite recipes we have all enjoyed. Recipes that Suzanne has come across on our travels, from cookery books and some of her in-house creations

From a career as a lecturer in Beauty therapy, with a licence to fly her own Cessna aeroplane, G-BGIZ (winner of Jersey to Dijon air rally), to her garden in later years and on to her main love of creating exceptional culinary dishes, she brings so much pleasure to us all.

We hope that you enjoy these recipes as much as we have

The compilation of this cookbook was the work of Roger's good friend Barry, who lives in Boston.

With Love From Your Family
March 30, 2025